Applied Biostatistical Principles and Concepts

The past three decades have witnessed modern advances in statistical modeling and evidence discovery in biomedical, clinical, and population-based research. With these advances come the challenges in accurate model stipulation and application of models in scientific evidence discovery regarding patient care and public health improvement.

Applied Biostatistical Principles and Concepts provides practical knowledge on evidence discovery in clinical, biomedical, and translational science research. Biostatistics is conceived as an information science aimed at assessing data variation, which may arise from natural phenomenon such as sex, age, race, and genetic variations or due to measurement or observation errors. The process of quantifying sample variations requires random variable, implying probability or unbiased sample, exploratory or descriptive statistics, and inferential statistics in quantifying uncertainties through estimation, confidence interval method, as well as hypothesis testing via *p* value method. Since reliable and valid data are required for setting clinical guidelines in enhancing therapeutics and improving patient and public health, clinicians and healthcare providers who play a fundamental role in the task force for clinical and public health guidelines development require basic knowledge of research methodology, namely, design, conduct, analysis, and interpretation. The concepts and techniques provided in this text will facilitate researchers'/clinicians' design and conduct studies, then translate data from bench to clinics in an attempt to improve the health of patients and populations. Suitable for both clinicians and health or biological sciences students, this book presents the reality in the statistical modeling of clinical, biomedical, and translational data with emphasis on clinically meaningful difference as effect size prior to random error quantification through *p* value, since *p* value, no matter how small, does not rule out uncertainties in our findings, and is not the measure of evidence but remains in large part a function of sample size, thus enhancing findings generalizability.

Laurens Holmes Jr. was trained in internal medicine, specializing in immunology and infectious diseases prior to his expertise in epidemiology-with-biostatistics. Over the past two decades, Dr. Holmes had been working in cancer epidemiology, control, and prevention. His involvement in evidence discovery emphasizes reality in statistical modeling of clinical, biomedical, and translational research data. With his concentration in survival data modeling, he is committed to clinical and biologic relevance of data prior to statistical significance as evidence against the null hypothesis and not the measure of evidence. In survival modeling, he advocates and stresses the importance of treatment effect heterogeneity and its application in drug development and therapeutics.

Applied Biostatistical Principles and Concepts

Clinicians' Guide to Data Analysis and Interpretation

Laurens Holmes Jr., MD, DrPH

Routledge
Taylor & Francis Group
LONDON AND NEW YORK

First published 2018
by Routledge
605 Third Avenue, New York, NY 10017

and by Routledge
2 Park Square, Milton Park, Abingdon, Oxon, OX14 4RN

Routledge is an imprint of the Taylor & Francis Group, an Informa business

Library of Congress Cataloging-in-Publication Data

Names: Holmes, Larry, Jr., 1960- author.
Title: Applied biostatistical principles and concepts : clinicians' guide to data analysis and interpretation / Laurens Holmes Jr.
Description: Abingdon, Oxon ; New York, NY : Routledge, 2017. | Includes bibliographical references and index.
Identifiers: LCCN 2017023417| ISBN 9781498741194 (hardback) | ISBN 9781315369204 (ebook)
Subjects: | MESH: Biometry | Research Design | Biostatistics | Data Interpretation, Statistical
Classification: LCC R853.S7 | NLM WA 950 | DDC 610.1/5195--dc23
LC record available at https://lccn.loc.gov/2017023417

ISBN: 978-1-4987-4119-4 (hbk)
ISBN: 978-1-315-36920-4 (ebk)

Dedicated to Jay Kumar, MD (Distinguished Orthopedic Surgeon and Scientist, in memoriam); and Richard Bowen, MD (Distinguished Orthopedic Surgeon and Scientist, Former Chair, Orthopedic Department, Nemours Alfred I. duPont Hospital for Children, Wilmington, Delaware)

Contents

Foreword xi
Preface xv
Acknowledgments xvii
Author xix
Introduction xxi

SECTION I
Design process

1 Basics of biomedical and clinical research 3
1.1 Introduction 3
1.2 Why conduct clinical research? 5
1.3 Study subjects 6
1.4 Subject selection 6
1.5 Sampling 7
1.6 Generalization 7
1.7 Sample size and power estimations 8
1.8 Screening (detection) and diagnostic (confirmation) tests 8
1.9 Balancing benefits and harmful effects in medicine 21
1.10 Summary 22
Questions for discussion 24
References 25

2 Research design: Experimental and nonexperimental studies 27
2.1 Introduction 27
2.2 Epidemiologic study designs 28
2.3 Nonexperimental designs 30
2.4 Experimental designs (clinical trials) 32
2.5 Nonexperimental versus experimental design 34
2.6 Measures of disease association or effect 36
2.7 Precision, random error, and bias 37

2.8 Confounding, covariates, effect measure modifier, interaction 39
2.9 Summary 41
Questions for discussion 42
References 43

3 Population, sample, probability, and biostatistical reasoning 45
3.1 Introduction 45
3.2 Populations 46
3.3 Sample and sampling strategies 47
3.4 Biostatistical reasoning 48
3.5 Measures of central tendency and dispersion 49
3.6 Standardized distribution—z score statistic 68
3.7 Basic probability notion 69
3.8 Simple and unconditional probability 69
3.9 Conditional probability 70
3.10 Independence and conditional probability 71
3.11 Probability distribution 72
3.12 Summary 72
Questions for discussion 73
References 74

SECTION II
Biostatistical modeling

4 Statistical considerations in clinical research 77
4.1 Introduction 77
4.2 Types of variables 82
4.3 Variables and sources of variation (variability) 82
4.4 Sampling, sample size, and power 84
4.5 Research questions, hypothesis testing, and statistical inference 87
4.6 Summary 100
Questions for discussion 101
References 102

5 Study size and statistical power estimations 107
5.1 Introduction 107
5.2 Sample size characterization 110
5.3 Purpose of sample size 110
5.4 Sample size computation 110
5.5 Sample size estimation for single- or one-sample proportion hypothesis testing 114
5.6 One-sample estimation of sample size with outcome mean 116
5.7 Two independent samples: Proportions 117

5.8 Two independent group means 119
5.9 Prospective cohort or two-group comparison in clinical trials 120
5.10 Case–control study 121
5.11 Summary 122
Questions for discussion 123
References 123

6 Single sample statistical inference 125
6.1 Introduction 125
6.2 One-sample group design 130
6.3 Hypothesis statement 130
6.4 Test statistic 130
6.5 Inference from a nonnormal population—One-sample t *test 136*
6.6 Other types of t *tests 138*
6.7 Summary 145
Questions for discussion 148
References 148

7 Two independent samples statistical inference 151
7.1 Introduction 151
7.2 Independent (two-sample) t *test and nonparametric alternative (Mann–Whitney* u *test) 152*
7.3 z *Test for two independent proportions 162*
7.4 Chi-square test of proportions in two groups 164
7.5 Summary 168
Questions for discussion 169
References 170

8 Statistical inference in three or more samples 171
8.1 Introduction 171
8.2 Analysis of variance (ANOVA)? 173
8.3 Other hypothesis tests based on ANOVA 182
8.4 Summary 188
Questions for discussion 189
References 190

9 Statistical inference involving relationships or associations 191
9.1 Introduction 191
9.2 Correlation and correlation coefficients 202
9.3 Simple linear regression 209
9.4 Multiple/multivariable linear regression 217
9.5 Logistic regression technique 219
9.6 Model building and interpretation 222
9.7 Survival analysis: Time-to-event method 229

9.8 Poisson regression 237
9.9 Summary 241
Questions for discussion 243
References 243

10 Special topics in evidence discovery 247
10.1 Introduction 247
10.2 Big data and implication in evidence discovery 248
10.3 Reality in statistical modeling of translational and clinical science data 251
10.4 Tabulation versus regression analysis: When and when not to use regression 254
10.5 Summary 262
Questions for discussion 262
References 263

Appendix 265
Index 269

Foreword

Clinical medicine or surgery continues to make advances through evidence that is judged to be objectively drawn from the care of individual patients. The natural observation of individuals remains the basis for our researchable formulation of questions and the subsequent hypothesis testing. Evidence-based medicine or surgery depends on how critical we are in evaluating evidence in order to inform our practice. These evaluations, no matter how objective, are however never absolute but probabilistic, as we will never know with absolute certainty how to treat future patients who were not a part of our study. Despite the obstacles facing us today in attempting to provide an objective evaluation of our patients since all our decisions are based on the judgment of some evidence, we have progressed from relying on expert opinion to using the body of evidence collected from randomized, controlled clinical trials, as well as prospective and retrospective cohort investigations.

Conducting a clinical trial is termed the "gold standard," as it yields more reliable and valid evidence from the data relative to nonexperimental or observational designs; however, its reliability and validity depend on how well the trial is designed and conducted before outcomes from data collection, analysis, results, interpretation, and dissemination. The designs and the techniques used to draw statistical inferences are often beyond the average clinician's understanding. A text that brings hypothesis formulation, analysis, and interpretation of the results of the findings is long overdue and highly anticipated. Statistical modeling, which is fundamentally a journey from sample to the application of findings, is essential to evidence discovery.

The text *Applied Biostatistical Principles and Concepts* has filled this gap, not only in the way complex modeling is explained but in the simplification of statistical techniques in a way that has never been presented before. This text has been prepared intentionally at the rudimentary level so as to benefit clinicians who do not have sophisticated mathematical backgrounds or previous advanced knowledge of biostatistics as applied statistics in health and medicine. Biomedical researchers who want to conduct clinical research, as well as consumers of research products, may also benefit from the sampling techniques, estimation, confidence interval method and hypothesis testing with *p* value method and their relevance to scientific evidence discovery, as well as the simplified approach to statistical modeling of clinical and biomedical research data. It is with this expectation and enthusiasm that we recommend this text to clinicians in all fields of clinical and biomedical research. Our experience with biomedical research and how the findings in this arm are translated to the clinical environment signals to us the need for the application of biologic and clinical relevance of findings before statistical inference. The examples provided by the authors to simplify research methods are familiar to orthopedic surgeons as well as clinicians in other specialties of medicine and surgery.

Though statistical inference is essential in our application of the research findings to clinical decision-making regarding the care of our patients, without clinical relevance or importance, it can be very misleading and even meaningless. The authors have attempted to deemphasize p value in the interpretation of clinical and biomedical research findings by stressing the importance of confidence intervals, which allow for the quantification of evidence. For example, a large study, because of a large sample size that minimizes variability, may show a statistically significant difference while in reality the difference is too insignificant to warrant any clinical importance. In contrast, a small study, as frequently seen in clinical trials or surgical research, may have a large effect of clinical relevance but not be statistically significant at ($p >$ 0.05). Thus, without considering the magnitude of the effect size with the confidence interval, we tend to regard these studies as negative findings, which is erroneous, since absence of evidence, simply on the basis of an arbitrary significance level of 5%, does not necessarily mean evidence of absence.[1] In effect, clinical research results cannot be adequately interpreted without considering the biologic and clinical significance of the data before the statistical stability of the findings (p value and 95% confidence interval), since p value, as observed by the authors, merely reflects the size of the study and not the measure of evidence.

In recommending this text, it is our hope that this book will benefit clinicians, research fellows, clinical fellows, postdoctoral students in biomedical and clinical settings, nurses, clinical research coordinators, physical therapists, and all those involved in clinical research design and conduct and the analysis of research data for statistical and clinical relevance. We are convinced that knowledge gained from this text will lead to the improvement of our patients' care through well-conceptualized research. Therefore, with the knowledge that no book is complete, no matter its content or volume, especially a book of this nature, which is prepared to guide clinicians on sampling, statistical modeling of data, and interpretation of findings, we assert that this book will benefit clinicians who are interested in applying appropriate statistical technique to scientific evidence discovery.

Finally, we are optimistic that *Applied Biostatistical Principles and Concepts for Clinicians* will bridge the gap in knowledge and practice of clinical and biomedical research, especially for clinicians in busy practices who are passionate about making a difference in their patients' care through scientific research initiatives.

Freeman Miller, MD
Director, Cerebral Palsy Program and Gait Analysis Laboratory
Nemours/A.I. DuPont Hospital for Children, Wilmington, Delaware

Reference

1. D. G. Altman, J. M. Bland, Absence of evidence is not evidence of absence, *BMJ* 311 (1995):485.

Preface

The past three decades have witnessed modern advances in statistical modeling and evidence discovery in biomedical, clinical, and population-based research. With these advances come the challenges in accurate model stipulation and application of models in scientific evidence discovery. While application of novel statistical techniques to our data is necessary and fundamental to research, the selection of the sample and the sampling method that reflects the representativeness of that sample to the targeted population is even more important. Since one of the rationales behind conducting research is to generate new knowledge and apply it to ameliorate life situations, including the improvement of patient and population health, sampling, sample size, and power estimations remain the basis for such inference. With the essential relevance of sample and sampling technique to how we come to make sense out of data, the design of a study transcends statistical technique, since no statistical tool, no matter how sophisticated, can correct the errors of sampling.

This text is written to highlight the importance of appropriate design before analysis by placing emphasis on subject selection and probability sample, and of the randomization process (when applicable) before selection of the analytic tool. In addition, it stresses the importance of biologic and clinical significance in the interpretation of study findings. The basis for statistical inference, implying the quantification of random error, is a random sample. When studies are conducted without a random sample—as often occurs in clinical and biomedical research—it is meaningless to report the findings with a *p* value. However, in the absence of a random sample, the *p* value can be applied to designs that utilize consecutive samples and a disease registry, since these samples reflect the population of interest and hence present a representative sample, justifying inference and generalization.

Essential to the selection of the test statistic is the understanding of the scale of the measurement of the variables, especially the response, outcome, or dependent variable, the type of sample (independent or correlated), the hypothesis, and the normality assumption. In terms of the selection of a statistical test, this task is based on the scale of measurement (binary), type of sample (single, independent), and the relationship (linear). For example, if the scale of the measurement of an outcome variable is a binary and repeated measure, but normality is not assumed, the repeated-measure logistic regression model remains a feasible model for evidence discovery in using the independent variables to predict the repeated outcome.

This book presents a simplified approach to evidence discovery by recommending the graphic illustration of data and normality tests for continuous (ratio/interval scale) data before the statistical test selection. Unlike current texts in biostatistics, the approach taken to present these materials is very simple. First, this text uses applied statistics by illustrating what, when, where, and why a test is appropriate. Where a selected parametric test violates the normality assumption, readers are presented with a nonparametric alternative. However, the use of non-parametric test remains a misnomer since all samples no matter the test involves inference from the population parameter. The rationale for the test is explained with limited mathematical formulae and is intended to stress the applied nature of biostatistics in biomedical and applied research.

Attempts have been made in this book to present the most commonly used statistical model in biomedical or clinical research. We believe that, while no book is complete, we have covered the basics that will facilitate the understanding of scientific evidence discovery. We hope this book remains a useful guide. It is our intention to bridge the gap between theoretical statistical models and reality in the statistical modeling of biomedical and clinical research data. As researchers, we all make mistakes; we believe we have learned from our mistakes during the past three decades and hence the need to examine the flaws and apply reality in the statistical modeling of biomedical and clinical research data. We hope this text results in increased reliability in conduct, analysis, and interpretation of clinical and translational research data, which is our intent and primary goal.

Acknowledgments

In preparing this book, so many people contributed directly or indirectly to the materials provided here. For this book to be practical, we used data collected from different research projects. We wish to express sincere gratitude to those who permitted the use of their data to illustrate the several statistical techniques used in this book.

An attempt at a simplified book in biostatistics remains challenging because of the variability in statistical reasoning of those who require such materials. The simplification, so to speak, of evidence discovery in clinical and biomedical research came from my interaction with research fellows at the Nemours orthopedic department who worked with me and gave me the reason to write this book. They are Drs. K. Durga, M. Ali, S. Joo, T. Palocaren, T. Haumont, M. J. Cornes, A. Tahbet, A. Atanda, P. Sitoula, B. Pruszczynski, S. Pourtaheri, M. Oto, and A. Karatas. The clinical fellows and surgical residents in the orthopedic department also motivated the preparation of this text. Finally, the invitation to the CTSI, MCW, Milwaukee to mentor the translationists of the future in clinical statistics and epidemiology motivated in a special way the preparation of the last two chapters of this text. In this vein, thanks are due to Drs. Reza Shaker (CTSI Director & Senior Associate Dean), Dorel Ward (executive director and faculty), and Joseph Kreshner (Executive Vice President and Dean, School of Medicine) of the Medical College of Wisconsin.

My colleagues at the Nemours Orthopedic Department, Nemours Center for Childhood Cancer Research, Nemours Health Equity and Inclusion Office, and the University of Delaware, College of Health Sciences and Department of Biological Sciences also inspired this preparation via questions on sample size and power estimations, *p* value and confidence interval interpretation, and the preference of a 95% confidence interval to *p* value in terms of statistical stability. They are Drs. Richard Bowen, Kirk Dabney, Suken Shah, Tariq Rahman, George Dodge, Pete Gabos, Freeman Miller, Richard Kruse, Nahir Thacker, Kenneth Rogers, William Mackenzie, Sigrid Rajaskaren, Raj Rajasekaren, Paul Pitel, Jennifer Ty, K. Obrien, Jim Richards, Stephen Stanhope, and Nancy Lenon, MA. I am very grateful to Jobayer Hossain, PhD, for his assistance in the preparation of the normal distribution curve figure used in this book.

I am unable to express adequately my gratitude to my kids (Maddy, Mackenzie, Landon, Aiden, and Devin) for allowing me the time away from them to work on this book. To my siblings, cousins, nephews, aunts, and uncles, I sincerely acknowledge what you all mean to me and will continue to mean to me in my aggressive intellectual search to make sense out of data by dedicating time and effort to training, educating, mentoring, and informing those in clinical research on how to draw inference and combine this with clinical importance in decision-making involving patient care.

Author

Educated at the Catholic University of Rome, Italy; University of Amsterdam, Faculty of Medicine; and the University of Texas, Texas Medical Center, School of Public Health, Laurens (Larry) Holmes, Jr., is a professor of epidemiology and biostatistics at the Medical College of Wisconsin, Clinical & Translational Science Institute (CTSI), Milwaukee, WI and a former professor of clinical trials and molecular epidemiology in the Department of Biological Sciences, University of Delaware, Newark, Delaware. He is recognized for his work on epidemiology and control of prostate cancer but has also published papers on other aspects of hormone-related malignancies and cardiovascular and chronic disease epidemiology utilizing various statistical methods, including the log binomial family, exact logistic model, and probability estimation from the logistic model by margin. Dr. Holmes is a strong proponent of reality in the statistical modeling of cancer and nonexperimental research data, where he presents on the rationale for tabular analysis in most nonexperimental research data, which are often not randomly sampled (probability sampling), rendering statistical inference application meaningless to such data. Since controlling for known confounding of variabilities in subgroup health and healthcare outcomes often fails to remove or explain these imbalances, a feasible alternative is to consider subgroup biologic/cellular events/molecular level variances or differences. One of the biostatistical approaches to addressing valid inference in biomedical and clinical research is a model proposed by Dr. Holmes that amplifies signals in the data before risk stratification, implying the role of biostatistics as a tool in scientific evidence discovery—"*data signal amplification and risk stratification.*" Professor Holmes serves as a voice of reason in statistical modeling in translational epidemiology, where he advocates knowledge transfer from unbiased sample from bench to bedside and the population, with the unique intent to improve patient care and public health.

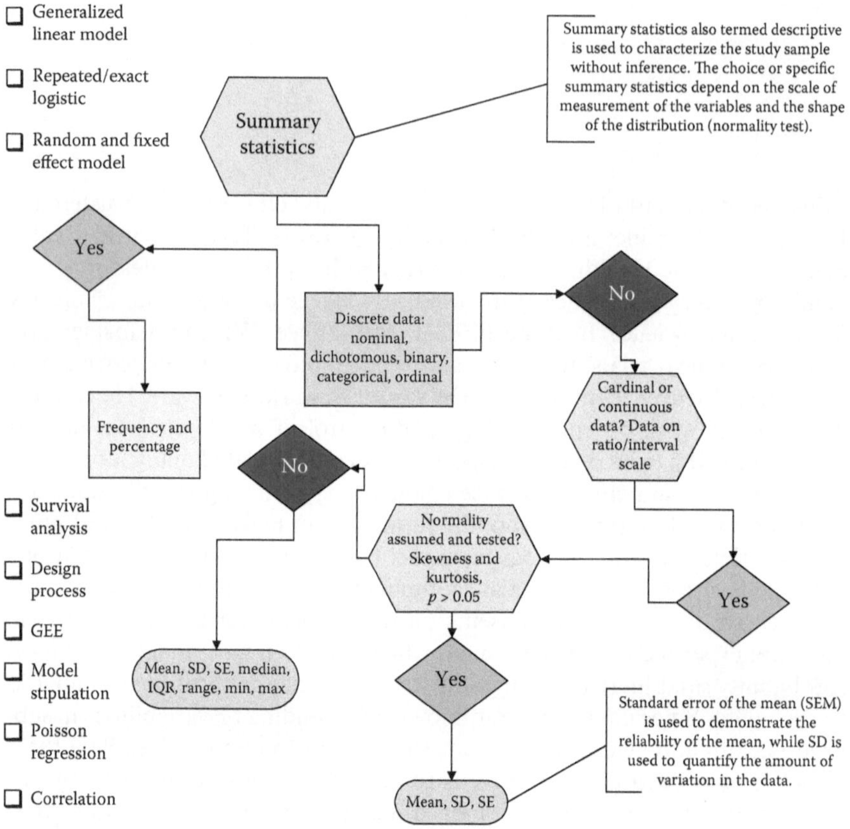

Reality in statistical modeling of biomedical and clinical research data remains the focus of scientific evidence discovery. This text is written to highlight the importance of appropriate design before analysis by placing emphasis on subject selection and probability sample and the randomization process when applicable before the selection of the analytic tool. In addition, this book stresses the importance of biologic and clinical significance in the interpretation of study finding. The basis for statistical inference, implying the quantification of random error, is random sample, which had been perpetually addressed in this book. When studies are conducted without a random sample, except when disease registries/databases or consecutive subjects are utilized, as often encountered in clinical and biomedical research, it is meaningless to report the findings with p value.

Introduction

Scientific evidence discovery "Statiscalase": Inference, *p* value, and statistical significance

The notion of applied biostatistics reflects an information science. In this application, biostatistics or statistics in general fundamentally involves the principles and procedures or methods utilized in collecting, processing, classifying, summarizing, and analyzing data, as well as inference from the sample. As an information science, biostatistics is concerned with generating reliable and valid information termed inference, implying drawing conclusions on the population based on the sample studies (measurements and observations).

In clinical, medical, and translational research, we are interested in improving the care of our patients as well as the health of the public through reliable and valid evidence discovery, implying drawing valid and reliable inference from the sample studied. While the target population comprises all patients, our samples represent a subpopulation but our intent is to apply the conclusion of our findings to the target population or all patients (past, present, and future). Therefore, a reliable inference implies that we select subjects who meet the study criteria to be included in the sample. The requirement is indicative of a need to assess an unbiased sample, implying equal and known chance or probability for patients to be included in the sample termed "representative sample." With such sample, we ensure the generation of a random variable that allows for the quantification of random error through probability value (p).

Clinical and biomedical researchers often ignore an important aspect of evidence discovery from their funded or unfunded projects. Since the attempt is to illustrate some sets of relationships from the data set, researchers often do not exercise substantial time in assessing the reliability and validity of the data to be utilized in the analysis. However, the expected inference or the conclusion to be drawn is based on the analysis of the unassessed data. It is after overcoming the reliability and validity limitations that one should begin to contemplate the analytic procedures, which again depends on the scale of measurements of the outcome and independent or predictor variables. The basic steps to be applied to statistical analysis must include though not limited to (a) assessment of data for reliability and validity; (b) variables definition including measurement scale;

(c) examination of the distribution of the variables and establishment of univariable, also termed univariate distribution pattern; and (d) examination of the basic associations among variables, also termed bivariate association. This final step, which could be time-consuming, allows us to understand the data structure upon which the complex associations such as multivariable regression model will depend. These steps are valuable given that researchers who advance to regression model without examining their data lose substantial information that is necessary in presenting useful argument on the performed study in relation to similar initiatives in the past.

Biostatistics is about health and biological samples, and presenting a book in this field to clinicians is challenging, especially given the limited involvement of clinicians in understanding how evidence from the studies they have directed is derived. We can improve biomedical and clinical knowledge by involving key personnel in such research into how evidence is derived from the collected data of the studies with which we are affiliated. This disinterest is constantly reflected in how proposals are written and submitted for funding as well as how manuscripts on inferential studies are submitted to peer-reviewed journals for consideration for publication.

Biostatistical involvement in evidence discovery in identifying risk factors in diseases and in examining the effectiveness or efficacy of treatment in improving care requires appropriate inference from the data. In this context, a biostatistical technique is required for the test of hypothesis and for random error quantification, implying the degree of precision or the degree of risk one is taking in drawing conclusions from the data. Additionally, biostatistical thinking enables the formulation of appropriate probability distributions based on the assumption of stochastic behavior, implying chance, probability, or randomness. As clinicians and biomedical researchers involved in statistical analysis, our data have inherent error (systematic or random), and the intent of analysis remains the assessment of information that contains error and to examine precision by assessing the chance or likelihood or erroneous inference and to quantify random error or the rule played by chance. Therefore, all attempts at analysis are to make sense of data. For example, if asthma symptoms occur in patients with higher IgE and lower IgG4 concentration, it is possible for the IgE level to be elevated and IgG4 to be depressed without asthma symptoms. With appropriate biostatistical reasoning, one can identify certain patterns in the data with frequencies and percentages and observe associations with bivariate approach, thus making sense of the data before complex modeling.

The desire to improve evidence discovery is what motivated this book and specifically the growing lack of understanding of the function of p value in evidence discovery among clinical and biomedical researchers. Statistics is about sampling, since it is not feasible to study the entire population. We assume that a random sample represents our study population, enabling us to draw inferences about the target or source population.

Whatever the approach utilized to obtain evidence from the observed data, the central tendency theorem holds true to our observations. This theory is addressed in this book as *measures of central tendency* or location and dispersion. The rationale behind summary statistics, such as mean, median, and mode, is presented with clear distinction on when to apply variance, standard deviation (SD), and standard error of the mean (SEM) to the summarized data. Interestingly, the relationship between SEM and sample size is illustrated using hypothetical data.

Sample characterization: Data visualization

Appropriate data collection is necessary for a valid estimation, implying the knowledge of the population, sample, parameter (population characteristics), and statistic, which reflects the feature or characteristics of the sample. Specifically, statistic remains the estimate of population parameter. While investigators have a tendency of testing hypothesis without examining the data graphically, one recommends the visual examination of the data via graphs, tables, as well as descriptive or summary statistics before hypothesis-specific analysis. The selection of the hypothesis testing technique (parametric vs. nonparametric) depends, as stressed throughout in this book, on rationale and assumptions on the distribution (normal or nonnormal probability) of the random (probability sample) variable of interest as well as on the assumed relationship between variables and the scale of measurement of the random variable. These criteria for hypothesis testing are described in detail later in the text.

Random sample

With unbiased or random sampling, we can ensure that our sample is representative of the targeted population, provided a sufficient number of samples are drawn. This observation implies that while randomization balances the baseline prognostic factors between treatment groups in an experiment, imbalance is expected to remain unless the sample size is sufficient to balance the between-group confounding factors. Unless sampling is appropriate and unbiased, statistical tests remain meaningless. *Applied Biostatistical Principles and Concepts* delves into sampling techniques and cautions against the use of a statistical model without thoughtful consideration of sampling. We need to clearly describe the method used to recruit patients/subjects into our study and apply a feasible sampling technique and randomization process or use consecutive samples in our attempt to examine the hypothesis of interest.

Sampling, p *value, and confidence interval*

Where sampling was not applied and consecutive samples were not used in the selection of study subjects, this text recommends clinicians and biomedical researchers describe the results of the study without reference to random error quantification with p value or confidence interval for precision. Such studies are classified as descriptive, implying an inability to generalize such findings to the targeted population, given the assumption of a nonrepresentative sample.

While analysis of the data used to draw inferences requires a systematic process in the collection, the scales of measurement are extraordinarily important before the selection of the statistical technique. Equally important in the consideration of the test statistic is the distribution, implying the shape and spread of the data as well as the effect size expected to be detected. This text examines the normality of the data before the technique to be applied in the evidence discovery. Since clinical studies are conducted to improve the care of patients and small sample sizes often result in the inability to detect an effect difference that is not due to chance, having adequate statistical power is extremely important before conducting a study. We recommend a priori power analysis before the prospective study and nested case–control studies and reserve post hoc power analysis for retrospective designs.

Factors influencing statistical power (sample size, effect size, variability)

This text considers the factors that influence power estimation, namely, sample size, effect size, and variability. Simply, as the sample size increases, power increases. Therefore, as effect size decreases, we need to increase the sample size in order to achieve a sufficient power, while decreasing the variability around the data results in an increase in the statistical power.

BOX 0.1 NEGATIVE RESULTS AND THE POWER OF A STUDY

- Power and sample size estimations are necessary in inferential designs or studies—absence of evidence does not mean evidence of absence.
- The statistical power of a study can be increased not only by increasing the sample size but also by reducing the measurement error, hence reducing variability (SEM, SD).
- Small studies are likely to yield negative results.
  - Negative results should not be reported with statistical significance without the power estimation.

Hypothesis testing

Hypothesis testing is central to inferential statistics. The test depends on the type of design, the relationship, the groups, and the sample independence. The organization of this text reflects the importance of sampling architecture in evidence discovery.

Single-sample hypothesis testing

This text deals with hypothesis tests involving a single sample. For example, if a study is conducted to determine whether or not vitamin D serum concentration in children with osteogenesis imperfecta is comparable to the general population of children, a single-sample *t* test is considered appropriate, assuming continuous (interval/ratio) scale of measurement of vitamin D and normally distributed data. Violations of normality require the appropriate inference to be drawn using a nonparametric alternative to a single-sample *t* test, which is a signed-rank test.

Two-sample hypothesis testing

Hypothesis testing involving two samples is common in clinical and biomedical research. The choice of appropriate technique will depend on the normality of the test, the scales of measurement of the outcome or the dependent variable, and the sample independence.

Independent sample

Consider a study conducted to examine the effect of drug A or serum lipid concentration in children. Assume the serum lipid is measured on a continuous scale, the two groups (drug A vs. placebo) are independent samples, and the serum lipid concentration meets the normality assumption. What would be the appropriate test to use in this design? The appropriate statistical test is the *independent sample t test*; however, if the normality assumption is violated, as would likely be observed with small sample size, and the data tend to be ordinal, a nonparametric alternative is required—namely, the *Mann–Whitney U test*. In addition, since the independent sample *t* test is computed by dividing the difference between the two means by the standard error of the mean difference, equal variance is assumed. The violation of the equal variance assumption requires the result of the independent sample *t* test to be reported with *unequal variance*.

Correlated or paired sample

If the sample is a paired sample, implying a single sample with data on serum lipid concentration obtained before and after treatment (within-sample effect), then the appropriate test is *paired sample or correlated t test* provided the normality assumption is not violated. The violation of the normality assumption requires the use of a ranking test—namely, the nonparametric equivalent to a paired *t* test, mainly the Wilcoxon rank-sum test. If the serum lipid level is measured on a dichotomous scale (upper and lower concentration), a *chi-square test* of independence remains an appropriate test statistic. However, if the expected cell count is less than two, a small expected cell count compensation is required using *Fisher's exact* or Yates.

More-than-two-samples hypothesis testing

Consider a study proposed to examine the effect of drug X, drug Y, and a placebo on urinary insufficiency in older men with prostate cancer. If creatinine urine concentration is measured on a continuous scale and normality is assumed, then the *analysis of variance (ANOVA)* is an adequate test. The violation of the normality test or the ordinal scale of measurement justifies the use of a nonparametric alternative, namely, the Kruskal–Wallis test. If a single sample is involved (drug X only is tested for urinary insufficiency) and normality is assumed, a repeated-measure analysis of variance (RANOVA) is the required test. When RANOVA is not possible because of the normality assumption or ordinal nature of the scale of measurement, the Friedman test remains a nonparametric alternative to RANOVA.

Linear relationship hypothesis testing

The hypothesis test pertaining to a linear relationship involves both normal and nonnormal data. Consider a study conducted to examine the correlation between vitamin D and calcium serum concentration; if both variables are normally distributed and there is no prespecified independent and dependent variable, the *Pearson correlation coefficient* is the required test to determine whether or not the correlation coefficient (r) is significantly different from zero (0). If one of the variables violates the normality assumption and the log transformation of the variables fails to achieve normality, a nonparametric alternative to the Pearson correlation coefficient is recommended, namely, the *Spearman rank correlation coefficient (rho)*. This text stresses the importance of correctly interpreting correlation coefficient findings, implying that the lack of significant r or rho does not necessarily imply a lack of relationship but that the relationship is not linear. A graphic illustration of the data will reveal the nature of the relationship.

A linear relationship may also involve a prediction, implying a regression model requiring the use of X (independent/predictor variable) to predict Y (outcome/response variable). Consider a study performed on the effect of a drug Z in lowering plasma glucose level. If normality is assumed, especially of the plasma glucose level (response variable), a *simple linear regression model* is an appropriate inferential statistical tool. Where the normality assumption is violated, a *robust simple linear regression model* is recommended. Where more than one independent variable is required in the linear prediction of the outcome, a *multiple linear regression model* (not a *multivariate* linear regression) is required. Because of multiple comparisons, caution is required in the building of this model, especially the role of type I error tolerance in addressing multiple comparisons, as well as the interpretation.

Binary outcome

Consider a study proposed to examine the effect of a drug A in treating angina pectoris, with angina coded as 0 = absence and 1 = presence representing the outcome or response variable, while drug A is measured in a categorical scale (low, moderate, and high dosage). If the intent of the study is to predict the odds of recovery or improvement after administration and follow-up, then the design requires the use of a statistical tool with a binary outcome and independent binary, dichotomous, categorical, or continuous variables. The appropriate regression model in this vignette is the unconditional univariable logistic regression model. This test does not assume the shape of the distribution of the data—hence, the sigmoid model categorized as the generalized linear model. Other logistic regression models that are feasible depending on the organization of the data and specific designs include conditional, ordinal, multinomial, and polynomial logistic regression models.

Repeated-measure logistic regression is performed if the outcome variable is repeated for each participant in a study and the intent is to account or adjust for multiple measure from each participant. An example of this can be illustrated in a study conducted to determine the effect of drug A on heart rate; heart rate is recoded into a binary variable, and measurement is obtained six times from each participant. In gait analysis studies, it is not uncommon to obtain multiple measures of knee gait velocity or knee range of motion, and so on. To determine the effect of intervention on these gait parameters, dichotomized into normal and abnormal, the repeated-measure logistic regression model is adequate, correcting or accounting for multiple measures. STATA fits this model by setting the repeated-measure variable with `xtset var` and then `xtgee var var`, reflecting the binomial as probability distribution and logit as the link function in the model. For example, in the previous illustration with knee gait velocity being predicted by cerebral palsy geography: `xtset cp` (panel variable), then `xtgee KneeRom i.cpGeo, family (binomial) link (logit)`. These models are discussed in this text, given the wide use and reporting of logistic regression in medical literature.

Time-to-event data (survival analysis)

Often, biomedical and clinical researchers attempt to examine the outcome of cancer treatment using survival as the response variable, and such design requires the use of time-to-an-event data. L. Holmes, Jr. et al. (2008) performed a retrospective cohort study to determine the effectiveness of androgen-deprivation therapy (ADT) in prolonging the survival of older men with locoregional prostate cancer.[1] Since the response variable was measured on a binary scale and the independent variable (ADT) was measured on a binary scale, a *univariable Cox proportional hazard* model was used to determine the crude and unadjusted effect of ADT on CaP survival. This is a semiparametric model, and the shape of the distribution of the data is not assumed. As is often the case, a meaningful model involves the examination of other variables that might also contribute to survival. To address this situation, a multivariable Cox regression proportional hazard model is required with the purpose of simultaneously controlling for the effect of potential confounders, such as tumor size, Gleason score, tumor stage, and primary therapy (radical prostatectomy) in the association between ADT and prostate cancer survival.

Time series analysis

Forecasting is not common in biomedical and clinical research. Time series are used to predict the response variable from the independent variable and to establish time trends. Consider a study to determine prostate cancer screening and treatment outcomes based on the presence of male physicians in the US Senate and the House of Representatives from 1966 to 2012. This evidence could be discovered using a time series regression, such as the ARIMA model. This is a regression model with the number of male physicians over time as the independent variable and the number of men screened for prostate cancer as the dependent variable. The multivariable model is built to account for other factors that may influence screening besides physician presence in the US Senate or House of Representatives. As it is an uncommon model in medicine, this topic is not discussed in this book; there are specific texts in biostatistics wherein the time series is discussed in detail.

Panel/Longitudinal/Cross-Sectional Time-Series Data Analysis/Modeling: Poolability, Fixed and Random Effect

We often encounter data with multiple entries, such as repeated measures at different time periods. In effect such data have individual (group) effect, time effect or the combination, implying fixed effect, random effect, and both, respectively. Panel data examine the group that reflects individual-specific effects, time effects, or the combination in order to assess heterogeneity or subgroup effect that may not be observed in poolability context. The referenced effects are either fixed or random. In a fixed effect model, we assess if the intercepts vary across group or time period. However, the random effect examines the differences in error variance component across individual or time periods. The poolability application, implying the absence of individual effect or time-specific effect ($\mu_i - 0$) uses the ordinary least square method (OLS), which generates the parameter estimates: $y_\mu = \alpha = X_\mu \beta + \varepsilon_\mu$. ($\mu_i - 0$). Where the data violates exogeneity assumption, that the expected value of disturbance is zero or that disturbances are not correlated with regressor, then the random effect estimator is biased, requiring the application of panel data model, thus the use of fixed and random effect models.

Stata, a statistical software used to perform all the analyses in this text, fits the model for both panel and pooled estimator: xtpois and xtbreg are used to provide these estimators.

Confounding

One of the issues in validation of a biomedical and clinical research is to assess whether associations between exposure and disease derived from the observed data are of a causal nature or not (due to systematic error, random error, or confounding). Confounding refers to the influence or effect of an extraneous factor(s) on the relationships or associations between the exposure and the outcome of interest. Nonexperimental studies are potentially subject to the effect of extraneous factors, which may distort the findings of these studies. To be a confounder, the extraneous variable must be a risk factor for the disease being studied and associated with the exposure being studied but not be a consequence of exposure. Consequently, confounding occurs

a When the effects of the exposure are mixed together with the effect of another variable, leading to a bias.
b If exposure X causes disease Y; Z is a confounder if Z is a known risk factor for disease Y, and Z is associated with X, but Z is not a result of exposure X.

p *Value and measure of evidence*

While statistical inference is essential in our application of the research findings to clinical decision-making regarding the care of our patients, statistical inference without clinical relevance or importance can be very misleading and even meaningless. This textbook has attempted to deemphasize the p value in the interpretation of epidemiologic or research findings by stressing the importance of confidence intervals, which allow for the quantification of evidence. For example, a large study due to a large sample size that minimizes variability may show a statistically significant difference, while in reality, the difference is too insignificant to warrant any clinical importance. In contrast, a small study, as frequently seen in clinical trials or surgical research, may have a large effect size of clinical relevance but not be statistically significant at $p > 0.05$. Thus, in not considering the magnitude of the effect size with the confidence interval, we tend to regard these studies as negative findings, which is erroneous, since absence of evidence, simply on the basis of an arbitrary significance level of 5%, does not necessarily mean evidence of absence.[2] In effect, clinical research results cannot be adequately interpreted without first considering the biologic and clinical significance of the data before the statistical stability of the findings (p value and 95% confidence interval), since p value, as observed by the authors, merely reflects the size of the study and not the measure of evidence.

Role of random error

Assuming a random sample was taken from the population studied, is this sample representative of the population? Is the observed result influenced by sampling variability? Is there a recognizable source of error, such as the quality of questions, a faulty instrument, and so on? Is the error due to chance, given no connection to a recognizable source or error? Random error can be minimized by

1 Improving design
2 Enlarging sample size
3 Increasing precision, as well as by using good quality control during the study implementation

It is important to note here that the sample studied is a random sample and that it is meaningless to apply statistical significance to the result designs that do not utilize random samples.

Null hypothesis and types of errors

The null hypothesis states that there is no association between the exposure and the disease variables, which, in most instances, translates to the statement that the ratio measure of association = 1.0 (null), with the alternate hypothesis stated to contradict the null (one-tail or two-tail)—that the measure of association is not equal to 1.0. The null hypothesis implies that the statistics (mean, odds ratio [OR], relative risk [RR]) being compared are the results of random sampling from the same population and that any difference in OR, RR, or mean between them is due to chance. There are two types of errors that are associated with hypothesis testing: type I (rejecting the null hypothesis when it is in fact true) and type II (failing to reject the null hypothesis when it is in fact false).[3]

Significance level (alpha)

The test statistics that depend on the design as well as the measure of the outcome and independent variables yield a *p* value. The significance level, or α (alpha), is traditionally set at 5% (0.05), which means that if the null hypothesis is true, we are willing to limit type I error to this set value.[4] The *p* value (significance level) is the probability of obtaining the observed result and more extreme results by chance alone, given that the null hypothesis is true. The significance level is arbitrarily cut off at 5% (0.05). A $p < 0.05$ is considered statistically significant, implying that the null hypothesis of no association should be rejected in favor of the alternate hypothesis. Simply, this is indicative of the fact that random error is an unlikely explanation of the observed result or point estimate (statistically significant). With $p > 0.05$, the null hypothesis should not be rejected, which implies that the observed result may be explained by random error or sampling variability (statistically insignificant).[5]

Confidence interval and precision

Confidence interval (CI) is determined by quantification of precision or random error around the point estimate, with the width of the CI determined by random error arising from measurement error or imprecise measurement and sampling variability and some cutoff value (95%). CI simply implies that if a study were repeated 100 times and 100 point estimates and 100 CIs were estimated, 95 out of 100 CIs would contain the true point estimate (measure of association). It is used to determine statistical significance of an association. If the 95% fails to include 1.0 (null), then the association is considered to be statistically significant.

The CI reflects the degree of precision around the point estimate (OR/RR/HR). If the range of RR or OR (point estimate) values consistent with the observed data falls within the lower and upper CI, the data are consistent with the inference, implying the rejection of the null hypothesis. Therefore, when the null value (1.0), implying no association, is excluded from the 95% CI, one can conclude that the findings are statistically significant. Consequently, such data are not consistent with the null hypothesis of no association, implying that such an association cannot be explained solely by chance.

BOX 0.2 REALITY IN STATISTICAL MODELING OF BIOMEDICAL AND CLINICAL RESEARCH DATA

- Descriptive statistics should be applied when data violate the probability sampling assumption.
- One should simply describe the data without *p* value and/or CI.
- A nonparametric test should be used when data are distribution-free and when study size is small, even with ratio or interval scales data (cardinal or continuous variables).
- It is meaningless to apply a *p* value to studies that did not apply probability sampling (random sample) in the selection of study participants and hence did not assess random variables.
    - Exceptions are large sample claims/administrative data, research registries, disease registries, and consecutive sample.
    - These data are assumed to be representative of the population of interest.

Application of CI in assessing evidence

Whereas large studies may not necessarily convey clinical importance, small studies are often labeled "nonsignificant" because of the significance level being greater than 0.05. This is attributed to the low power of these studies, which preclude a detection of statistically significant difference. The magnitude of effect (quantification of the association) and 95% CI, which may appear to be wide, indicating considerable uncertainty, are reliable interpretations of small and negative findings. The *p*-value interpretations of such studies are misleading, clearly wrong, and foolhardy.[6]

Biostatistical reasoning reflects the degree upon which evidence discovered from the observed data is generalizable across targeted populations. Being able to use appropriate test statistics or statistical techniques/procedures to make sense of the data collected during the course of our research is fundamental to evidence discovery. This ability depends on a careful understanding of the scale of measurement of our variables, especially the response variable, the sampling technique used, the type of study design (experimental or nonexperimental), and the power of the study. Where probability sampling was not applied or consecutive patient studies undertaken to reflect the sample representativeness, it is not meaningful to quantify random error (*p* value) and estimate precision (confidence intervals).

BOX 0.3 MODEL SPECIFICATION

- Tabular analysis, such as M-H or chi-square, should be performed before the regression model.
- Appropriate model specification is required for credible evidence from data.
- Background knowledge of exposure, disease, confounders, effect measure modifiers, and the relationship between exposure and disease are essential for model selection.
- Model check is necessary for appropriate interpretation of evidence.

BOX 0.4 REALITY IN STATISTICAL INFERENCE AND RESULTS INTERPRETATION

- *p* Values should not be overemphasized in the presentation of epidemiologic study findings.
    - The *p* value, no matter how small, does not rule out alternative explanations for the obtained results—bias and confounding.
    - *p* Values do not measure evidence but partially reflect the size of the study.
- The interpretation of the biologic and clinical relevance of the findings precedes statistical inference or stability.
    - One should examine the magnitude of effect or point estimate and provide a clinical/public health interpretation before random error quantification.
- Results should be presented with the point estimate, such as HR, RR, OR, and confidence interval (lower and upper 95% or 99%).
    - Why is the preference for CI to *p* value in reporting precision or random variability?

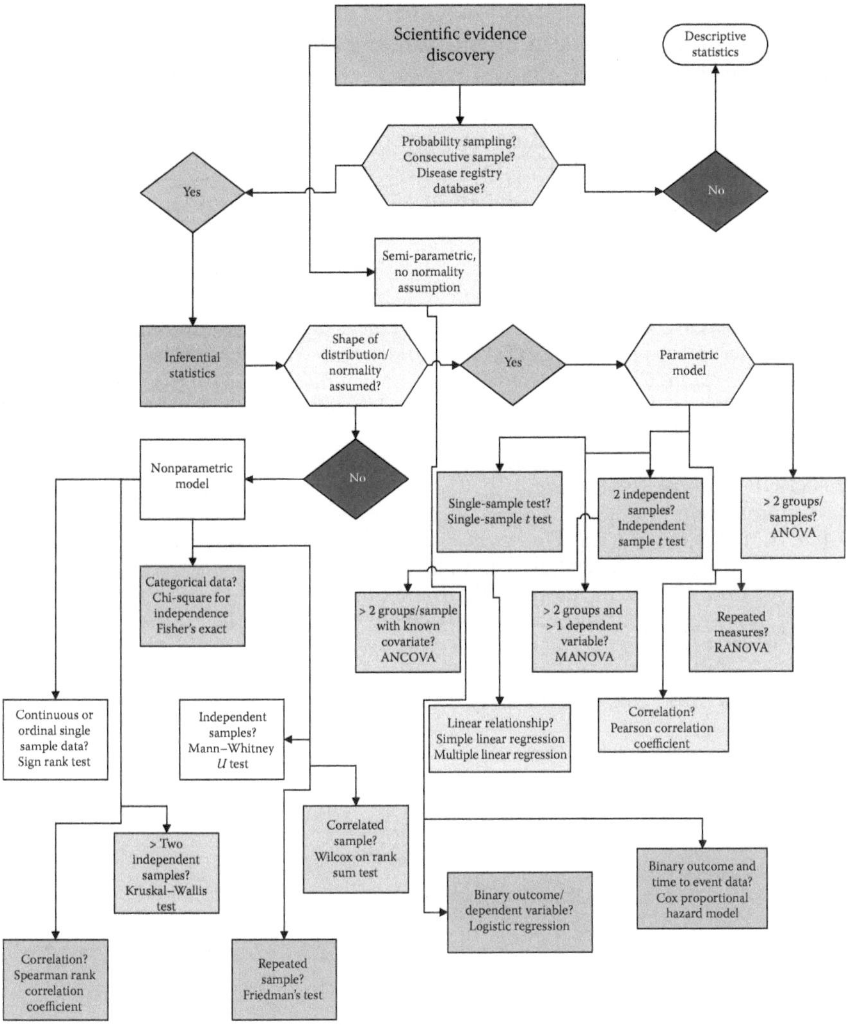

Selection of statistical technique.

The fundamental thinking in inferential statistics is the assumption that observations represent random samples drawn from the population of patients, implying known and equal probability for all patients in the population to be included in our samples. This is important in deciding the targeted population to whom the study findings should apply, implying knowledge of the actual population the samples represent. The source of the sample is important for adequate generalization since in/outpatient subjects in a clinical investigation rarely represent the random sample of the population of patients with a given condition as a whole.

This book presents the tools for evidence discovery by appealing to reality in the statistical modeling in biomedical and clinical research. The chapters that follow should assist you as a reader in understanding design and inference in order to appraise published medical and biomedical literature as well as facilitate the implementation of your own research protocol and making sense of your data. It will remain our hope that these words are not dead but active in the process of the acquisition of knowledge of evidence discovery.

References

1. L. Holmes Jr., W. Chan, Z. Jiang, X. L. Du, Effectiveness of androgen deprivation therapy in prolonging survival of older men with locoregional prostate cancer, *J. Prostate Cancer*, Prostatic Dis. 10 no. 4 (2007):388–395.
2. D. G. Altman, J. M. Bland, Absence of evidence is not evidence of absence, *BMJ* 311 (1995):485.
3. G. D. Murray, Statistical guidelines for *British Journal of Surgery*, *Br. J. Surg* 78 (1991):782–784; S. M. Gore et al., *The Lancet*'s statistical review process: Areas for improvement by authors, *Lancet* 340 (1992):100–102.
4. E. L. Lehmann, *Testing Statistical Hypothesis*, 2nd ed. (New York: Wiley, 1989).
5. G. D. Murray, Statistical guidelines for *British Journal of Surgery*, *Br. J. Surg* 78 (1991):782–784; S. M. Gore et al., *The Lancet*'s statistical review process: Areas for improvement by authors, *Lancet* 340 (1992):100–102; E. L. Lehmann, *Testing Statistical Hypothesis*, 2nd ed. (New York: Wiley, 1989).
6. M. Elwood, *Critical Appraisal of Epidemiological Studies in Clinical Trials*, 2nd ed. (New York: Oxford University Press, 2003).

Section I

Design process

The design process that involves the type of study based on the research question or the clinical or biological phenomenon to be investigated and the sample is extremely important in accurate and valid evidence discovery. The clinicians' or researchers' inability to apply a representative and unbiased sample tends to create inconsistent findings across studies. In effect, design transcends statistical models, and no matter the statistical tool used in the data analysis, the errors of sampling cannot be corrected. This section deals with the types of research designs and their applications in the selection of test statistic.

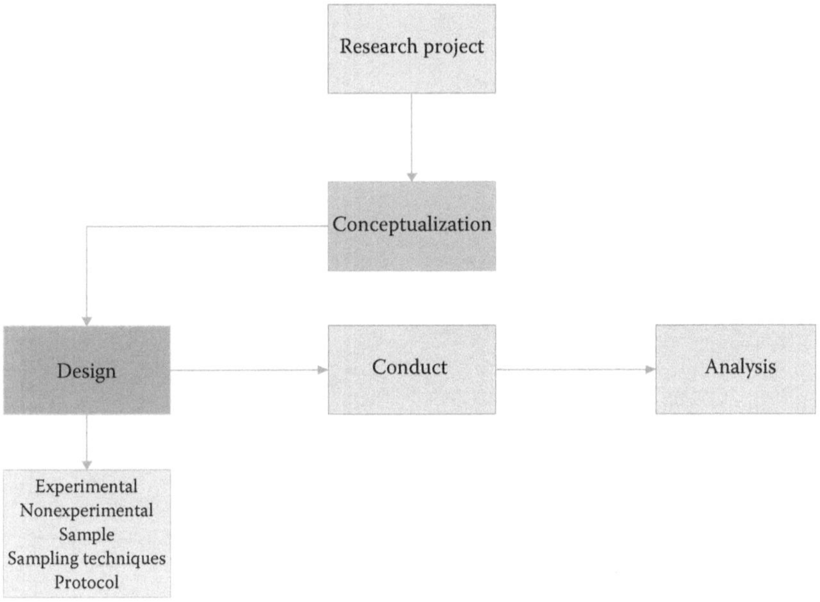

1 Basics of biomedical and clinical research

1.1 Introduction

Biomedical and clinical research remain tools to understanding disease pathways, treatment modalities, and outcomes of care. While knowledge of biomedical sciences and clinical medicine is significant for advances in this field, the generation of such knowledge requires solid and reliable design processes as well as adequate statistical techniques. Biomedical and clinical research is conducted primarily to enhance therapeutics, implying the intent to improve patients' care. The application of this concept in biomedical sciences, public health, and clinical medicine signaled a departure from nihilism, which claimed that disease improved without therapy. The scientific medical discoveries on pellagra, diabetes mellitus, and antibiotics like penicillin and sulfonamide provide reliable data on medicinal benefits in therapeutics. Today, with biomedical and clinical research, clinical investigators applying reliable and valid research methodologies can demonstrate the efficacy and effectiveness of agents and devices, competing therapies, combination treatments, comparative effectiveness, and diagnostic and screening criteria for most diseases.

In claiming the advantage of therapeutics in medicine (complementary versus traditional), there is a need to understand the biological theories and the complexities of disease among clinical investigators, who may be expert physicians, as well as other healthcare providers and those who are indeed researchers. While understanding the biological and clinical importance of a disease is essential in formulating the research question, the clinician is also expected to acquire statistical reasoning. The combination of these two models enhances the analysis and the interpretation of the data from clinical research. Therefore, in clinical research, there is an investigator (clinical) who examines the formal hypothesis or establishes the biology based on work in the clinical settings (experience, observation, and data), as well as another investigator (biostatistician/epidemiologist) whose contribution is to generalize observations from sample to target population, as well as combine empirical (observation and data) and theory-based knowledge (probability and determinism) with the understanding of the results of the study. Despite these distinctions, effective clinical and biomedical research involves the understanding of these two models of thinking or reasoning by the investigators, clinicians, and epidemiologists/biostatisticians. Without this integration, our effort toward the design and interpretation of research findings is limited, since making reasonable, accurate, and reliable inferences from data in the presence of uncertainty remains the cornerstone of clinical research results utilization for improving the healthcare of future patients. In stressing the essence of this integration, one is not claiming the relevance of statistical reasoning over biological and clinical importance, since clinical research thinking is fundamentally biologic, clinical, and statistical.

The approach to biomedical and clinical research involves research conceptualization, the design process, and statistical inference. In biomedical sciences, for example, the research conceptualization may involve therapeutics in mice or rats with cancer, and because of the similarities to human malignancies, these findings would be translational, and hence generalization (biologic) to human malignancies without a formal statistical model can be made. The design process may involve treated and untreated mice, with a follow-up time to determine the survival difference in the two groups. The statistical inference, given that adequate numbers (sample size and power estimations) of mice were studied, involves the use of Kaplan–Meier's survival estimates, as well as the log-rank test for the equality of survival in these two groups. Finally, statistical stability is examined in ruling out random variation using p value (significance level) and 95% confidence interval (precision). A similar approach is utilized in clinical research that involves human subjects or patients in clinical settings. The research conceptualization in this context involves the clinical investigator or clinician utilizing his or her experience in the management of patients with malignancy (e.g., leukemia), observation, and data to formulate hypotheses regarding therapeutics. A case–comparison/control design could be applied here in which the treated group (cases) is placed on the new drug X, while the comparison group (control) is placed on a standard care drug Y and both are followed for the assessment of outcome (death or biochemical failure). The statistical inference and the interpretation of the results are similar to the example with mice and malignancy therapeutics. There are excellent books in study designs, including one by the author of this book.

Historically, central to clinical research and therapeutics is the concept of disease screening and diagnostic testing. We can view the disease diagnosis as well as the diagnostic test as key elements in the ascertainment of subjects for clinical research. Inappropriate patient ascertainment may result in selection, information, and misclassification biases (discussed in subsequent chapters). This historical concept remains valid in research conduct and is the main material elaborated in this chapter. The sensitivity, specificity, predictive values, and likelihood ratios are described with examples. Thus, the validity of the results obtained in clinical research depends on how adequately the subjects were identified and assigned to treatment (experimental design or clinical trial) or followed after exposure (nonexperimental design).

1.2 Why conduct clinical research?

Conducting research in biomedical, clinical, and public health involves a response to a health or health-related issue. Thus, research conducted commences with question formulation, which is followed by design plans to answer the question, data collection and analysis, the drawing of conclusions from the results or findings, and then information sharing through publication or dissemination. For example, a reason to conduct research may be to understand the natural history of a disease, such as unicameral bone cyst, which is a benign tumor of the bone. Another example of the natural history of a disease is the Swedish prospective cohort study of men diagnosed with prostate cancer (CaP) and followed for 10 years without specific treatment (watchful waiting or observational management) for CaP. In the latter example, with the primary end point being cause-specific mortality (prostate cancer dead), the experience of this group was compared and a 10-year relative survival of 87.0% was reported.[1] The natural history of disease refers loosely to the collectivity of the actual sequence of events since this phenomenon (actual sequence of events) can vary widely among patients.[2] In more concrete terms, we normally refer to the natural history of a disease as the assessment of the actual sequence of events for many patients in order to obtain some estimates of these events. In this respect, the natural history of a disease can be characterized using measures of disease occurrence, such as case fatality, mortality rate, median survival time, and so on. Research may also be conducted to relate laboratory data or information with screening, diagnosis, treatment, and prognosis. A researcher/investigator may wish to use the laboratory value for blood glucose level, for example, to screen, diagnose, and determine the prognosis of diabetes mellitus. Finally, a natural history of a disease may be studied in a randomized, placebo-controlled clinical trial, where treatment is allocated to one group, while the other group (control) is given the placebo. The result in the control group without the treatment represents the natural history of the disease studied.

The primary reason to conduct research in clinical medicine is to address questions pertaining to screening, diagnosis, treatment, and outcome of care (prognosis), with the ultimate goal being the improvement of patients' care (Figure 1.1). This effort involves protocol development and management/coordination, recruitment and data collection/entry, data management and analysis, and making sense of the data through interpretation and inference.

The biomedical or clinical researcher should have a clear idea of the concept to be measured. This step allows the investigator to clearly address the research questions. The statement of such questions must reflect the scale of measurement of the variable—such as nominal, ordinal, interval, or ratio. The reliability of the variables to be measured (if questionnaires are used to collect information) has to be examined on the basis of the stability of the response to the question over time—a sort of test and retest reliability. As is often seen in clinical research involving radiographic measures, reliability

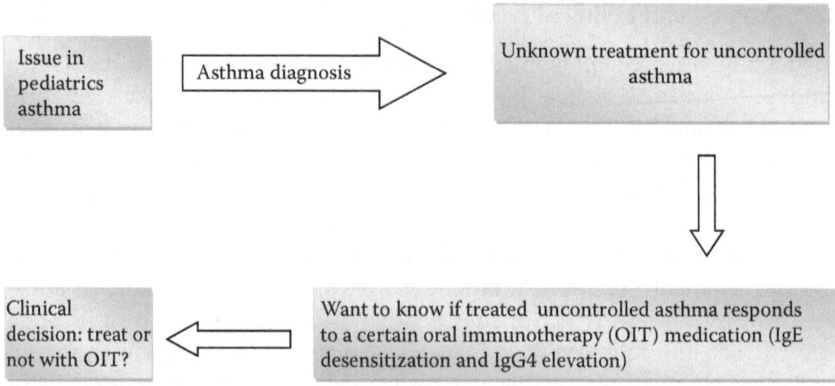

Figure 1.1 Rationale for research conduct and process.

could be measured by examining the agreement between two observers or surgeons (interrater reliability). Very important is the validity or accuracy of the measure, which is simply the extent to which the empirically observed association between measures of the concepts agree with the testable hypothesis about the association between variables assessed.

1.3 Study subjects

Biomedical research may involve animals as well as human subjects. For example, biomedical researchers may be interested in finding out if a certain drug (n34) enhances programmed cell death (apoptosis) in transgenic mice induced with neuroblastoma. A case–control nonexperimental epidemiologic design may be proposed for this investigation. The issues to be addressed include study subject selection since the control (mice not administered n34) must be comparable to the treatment mice (n34 mice). Since these mice are genetically homogeneous, such selection is feasible, minimizing selection bias, sampling, and generalization errors.

1.4 Subject selection

Investigators must select samples that are representative of the patient population, implying performing the investigation on number of patients large enough to minimize random error (increased sample representativeness) in the generalization of the study findings to the targeted population of patients. One must stress the importance of sampling design since the generalizability of the results of a study is dependent on the accuracy of the sampling design. Additionally, inference remains invalid if drawn from an erroneous sampling design. An example of a study sample would be children with adolescent idiopathic scoliosis (AIS) who have undergone posterior spinal fusion for curve deformities correction between 2000 and 2011. Well-structured inclusion and exclusion criteria are essential in appropriate subject selection. The purpose of this is to ensure that the study findings are reasonably generalized. Therefore, criteria should be selected in such a manner that the generalization of the study findings to the targeted population is feasible.

1.5 Sampling

Biomedical and clinical researchers must determine a priori who should be in the sample. Reason behind sampling, among others (research complexity and efficiency, limited resources), include increasing precision (minimize sampling variability) and ensuring accuracy of the estimates, such as the mean or proportion. Commonly used probability sampling techniques include the simple random sample, systematic random sample, and stratified sample, as well as the cluster sample. It is, however, important to note that while appropriate probability sampling technique is essential in lessening sampling variability, completely eliminating it is impossible, and there remains the possibility of random variability, hence the need to quantify such errors (random) by probability value (p).

The utility of findings from an inferential study depends on appropriate sampling. Sampling as a desirable approach in research is based on the rationale of appropriate samples representing the target population. While study size may be influenced by the available resources, the study sample must reflect the characteristics of the targeted population. A *sample* is described as a subset of the targeted population, which is always desirable, given the impossibility of studying the entire population. In clinical research, the study sample rarely meets the requirement for probability sampling. In this context, convenient (subjects who meet criteria and are accessible to investigators) and consecutive (the entire patient population over a long period of time) samples are often used.

Inferential studies that quantify random error require probability sampling. This approach ensures that the study sample represents the targeted population and that data derived from such sampling techniques reflect the true experience in the population that the study sample was drawn from. These techniques include the simple random sample, stratified sample, systematic sample, and cluster sample.

1.6 Generalization

When studying physical phenomena, we can apply the findings easily without determining how to reasonably apply the findings to geographic locations in which the phenomena were not observed. However, biologic or biomedical studies differ because of the heterogeneity of species and the changing environmental conditions. Can we generalize the findings of a study based on a consecutive sample? This question requires the investigators' determination as to whether the sample is comparable to the probability sample to justify generalization. For example, if the investigator estimates that the consecutive sample was large enough to minimize random error (representative sample), then such a study finding could be generalized to the target population with the assumption that the sampling technique used is similar to the probability sampling technique. In contrast, if the consecutive sample is judged not to minimize random error, such a finding should not be generalized. These studies' results should be presented with descriptive statistics, without any attempt to quantify random error.

1.7 Sample size and power estimations

While this issue is discussed in detail in subsequent chapters, the importance of understanding the essence of the study size needed for a research project needs to be mentioned early. Sample size estimation is important at the beginning of the design of a research project. In inferential or analytic studies, the findings require generalization. This process involves a clear statement of the null and alternative hypotheses, indicating the direction of the test, selecting the test statistic based on the scale of measurement of the outcome and independent or predictor variables, clinically reasonable effect size, variability, and the statement of type I error tolerance and type II error. Given the importance of power, adequate sample size is necessary in order to avoid missing a real difference and concluding that there is no difference. Subsequent chapters will provide details in specific statistical test settings (*t* test, chi-square, correlation coefficient, logistic regression, and survival analysis) for how to estimate the study size. However, researchers must plan to address loss to follow-up by compensating for the attrition rate, as well as to increase the study size while utilizing multivariable statistical modeling to adjust for confounding at the analysis phase of the research.

1.8 Screening (detection) and diagnostic (confirmation) tests

Clinical or medical research also involves designs that examine the effect of testing on outcome. Simply, a screening or diagnostic test is beneficial if survival is prolonged among those screened for the disease compared to those who are not screened. Remarkably, the outcome of diagnostic tests is not the mere diagnosis or disease stage or grade of tumor, as in the Gleason score used in prostate cancer clinical assessment, but involves the mortality or morbidity that could be prevented among those who tested positive for the disease.

The benefit of a diagnostic test depends on whether or not there are procedures and treatment in place to follow up the true positives (patients or individuals with the symptoms who test positive for the disease). For example, to determine whether or not screening for prostate-specific antigen (PSA) prolongs survival or reduces the risk related to prostate cancer, investigators may compare the rates of PSA among patients who died of prostate cancer with controls who did not.

Medicine is a conservative science, and the practice of clinical medicine involves both art and science. The process upon which clinical diagnosis is achieved remains complex, involving history, a review of the system, physical examination, laboratory data, and neuroimaging, as well as probability reasoning. The screening test is performed in individuals who do not have the symptoms or signs of a disease or a specific health condition[3]—for example, the use of PSA in asymptomatic (no signs or symptoms of prostate cancer disease) African-American men, 40 to 45 years of age, to assess the presence or absence of prostate cancer in this population. A diagnostic test is performed in clinical medicine to acquire data on the presence (+ve) or absence (−ve) of a specific condition.[4] The questions are as follows.

1.8.1 Why conduct a diagnostic test?

A diagnostic test is performed to confirm the presence of a disease following symptoms of an illness. For example, a 21-year-old Caucasian female presents with mild fever and frequent and painful urination that is relieved after voiding the bladder. The physician suspects cystitis and recommends urinalysis for bacterial pathogen isolation. The test confirms *E. coli* (Gram-negative bacterial pathogen). The above example is illustrative of a diagnostic test, which simply confirms the diagnosis of bacterial cystitis in this hypothetical illustration.

1.8.2 When is a diagnostic test performed?

A diagnostic test could also be performed (1) to provide prognostic information for patients with a confirmed diagnosis of a disease, such as diabetes mellitus (DM), for example, a blood glucose level in patients with DM; (2) to monitor therapy to assess benefits or side effects, for example, to assess pseudoarthrosis among patients with AIS who underwent spine fusion to correct curve deformities; (3) to confirm that a person or patient is free from a disease, for example, though not a very reliable marker of prostate cancer prognosis, PSA level to assess prostate cancer remission in men diagnosed with locoregional CaP and treated for the disease with radical prostatectomy and radiation therapy.

1.8.3 What is a screening test, and what are the possible results?

Screening is an effort to detect disease that is not readily apparent or risk factors for a disease in an at-risk segment of the population. This test can result in four possible outcomes or results: (1) true-positive—positive test result given the presence of disease; (2) false-positive—positive test in the absence

Table 1.1 A 2 × 2 contingent table illustrating diagnostic test results

	Population (target)	
Test result	*Disease*	*Nondisease or disease-free*
Positive	a	b
Negative	c	d

Abbreviations: a = true positive, b = false positive, c = false negative, and d = true negative. Sensitivity = a/a + c; specificity = d/b + d; positive predictive value (PPV) = a/a + b; negative predictive value = d/c + d; false-positive rate = c/a + c; false-negative rate = b/b + d.

of disease; (3) false-negative—positive test in the absence of disease; and (4) true-negative—negative test in the absence of disease.

Diagnostic tests, results, and implications of screening depend on both the prevalence of the disease and test performance (Table 1.1). For example, rare diseases are associated with relatively frequent false positives relative to true negatives, and common diseases are associated with relatively frequent false negatives relative to true negatives. A screening test is generally inappropriate when the disease is either exceedingly rare or extremely common.

1.8.4 What are the measures of a diagnostic and screening test?

Measures of the diagnostic value of a test are its *sensitivity* and *specificity*. These parameters have important implications for screening and clinical guidelines.[5]

Sensitivity refers to the ability of a test to detect a disease when it is present. This measures the proportion of those with disease who are correctly classified as diseased by the test

$$\text{Sensitivity} = a \div (a + c)$$

This implies subjects with true-positive test results: (a)/(subjects with true-positive results + subjects with false-negative test result (a + c)). A test that is not sensitive is likely to generate a false-negative result (c). The false-negative error rate is given as follows:

$$\text{False-Negative Error Rate} = \Pr(T- \mid D+) = c \div (a + c)$$

This is otherwise termed *beta error rate* or type II error.

There is a relationship between sensitivity and false-negative error rate:

$$\text{Sensitivity } [a/(a + c)] + \text{False-Negative Error Rate} = \Pr(T- \mid D+)$$
$$= [c \div (a + c)] = 1.0\ (100\%)$$

Specificity refers to the ability of a test to indicate nondisease (disease-free) when no disease is present. This is the measure of the proportion of those without disease who are correctly classified as disease-free by the test. Specificity is derived in this way:

$$\text{Specificity} = d/(b + d)$$

This implies subjects with true-negative test results (d)/(Subjects with true-negative result + Subjects with false-positive (b + d)). A test that is not specific is likely to generate false-positive results (b). The false-positive error rate is as follows:

$$\text{False-Positive Error Rate} = \Pr(T+ \mid D-) = b \div (b + d)$$

There is a relationship between specificity and false-positive error rate:

$$\text{Specificity } (d/b + d) + \text{False-Positive Error Rate } (b/b + d) = 1.0\ (100\%)$$

1.8.5 What are predictive values?

Predictive values refer to (1) the probability of having the disease being tested for if the test result is positive and (2) the probability of not having the diseases being tested for if the result is negative.[6]

BOX 1.1 RELATIONSHIP BETWEEN DISEASE PREVALENCE, SENSITIVITY, SPECIFICITY, AND PREDICTIVE VALUE

- There is a relationship between disease prevalence, sensitivity, specificity, and predictive values.
- The prevalence simply means the probability of the condition before performing the test (i.e., pretest probability).
- The predictive values refer to the probability of the disease being present or absent after obtaining the results of the test.
- Using the 2 × 2 table, positive predictive value (PPV) is the proportion of those with a positive test who have the disease (a /(a + b)) while the negative predictive value (NPV) is the proportion of those with a negative test who do not have the disease (d /(c + d)).
- The predictive values will vary with the prevalence of the disease or condition being tested for.
- Therefore, the probability of the diseases before (prevalence) and the probability of disease after (predictive value) will be interrelated, with the differences in predictive values driven by the differences in the prevalence of the disease.

1.8.6 What are the types of predictive values?

There are two types of predictive values used in diagnostic/screening tests:

Positive predictive value (PPV): the probability of a test being positive given that the disease is present. Mathematically, positive predictive value is as follows:

$$\text{PD+ or PPV} = a/\left\{a + \left[(pT+ \mid D-)pD-)\right]\right\} = a/\{a + b\}$$

where PD+ = True positives/{True positives + False positives}. Using Bayes's theorem, PPV is the probability that an individual with a positive test result truly has disease, which is the proportion of all positives (true and false) that are classified as true positives. PPV is thus the probability that a positive test result truly indicates the presence of disease.

Negative predictive value (NPV) or PD− is the probability of disease absence after a negative test result. Mathematically, negative predictive value is as follows:

$$\text{NPV} = \text{True negatives}/\{\text{True negatives} + \text{False negatives}\} = d/(d + b)$$

Using the Bayesian theorem: PD− = [Specificity × (1 − Prevalence)]/{[Specificity × (1 − Prevalence)] + [Prevalence × (1 − Sensitivity)]}.

1.8.7 What is disease prevalence, and how is it related to positive predictive value?

Prevalence is the probability of the disease, while sensitivity, in comparison, is the probability of a positive test in those with the disease:

$$\text{Prevalence} = \{a + c\}/\{a + b + c + d\}$$

Using the Bayesian theorem: PD+ = (Sensitivity × Prevalence)/{[Sensitivity × Prevalence] + [(1 − Specificity) (1 − Prevalence)]}. Remember that *sensitivity remains* the probability of a positive test in those with the disease − {a/a = c}.

1.8.8 What are likelihood ratios?

Likelihood ratio (LR) is the probability of a particular test result for an individual with the disease of interest divided by the probability of that test result from an individual without the disease of interest. There are two types of likelihood ratios:

1 *Likelihood ratio positive (LR+)* refers to the ratio of the sensitivity of a test to the false-positive error rate of the test. Mathematically:

$$\mathbf{LR+} = [a/(a+c)/[b/(b+d)]$$

The *LR*+ = Sensitivity/(1 − Specificity).

2 *Likelihood ratio negative (LR−)* refers to the ratio of the false-negative error rate to the specificity of the test. Mathematically:

$$\mathbf{LR-} = \{c/(a+c)\}/\{d/(b+d)\}$$

The LR− = (1 − Sensitivity)/Specificity.

1.8.9 What is the measure of the separation between positive and negative tests?

The ratio of LR+ to LR− refers to the measure of separation between the positive and negative test. Mathematically:

$$\text{LR+ to LR- ratio} = \text{LR+/LR-}$$

This is an approximation of the odds ratio: OR = ad/bc, using the two-by-two contingent table. *Odds ratio:* odds of exposure in the disease/odds of exposure in the nondisease. For example, the odds of disease (lung cancer) = probability that lung cancer will occur (*P*)/probability that it will not occur (1 − *P*).

Vignette 1.1: Consider 160 persons appearing in a deep-vein thrombosis (DVT) clinic for a lower extremities Doppler ultrasound study. If 24 out of 40 subjects with DVT tested positive for DVT, and 114 out of 120 without DVT tested negative, calculate (1) sensitivity, (2) specificity, (3) false-positive error rate, (4) false-negative error rate, (5) positive predictive value, (6) negative predictive value, (7) likelihood ratio positive, (8) likelihood ratio negative, (9) ratio of LR+ to LR−, and (10) the prevalence of DVT. Generate a two-by-two contingent table, and perform the computation.

Computation: (1) Sensitivity = 24/40 = 0.6 (60%); (2) Specificity = 0.95 (95%); (3) FP error rate = b/(b + d) = 6/120 = 0.05 (5%); (4) FN error rate = c/(a + c) = 16/40 = 0.4 (40%); (5) PPV = 24(a)/30(a + b) = 0.8 (80%); (6) NPV = 114(d)/130(c + d) = 0.88 (88%); (7) LR+ = {a/(a + c)} = Sensitivity/{b/(b + b)} (False-positive error rate) → 0.6/0.05 = 12.0; (8) LR− = False-negative error rate {(c/(a +c)/Specificity {d/(d + b)} → 0.4/0.95 = 0.42; (9) LR+ to LR− ratio = LR+/LR− = 12/0.42 = 28.57; and (10) Prevalence of DVT = (a + c)/(a + b + c + d) → 40/160 = 0.25 (25%). False-positive error rate (alpha error rate or type I error rate) simply refers to an error committed by asserting that a proposition is *true*, when it is indeed *not true* (false). If a test is not *specific*, this will lead to the test falsely indicating the presence of a disease in nondisease subjects. The rate at which this occurs is termed the false-positive error rate and is mathematically given by B/(B + D). The false-positive error rate is related to specificity: FP rate + Specificity = 1.0 (100%).

1.8.10 What is multiple or sequential testing?

Multiple or sequential testing refers to (a) *parallel testing* (ordering tests together). The idea is to increase sensitivity, but specificity is compromised. There are four possible outcomes in parallel testing:

1 T1 + T2+ (disease is present)
2 T1 + T2− (further testing)
3 T1 − T2+ (further testing)
4 T1 − T2− (disease is absent)[7]

(1) Sensitivity (net) = (Sensitivity T1 + Sensitivity T2) − Sensitivity T1 × Sensitivity T2. (2) Specificity (net) = Specificity T1 × Specificity T2. (3) Individual tested positive on either test is classified as positive. (4) Appropriate when false-negative is the main concern.

Serial testing refers to using two tests in a series, with test 2 performed only on those individuals who are positive on test 1.[8]

1.8.11 Disease screening: Principles, advantages, and limitations

Population screening refers to early screening and treatment in large groups to reduce morbidity or mortality from the specified disease among the screened. Screening for disease control or mortality reduction involves the examination of asymptomatic or preclinical cases to correctly classify the diseased as positive and nondiseased as negative (Table 1.2).[9]

Table 1.2 Screening and diagnostic test

Test parameters	*Estimation*	*Interpretation*
True positive (TP)	A (2 × 2 table)	Number of individuals with the disease who have a positive test result
True negative (TN)	D (2 × 2 table)	Number of individuals without the disease who have a negative test result
False positive (FP)	C (2 × 2 table)	Number of individuals without the disease who have a positive test result
False negative (FN)	B (2 × 2 table)	Number of individuals with the disease who have a negative test result
Sensitivity = True-positive rate (TPR)	TP/(TP + FN)	The proportion of individuals with the disease who have a positive test result
1 − Sensitivity = False-positive rate (FPR)	FN/(TP + FN)	The proportion of individuals with the disease who have a negative test result
Specificity = True-negative rate (TNR)	TN/(TN + FP)	The proportion of individuals without the disease who have a negative test result
1 − Specificity = False-negative rate (FNR)	FP/(TN + FP)	The proportion of individuals without the disease who have a positive test result
Positive predictive value	TP/(TP + FP)	The probability that a patient with a positive test result will have the disease
Negative predictive value	TN/(TN + FN)	The probability that a patient with a negative test result will not have the disease.
Likelihood ratio of a positive test result (LR+)	Sensitivity/(1 − Specificity)	The increase in the odds of having the disease after a positive test result
Likelihood ratio of a negative test result (LR−)	(1 − Sensitivity)/Specificity	The decrease in the odds of having the disease after a negative test result

Notes: This table is based on a 2 × 2 contingency table, where the disease is represented in the column, while the test results are on the row. *Bayes' theorem* refers to posttest odds, which are estimated by: pretest odds × likelihood ratio. These are the odds of having or not having the disease after testing. *Accuracy of the test* is measured by (TP + TN)/(TP + TN + FP + FN) and is the probability that the results of a test will accurately predict the presence or absence of disease.

1.8.12 Diagnostic or screening test accuracy/validity

This refers to the ability of the test to accurately distinguish those who do and do not have a specific disease.[10] Sensitivity and specificity are traditionally used to determine the validity of a diagnostic test (Figure 1.2). *Sensitivity* is the ability of the test to classify correctly those who have the disease or

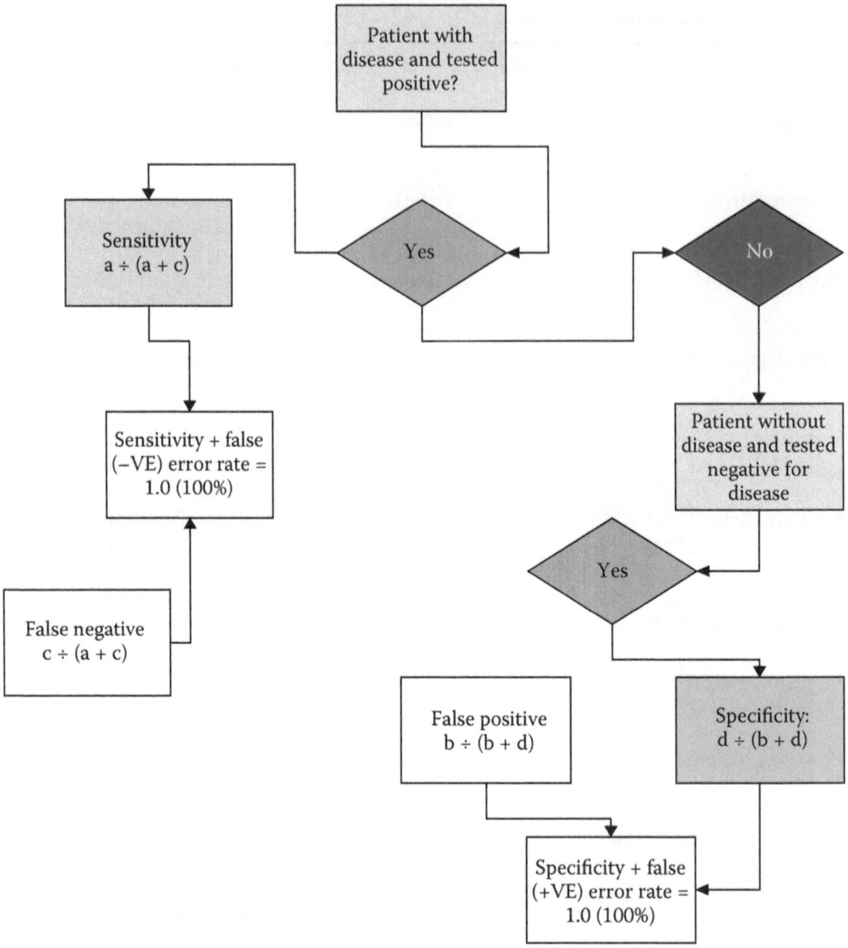

Figure 1.2 Screening and diagnostic test.

specific/targeted disorder. Sensitivity is represented by a/(a + c) in a two-by-two contingency table (Table 1.3). "SnNout" is used to describe sensitivity, meaning that when "sen"sitivity is high, a "n"egative result rules "out" diagnosis. *Specificity* is the ability of the test to classify correctly those without the disease as nondiseased. Specificity is represented by d/(b + d). "SpPin," which is used to describe specificity, implies that a very high specificity with a positive result effectively rules in the diagnosis.

The predictive value of the test addresses the effectiveness of the test in accurately identifying those with the disease and those without. The positive predictive value of the test addresses the following question: if the test result is positive in an individual, what is the probability that such individual has the disease? This is estimated by a/(a + b). The negative predictive value

Table 1.3 2 × 2 contingency table

	Disease (+)	*Disease (−)*
Test (+)	**(A)** TP	**(B)** FP
Test (−)	**(C)** FP	**(D)** TN

addresses the probability of an individual with a negative test being disease-free. This is estimated by d/(c + d). The false-positive error rate is estimated by 1 − specificity = b/(b + d). The false-negative error rate is estimated by 1 − sensitivity = c/(a + c). Prevalence = (a +c)/(a + b + c + d). LR+, which is the likelihood ratio for a positive test, is estimated by sensitivity/(1 − specificity). LR−, which is the likelihood ratio for a negative test, is estimated by (1 − sensitivity)/specificity. The posttest probability is estimated by posttest odds/(posttest odds + 1), where pretest odds are estimated by prevalence/(1 − prevalence) and posttest odds are estimated by pretest odds × likelihood ratio.

Vignette 1.2: Consider a population of 2000 people, of whom 200 have unicameral bone cysts and 1800 do not. If 160 with the disease were correctly identified as positive by the test, 40 were not. Of the 1800 who did not have the disease, 1600 were correctly classified as negative. Calculate (1) sensitivity, (2) specificity, (3) positive predictive value, and (4) negative predictive value.

Solution: (a) Sensitivity = a/(a + c); substituting: 160 ÷ 200 = 80%; (b) Specificity = d(d + b) =1600 ÷ 1800 = 89%; (c) Positive predictive value = a/(a + b) = 160 ÷ 360 = 44.4%; and (d) Negative predictive value = d/(c + d) = 1600 ÷ 1640 = 97.6%.

1.8.13 What is a receiver operating characteristic (ROC) curve?

The ROC, which is derived from electronics, was used to measure the ability of the radar operators to differentiate signals from noise. The ROC curve is the graphic approach to illustrating the relationship between the cutoff point that differentiates positive and normal results in a screening test. This curve is constructed by selecting several cutoff points and using them to determine the sensitivity and specificity of the test. The graph is then constructed by plotting the sensitivity (true positive) on the *Y* axis as a function of 1 − specificity (false-positive rate/proportion) on the *X* axis [sensitivity versus (1 − specificity)]. The area under the ROC curve provides some measure of the accuracy of the test as well as being useful in comparing the accuracy of two or more tests. Simply, the larger the area, the better or more accurate the test. In interpreting the area under the ROC curve (0.5–1.0), 1.0 is indicative of perfect test, while 0.5 represents a poor test; this implies that an ideal test is that which reaches the upper left corner of the graph (all true-positive without false-positive results).

1.8.14 What is the relationship between disease prevalence and predictive value?

There is a positive relationship between disease prevalence and predictive values; thus, the higher the prevalence in the population at risk or screened population, the higher the positive predictive value.

1.8.15 Advantages and disadvantages of screening

Screening is most productive and efficient if it is directed at a high-risk population. Screening of a high-risk population may motivate participants to follow recommendations after the screening and seek medical services given positive test results. In terms of *disadvantages of screening*, if the entire population is screened and the condition is infrequent (low prevalence), this will imply wasting resources, yielding few detected cases compared to the effort invested in the screening.

1.8.16 Issues in early disease detection

1.8.16.1 What are the benefits of screening?

Screening for a disease allows for detection, implying early diagnosis, timely treatment, and good prognosis. For example, the diagnosis of malignancy at an early disease stage or favorable tumor grade enhances and prolongs survival.

1.8.16.1.1 EARLY DISEASE DETECTION

The natural history of a disease involves (a) a *preclinical phase*, which is the phase that may be termed the biologic or psychological onset, but the symptoms have not yet occurred; (b) a *clinical phase*, which is the period after the symptoms have occurred; (c) a *detectable preclinical phase*, which is the natural stage of the disease where the disease is detected by screening; (d) *lead time*, which is the interval by which the time of diagnosis is advanced by screening and early detection of the disease relative to the usual time of diagnosis; and (e) a *critical point*, which refers to a point in the natural history of the disease in which the condition is potentially curable, implying optimal treatment potential. The inability to identify a critical point in natural history of disease, screening, and early detection calls into question the benefit of screening. Effectiveness of screening includes (a) mortality reduction in the high-risk population screened, (b) reduction in case fatality, (c) increase in the percentage of asymptomatic cases, (d) minimized complications, (e) reduction in recurrent cases or malignancies, and (f) improvement in the quality of life.[11]

Issues in screening include (1) sensitivity and specificity of the screening test as well as the predictive values, (2) false-positive test results, (3) cost of early detection, (4) emotional and physical adverse effects of screening, and (5) benefit of the screening.[12]

1.8.17 Biases in disease screening and detection

Biases include referral bias, also referred to as volunteer bias; length-biased sampling associated with prognostic selection, which refers to a selection bias in which screening involves the selection of cases of disease with better prognoses;[13] lead-time bias; and overdiagnosis bias.

1.8.17.1 What is lead-time bias?

Lead-time bias refers to the apparent increase in survival time after diagnosis resulting from earlier time of diagnosis rather than later time of death.

1.8.17.2 What is length bias?

This is a form of selection bias and refers to the tendency in a population screening effort to detect preferentially the longer, more indolent cases of any particular disease.

Vignette 1.3: Consider a new screening program for prostate cancer (CaP) in County X. The CaP screening program used a test that is effective in screening for early-stage CaP. Assume that there is no effective treatment for CaP, and as such, the screening results do not change the natural history or course of CaP. Second, assume that the rates observed are based on all known cases of CaP and that there are no changes in the quality of death certification for CaP. With these assumptions, what will be the influence of this screening test on the incidence and prevalence proportion during the first year of this program and what will be the influence of this screening on the case-fatality and mortality rates of CaP during the first year of CaP screening?

Solutions: (a) There will be an increase in both incidence rate and prevalence proportion. (b) There will be a decrease in case-fatality rate while the mortality rate will remain constant because of the assumption that changes have not been observed with respect to the quality of death certification.

1.8.18 Disease screening, diagnostic tests, and clinical reasoning

1.8.18.1 What is clinical reasoning?

The process by which clinicians channel their thinking toward probable diagnosis is classically thought of as a mixture of pattern recognition and "hypothetico-deductive" reasoning.[14] The reasoning process depends on medical knowledge in areas such as disease prevalence and pathophysiological mechanisms. Teaching on the process of reasoning, as diagnostic tests provide new information, has included modifications of Bayes's theorem in an attempt to get clinicians to think constructively about pretest and posttest possibilities.[15]

Clinical decision-making is guided by and large by statistical and epidemiologic principles, as well as biologic and clinical reasoning. The understanding of the former is the purpose of this book, which is not intended to place statistical stability in results interpretation over sound biologic theories and clinical judgment in clinical research conceptualization, design, conduct, and interpretation of results. A sound clinical judgment comes with experience, but such experience, in order not to be biased, ought to be guided by some statistical and epidemiologic principles, including though not limited to probability concepts (sensitivity, specificity, and predictive values), Bayes's theorem, and risk and predisposition to disease. Therefore, since clinical decision-making involves some risk acceptance, the understanding of probability serves to guide alternatives to treatment while assessing the risk and benefit of therapeutics.

Vignette 1.4: A forty-eight-year-old Asian-American woman presents with a hip fracture. She has a history of metabolic fracture and had been previously diagnosed with osteoporosis. The clinical scenario involves the estimation of the probability of hip fracture in this individual, and the clinical impression on previous cases indicates the common presentation of this condition in this subpopulation—age, concurrent diagnosis of osteoporosis. The probability of response to treatment is dependent on the response of similar patients in the past, indicative of statistical reasoning. Although not a very good example to illustrate the application of a diagnostic test, the risk inherent in this case could be seen in the diagnosis of hip fracture resulting in a false-positive or false-negative test result. Also, the natural history of hip fracture may influence the clinical judgment in terms of the planned therapeutics. Clinical reasoning is also brought into question when considering alternative treatment.[16]

As sound clinical reasoning (avoiding biases) continues to shape therapeutics, there remains the necessity of clinicians being able to appraise clinical and scientific literature for evidence; the volumes of clinical and epidemiologic studies become the basis of clinical decision-making. Clinicians must understand how outcome studies are conducted and how the results obtained from these studies can be used in clinical decision-making involving care improvement and patient safety. The intent is not to train physicians or clinicians to become statisticians but to refine the already available skills in order to provide evidence-based care that is optimal through the utilization of results from internally (biases, confounding, random error) and externally (generalizability) valid studies.[17]

1.9 Balancing benefits and harmful effects in medicine

Clinicians are interested in knowing about the impact of treatment or intervention on individual patients. A large impact, relative to a small one, is of interest to both the clinician and his or her patient. The relative risk (RR) and absolute risk (AR) are two concepts that are extrapolated to determine risk in the individual patients. The absolute risk reduction (ARR) is used to assess whether the benefit of treatment outweighs the adverse effects.

We present these concepts in detail in the chapter on the measure of disease association and effect, but it is sufficient to provide a basic understanding of relative risk reduction (RRR), ARR, number needed to treat (NNT), and number needed to harm (NNH) here. Simply, the RRR refers to the difference in event rates between two groups, implying a proportion of event rate in the control or untreated group.[18] Suppose 40 patients had recurrent cystitis out of 100 patients treated initially with erythromycin (control group) and 30 patients had recurrent cystitis out of 100 patients treated initially with erythromycin plus amoxicillin (treatment group). What is the RRR? The RRR is the absolute risk difference (40% to 30%) divided by the event rate in the control group (40%):

$$\text{RRR} = \text{Absolute risk difference (ARD)/Event rate in the control (ERC)}$$

where ARD = Event rate in the control − Event rate in the treatment group. Substituting: 40–30/40 = 25%. This means that recurrent cystitis was 25% lower in the treatment group compared to the control.

What is the ARR? Also termed *risk difference*, it is the arithmetic difference between two event rates expressed as the ERC minus the event rate in the treatment (ERT). Substituting, ARR = ERC − ERT = 40% − 30% = 10%.

The NNT simply reflects the consequences of treating or not treating patients, given a specified therapy. NNT may be described as the number of patients who would be treated for one of them to benefit. Mathematically, NNT is estimated by 100 divided by the ARR expressed as percentage (100/ARR). NNT could also be expressed as a proportion: 1/ARR. As ARR increases, NNT decreases, and inversely, as ARR decreases, NNT increases.

Vignette 1.5: If in diabetic patients treated for the disease with insulin, the risk of renal insufficiency is 1.65 and 1.46 among the controls, how many diabetic patients need to be treated (NNT)? What is the estimated ARR, RR, RRR, and NNT? Based on these data, what is the odds ratio? *Solution*: risk in controls − risk in treatment (cases), while NNT = 1/ARR. ARR = risk in control (p1) − risk in treatment group (p2): p1 − p2 = 1.46 − 1.65 = −0.19. Relative risk (RR) = p1/p2 = 1.46 ÷ 1.65 = 0.71. The RRR = (p1 − p2)/p1 − (1.46–1.65)/1.65 = −0.29. The NNH is expressed as the inverse of the absolute risk increase (1/ARI). The NNH represents the number of patients required to be treated for one of them to experience an adverse effect. Mathematically, NNH is estimated as: 100/ARI expressed as percentage. NNT could also be expressed as proportion: 1/ARI. NNT = 1/0.19 = 6. Odds ratio = p1(1 − p1) ÷ p2 (1 − p2). Substituting: (0.46/0.54)/(0.65/0.35) = 0.46.

Vignette 1.6: If the risk of developing postoperative infection in cerebral palsy children with scoliosis is 2.9 among those with rod instrumentation, and 1.9 among those who received spinal fusion without instrumentation, examine the risk associated with unit rod instrumentation. What is the estimated ARI and the NNH? *Solution*: ARI = Risk in cases (instrumented group) − Risk in control (noninstrumented group), while NNH is 1/ARI.

1.10 Summary

Clinical research is conducted primarily to improve therapeutics and prevent disease occurrence in clinical settings in contrast to population-based research. This effort involves adequate conceptualization, design process, conduct, analysis, and accurate interpretation of the results, which is achieved through a joint effort of a clinician and a biostatistician. The selection of patients depends on the accurate ascertainment of disease, implying a screening/diagnostic test that is capable of classifying those with the disease as test-positive (sensitivity) and those without as test-negative (specificity). Screening is a particular form of disease detection test and is applied to a population at risk for developing a disease, such as prostate cancer (PSA for men 50 years and older), in an attempt to diagnose CaP earlier than the natural history would manifest CaP. The intent is to diagnose early where CaP is treatable and curable. Diagnostic tests are performed to confirm the presence of a disease after symptoms of an illness.

The prevalence of disease simply means the probability of the condition before performing the test, meaning pretest probability. The predictive values refer to the probability of the disease being present or absent after obtaining the results of the test. Using the two-by-two table, positive predictive value (PPV) is the proportion of those with a positive test who have the disease [a/(a + b)], while the negative predictive value (NPV) is the proportion of those with a negative test who do not have the disease [d/(c + d)]. The predictive values will vary with the prevalence of the disease or condition being tested for. Therefore, the probability of the disease before (prevalence) and the probability of the disease after (predictive value) will be interrelated, with the differences in predictive values driven by the differences in the prevalence of the disease. Sensitivity and specificity are properties of a diagnostic test and should be consistent when the test is used in similar patients and in similar settings. Predictive values, although related to the sensitivity and specificity of the test, will vary with the prevalence of the condition or disease being tested. The difference in the sensitivity and specificity of the test is most likely a result of the test not being administered in similar conditions (patients and settings).[19] The screening test should be highly sensitive (sensitivity) while a diagnostic test should be highly specific (Specificity). As the cutoff point between positive and negative results changes, the sensitivity and specificity of the test will be influenced. This relationship is illustrated by the ROC and assesses the extent to which a screening test can be used to discriminate between those with and without disease, and to select the cutoff point to characterize normal and abnormal results.

The advantages and limitations of screening remind us of the balanced clinical judgment in a recommending large-population screening test. The common biases in screening include length-bias sampling, lead-time, overdiagnosis, and volunteer or referral bias (where those screened for the disease are healthier than the general population, thus influencing the conclusion regarding the benefit of screening). These systematic errors are all selection bias and, if not considered, have the tendency of affecting the conclusions regarding the benefits of screening.

Often, clinicians may want to know the benefits or risk of treating a future or potential patient. In assessing such a benefit versus risk ratio, the NNT and the NNH are practical alternatives to relative risk or ARR in assessing the treatment effect. NNT remains a concise and clinically more useful way of presenting intervention effect. The NNT simply reflects the consequences of treating or not treating patients, given a specified therapy. The question remains as to which NNT is clinically acceptable to clinicians and patients—the *NNT threshold*. To address this question, one must consider the cost of treatment, the severity of preventable outcomes, and the adverse or side effects of the treatment or intervention. NNT may be described as the number of patients who would have to be treated for one of them to benefit. The NNH is expressed as the inverse of the absolute risk increase (1/ARI).

The NNH represents the number of patients required to be treated for one of them to experience an adverse effect.

Questions for discussion

1 Suppose there is no good treatment for disease X. (a) What will be the advantages, if any, in performing a screening trial in this context? (b) What are the design issues in such a trial if you were to conduct one? (c) Survival is often seen as a definitive outcome measure in screening trials, would you consider population incidence of advanced disease and stage shifts as possible outcome measures? (d) Early detection induces a bias in the comparison of survival times that artificially makes screen-detected cases appear to live longer. What is this biased called, and how would you correct this in order to estimate the true benefit of screening?

2 Suppose that disease A is potentially detectable by screening during a window of time between its onset and the time when it would ordinarily become clinically manifest. (a) What is lead-time bias? (b) Would people with longer windows due to person-to-person variability in disease manifestation be more likely to be screened in the window? (c) Would you expect the "window of screening" to result in length-time bias?

3 Suppose that 82% of those with hypertension and 25% of those without hypertension are classified as hypertensive by an automated blood-pressure machine. (a) Estimate the positive predictive value and negative predictive value of this machine, assuming that 34.5% of the adult US population has high blood pressure. Hints: Sensitivity = 0.82, specificity = 1 − 0.25 = 0.75. Using Bayes's theorem: PV+ = (sen × prevalence)/(sen × prevalence) + (specificity × prevalence). Comment on these results, and state which is more predictive, positive or negative?

4 Suppose 8 out of 1000 cerebral palsy children operated on for scoliosis developed deep wound infection, and 992 did not, while 10 out of 1000 children who were not treated with surgery developed deep wound infection. What is the relative risk of deep wound infection associated with surgery? Estimate the RRR. Why is the ARR also called *absolute risk difference*? What is the NNT? Hints: RR = (a/a + b)/(c/c + d); ARR = (c/c + d) − (a/a + b); NNT = 1/(c/c + d) − (a/a + b). What is the 95% CI for ARR and NNT? Hint: CI for NNT = 1/UCI − 1/LCI of ARR. Hints: 95% CI for ARR = +1.96 [CER × (1 − CER)/number of control patients + EER × (1 − EER)/number of experimental or treatment patients].

5 In a cohort of 1069 children with cerebral palsy, 141 had severe mental retardation and were quadriplegic, while 420 of 13,525 nonquadriplegic had mental retardation (MR). What are the odds of developing MR among quadriplegics? What are the odds of developing MR among nonquadriplegics? What is the relative risk of developing MR, given quadriplegic CP? Estimate the odds ratio, given quadriplegic CP.

References

1. J. E. Johansson, H. O. Adami, S. O. Anderson et al., High 10-year survival rate in patients with early, untreated prostatic cancer, *JAMA* 267 (1992):216–219.
2. R. S. Greenberg et al., *Medical Epidemiology*, 4th ed. (New York: Lange, 2005).
3. D. L. Sackett, W. S. Richardson, W. Rosenberg, and R. B. Haynes, *Evidence-Based Medicine: How to Practice and Teach Evidence-Based Medicine*, 2nd ed. (Edinburg: Churchill Livingstone, 2000).
4. D. L. Sackett, W. S. Richardson, W. Rosenberg, and R. B. Haynes, *Evidence-Based Medicine: How to Practice and Teach Evidence-Based Medicine*, 2nd ed. (Edinburg: Churchill Livingstone, 2000); D. L. Katz, Clinical Epidemiology & Evidence-Based Medicine: Fundamental Principles of Clinical Reasoning & Research (Thousand Oaks, CA: Sage, 2001).
5. M. S. Kocher, Ultrasonographic screening for developmental dysplasia of the hip: An epidemiologic analysis (Part II), *Am J Orthop* 30 (2001):19–24.
6. J. F. Jekel, L. Katz, and J. G. Elmore, *Epidemiology, Biostatistics, and Preventive Medicine* (Philadelphia: Saunders, 2001).
7. D. L. Katz, *Clinical Epidemiology & Evidence-Based Medicine: Fundamental Principles of Clinical Reasoning & Research* (Thousand Oaks, CA: Sage, 2001).
8. D. L. Katz, *Clinical Epidemiology & Evidence-Based Medicine: Fundamental Principles of Clinical Reasoning & Research* (Thousand Oaks, CA: Sage, 2001); R. K. Riegelman and R. P. Hirsch, Studying a Test and Testing a Test, 2nd ed. (Boston: Little Brown & Company, 1989).
9. D. L. Sackett, W. S. Richardson, W. Rosenberg, and R. B. Haynes, *Evidence-Based Medicine: How to Practice and Teach Evidence-Based Medicine*, 2nd ed. (Edinburg: Churchill Livingstone, 2000); S. Greenland, Bias methods for sensitivity analysis of bases, *Int J Epidemiol* 25 (1996):1107–1116; G. D. Friedman, *Primer of Epidemiology*, 4th ed. (New York: McGraw-Hill, 1994); D. G. Altman, *Practical Statistics for Medical Research* (London: Chapman & Hall, 1991).
10. P. Armitage and G. Berry, *Statistical Methods in Medical Research*, 3rd ed. (Oxford, UK: Blackwell Scientific Publishing, 1994).
11. S. Greenland, Bias methods for sensitivity analysis of bases, *Int J Epidemiol* 25 (1996): 1107–1116; B. Rosner, *Fundamentals of Biostatistics*, 5th ed. (Duxbury, CA: 2000).
12. S. Greenland, Bias methods for sensitivity analysis of bases, *Int J Epidemiol* 25 (1996):1107–1116; J. A. Freiman et al., The importance of beta, the type II error and sample size in the design and interpretation of the randomized clinical trial, *N Engl J Med* 299 (1978):690–694.
13. J. F. Jekel, L. Katz, and J. G. Elmore, *Epidemiology, Biostatistics, and Preventive Medicine* (Philadelphia: Saunders, 2001); S. Greenland, Bias methods for sensitivity analysis of bases, *Int J Epidemiol* 25 (1996):1107–1116.
14. D. L. Sackett, R. B. Haynes, G. H. Guyatt, and P. Tugwell, *Clinical Epidemiology: A Basic Science for Clinical Medicine* (Boston: Little, Brown, 1991); J. Dowie and A. Elstein, *Professional Judgment: A Reader in Clinical Decision Making* (Cambridge: Cambridge University Press, 1988).
15. D. L. Sackett, R. B. Haynes, G. H. Guyatt, and P. Tugwell, *Clinical Epidemiology: A Basic Science for Clinical Medicine* (Boston: Little, Brown, 1991).
16. J. P. Kassirer, Diagnostic reasoning, *Ann Intern Med* 110 (1989):893–900.
17. J. P. Kassirer, B. J. Kuipers, and G. A. Gorry, Toward a theory of clinical expertise, *Am J Med* 73 (1982):251–259; A. Tversky and D. Kahnemann, Judgment under uncertainty: Heuristics and biases, *Science* 185 (1974):1124–1131.

18. G. Chatellier, E. Zapletal et al., The number needed to treat: A clinically nomogram in its proper context, *BMJ* 312 (1996):426–429.
19. D. L. Sackett, W. S. Richardson, W. Rosenberg, and R. B. Haynes, *Evidence-Based Medicine: How to Practice and Teach Evidence-Based Medicine*, 2nd ed. (Edinburg: Churchill Livingstone, 2000).

2 Research design

Experimental and nonexperimental studies

2.1 Introduction

Design process is fundamental to evidence obtained from biomedical and clinical research, since errors in sampling may adversely affect the evidence derived from the sample. Designs may be classified in several ways, including descriptive versus inferential and experimental versus nonexperimental. While a descriptive study design characterizes samples with respect to independent and outcome variables without any attempt at generalization to the population of interest, inferential studies test specific hypotheses in order to draw inferences on the population, implying those patients who were not studied with the sample.

The use of observational and nonobservational, or experimental, design was very popular in study designs classification, though this is an incorrect characterization of studies. All studies are observational in the sense that the outcomes of experimental and nonexperimental designs require the observation of subjects for the determination of the end point or outcome. Designs can be classified correctly as experimental or nonexperimental. In an experimental design, as we commonly use the term in biological sciences research, the investigator assigns the study subjects, for example, mice, to treatment with a certain therapeutic agent or to placebo control. Similarly, in an experiment involving humans, also termed a *clinical trial*, patients are allocated to the arms of the study by the investigator; however, the investigator does not manipulate the occurrence of the outcome but observes the event as it unfolds, such as the biochemical end point, recovery, deep wound or bone cyst healing, or mortality. The nonexperimental designs are also loosely termed *epidemiologic designs* despite the rigorous involvement of epidemiologic principles and methods in the design of clinical trials.

Epidemiologic study design is covered in most epidemiologic texts in detail, including the *Applied Epidemiologic Principles and Concepts for Clinicians*, which is a companion text to this volume. This chapter provides a brief overview of epidemiologic designs, namely, nonexperimental and experimental design involving humans (clinical trial). The design process that reflects the sampling provides the information required for the selection of the test statistic in an inferential study. In addition, the scale of measurement of the response or outcome variable guides the selection of the test statistic or model. For example, if the outcome of a study designed to assess the comparative effectiveness of botulinum toxin and baclofen in reducing spasticity in spastic cerebral palsy is measured on a binary scale (presence or absence of spasticity), then the logistic regression model is an adequate statistical technique. While a brief overview of the basics of these designs is essential in increasing one's knowledge of the designs, the selection of appropriate design will depend on the research question to be addressed, availability of exposed or case subjects, and timing of the study, as well as the advantages and disadvantages of the design. Also, the available research resources may influence the choice of the design as well as constrict the study size.

2.2 Epidemiologic study designs

Clinical research design is fundamentally epidemiologic. What is epidemiology? While there are many definitions of *epidemiology*, a simple approach is to consider epidemiology as the study of the distribution and determinants of disease, disabilities, injuries, and health-related events at the population level. Equally important to the understanding of epidemiology is the application of the results from epidemiologic research in implementing health programs to reduce health complications, decrease risk factors, maintain health, and promote and control disease at the population level. Since diseases do not occur randomly, epidemiologic principles are utilized to examine disease distribution, which may vary by sex, age, geography, and time. Therefore, descriptive epidemiology focuses on characterizing disease occurrence by person, place, and time (PPT).

Besides disease distribution, epidemiologists also attempt to establish a possible association between disease and exposure by answering the following questions: Is the exposure related to the disease? Is there any causal relationship between the exposure and the disease? This approach, though inappropriately characterized, has been classified as analytic epidemiology. Practically, epidemiologic designs are used in studying the natural course of the disease, characterizing diseases or events of interest by person, place, and time; identifying risk factors; assessing effectiveness and efficacy of treatment in routine use and closed laboratory environments, respectively; examine complications; and compare effectiveness and safety in treatment settings (Figure 2.1). Epidemiologic designs provide the building blocks for causal inference. Meta-analysis, which is the study of studies, is highly dependent on epidemiologic principles and methods for its conduct, analysis, and inference. However, for the purpose of simplicity, we will focus on nonexperimental and clinical trials as epidemiologic designs. Classified under nonexperimental epidemiologic designs are (a) case reports, (b) case series, (c) ecologic designs,

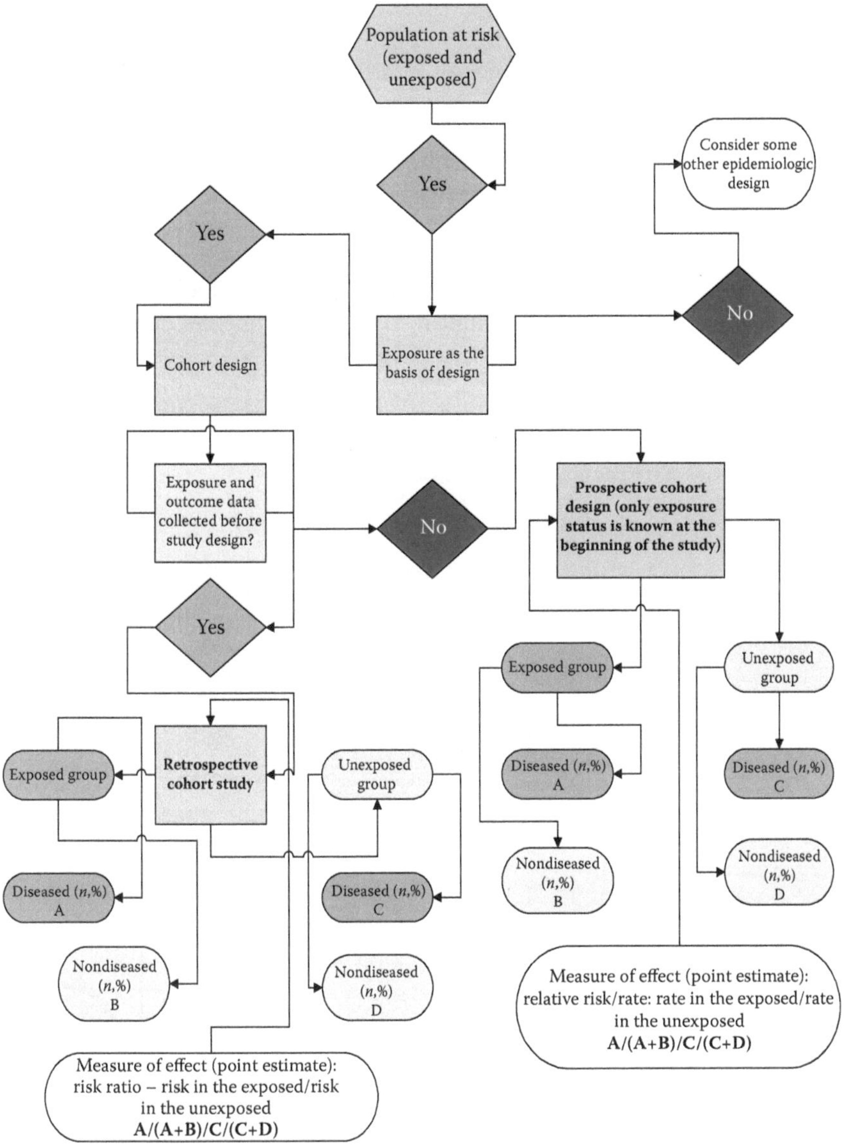

Figure 2.1 Design and measure of effect in biomedical, clinical, and population-based research.

(d) cross-sectional studies, (e) case–control studies, and (f) cohort studies (retrospective, prospective, and ambidirectional). Experimental designs involving human subjects (clinical trials) are classified into phases (I, II, III, and IV) and types of design (parallel, sequential, crossover, community intervention, cluster, factorial, etc.).

2.3 Nonexperimental designs

Epidemiologic designs are used in conducting clinical and biomedical research. The selection of an appropriate design is essential to the results, since no matter how sophisticated the statistics used in the analysis of the data, a study based on unsound or flawed design principles will generate an invalid result (Figure 2.2). There are two broad classifications of study designs: (a) nonexperimental, also loosely termed observational, and (b) experimental or the clinical trial, if the experiment is conducted in humans. What distinguishes these methods is the process of assignment or allocation of subjects to the study arms. Whereas the clinical trial or experimental design allocates

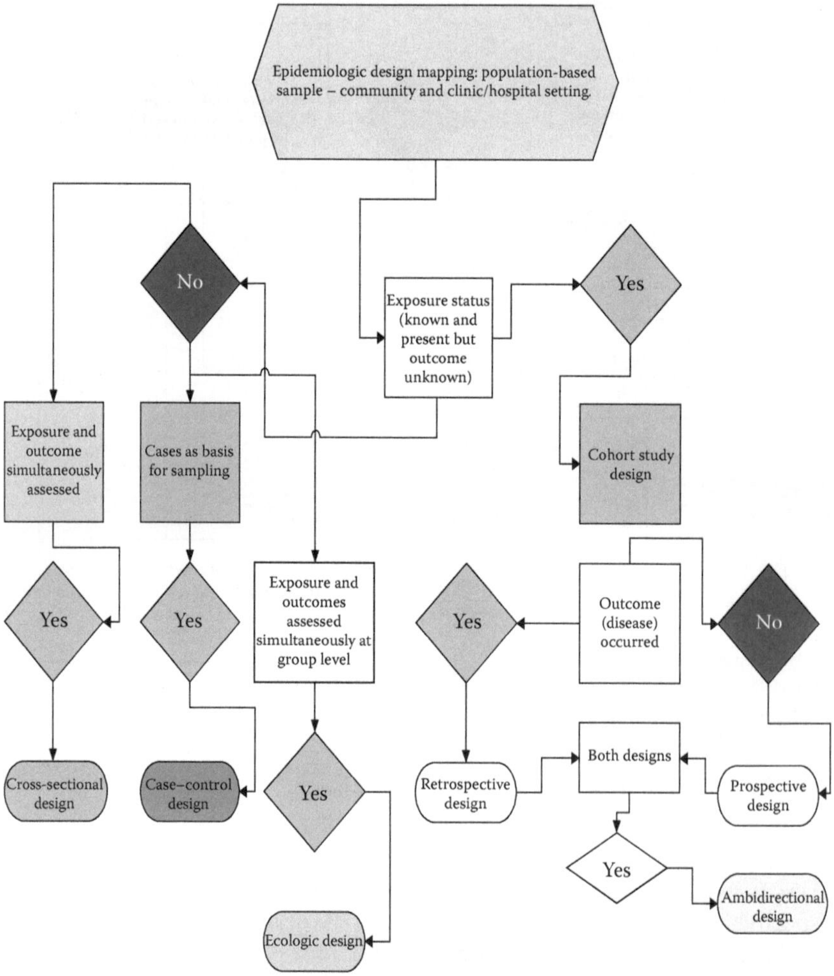

Figure 2.2 Selection of epidemiologic design.

subjects or eligible participants to the treatment or control arm of the study, based on the equipoise (collective uncertainty about the advantage or superior benefit of one treatment arm versus its alternative or control arm) principle, nonexperimental designs do not involve subject allocation to an exposure or nonexposure arm, but merely observe the exposed as well as the unexposed for the occurrence of the outcomes of interest (prospective cohort design if there is follow-up or cross-sectional in the absence of follow-up), such as symptoms, disease, or death.

Traditionally, there are two primary types of nonexperimental design: (a) cohort studies—study subjects are characterized by their exposure status and followed for a period of time to ascertain the outcome of interest, and (b) case–control studies—study subjects are characterized by their disease status, and the presence of exposure is ascertained in the cases as well as the controls or comparison group, who are comparable to the cases but do not have the disease of interest.

While cohort design provides information on the outcome of interest, case–control generates data on the exposure distribution among the cases and control groups. Cross-sectional and ecologic designs are other traditional designs often employed in epidemiologic methods. The former assesses the relationship between disease or outcome of interest and exposure among a well-defined group or population at a point in time. This design measures the prevalence of the exposure or exposures of interest in relation to the disease prevalence of interest—for example, a study to be conducted using the US National Health Interview Survey to assess the factors associated with ethnic/racial disparities in hypertension. Since information on the exposure and outcome were collected before the design of the study and there was no follow-up of participants, cross-sectional design remains a feasible approach to providing information on the disease prevalence (hypertension) in relation to exposure prevalence (exercise, diet, education, marital status, etc.). The ecologic design examines the association between exposure and disease at a group level and does not use individual (case) data as the unit analysis.

What is the most appropriate design depends on many factors, some of which include (a) the nature of the research question and hypothesis to be tested, (b) the current state of knowledge regarding the hypothesis to be tested or the research question to be answered, (c) the frequency of the exposure and disease in the specific population (rare disease for case–control and rare exposure for cohort design), (d) expected magnitude of association between the exposure and outcome of interest, (e) subjects' availability and enrollment, (f) financial and human resources, and (g) ethical considerations, if a clinical trial is planned. However, regardless of the design used, there are advantages and limitations in these designs in terms of the level of evidence (internal and external validity). Therefore, the intent is to increase the validity of the study by (a) minimizing bias, (b) controlling confounding, and (c) increasing precision by minimizing random error (Figure 2.3).

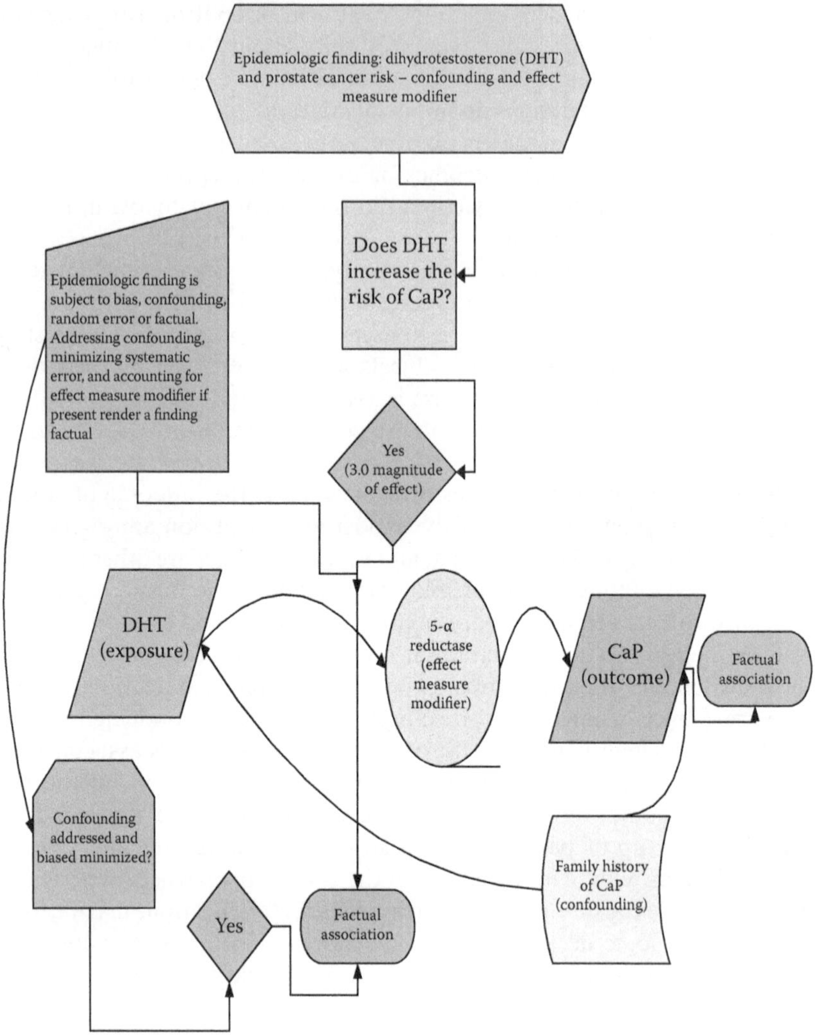

Figure 2.3 Epidemiologic confounding as statistical covariate.

2.4 Experimental designs (clinical trials)

The clinical trial remains the gold standard in terms of research design if an appropriate sample size is used, because of its distinctive features of randomization and placebo control. These features minimize baseline variability between the treatment and control groups, yielding a more accurate result of the effect of the treatment. But there is a price to these advantages, mainly enrollment issues, the high cost of conducting the trial, and ethical considerations. Therefore, despite the advantages of randomized placebo-controlled clinical trials, this design may not be feasible in certain contexts, requiring the use of nonexperimental designs.

The core of the *experimental design* is the allocation, which denotes the assignment of individuals or subjects/participants by the investigator and may involve randomization.[1] The distinct feature from nonexperimental or observational designs is that the investigator controls the assignment of the exposure or treatment, but otherwise, the symmetry of potential unknown confounders is maintained through randomization.[1] Properly executed experimental studies provide the strongest empirical evidence. The randomization of subjects to treatment or control arms also provides a better foundation for statistical procedures than do observational studies.

A *randomized controlled clinical trial (RCT)* is a prospective, analytical experimental study using primary data generated in the clinical environment to draw statistical inference on the efficacy of the treatment, device, or procedure (Figure 2.4). Subjects similar at the baseline are randomly allocated to two or more treatment groups and the outcomes from the groups are compared after a follow-up period.[1] This design, termed the gold standard, is the most valid and reliable evidence of the clinical efficacy of preventive and therapeutic procedures in the clinical setting. However, it may not always be feasible. *The randomized crossover clinical trial* represents a prospective, analytical, experimental design using primary data generated in the clinical environment to assess efficacy as in RCT. In this design, subjects, for example, with a chronic condition, such as low back pain, are randomly allocated to one of two treatment groups and, after a sufficient treatment period and often a washout period, are switched to the other treatment for the same period. This design is susceptible to bias if carried-over effects from the first treatment occur (sort of contamination).[2]

Clinical trials involve a huge amount of organization and coordination. Simply, the elements include the consideration of (a) study subject—clinical trials involve human subjects; (b) design direction—prospective in design; (c) comparison group—new treatment versus placebo/standard care; (d) intervention measure—primary outcome (death, recovery, progression, reduction in SE, etc.); (e) the effect of medication, surgery—relating to outcome; and (f) timing of the clinical trial—conducted early in the development of therapies.[3] Conducting the trial, which is the design and implementation, distinct from conceptualization, requires that the investigators (a) review existing scientific data and build on that knowledge, (b) formulate testable hypotheses and the techniques to test these hypothesis, (c) deal with ethical considerations, (d) determine the scientific merits of the study through statistical inference, and (e) resolve validity issues—biases and confounding.[4]

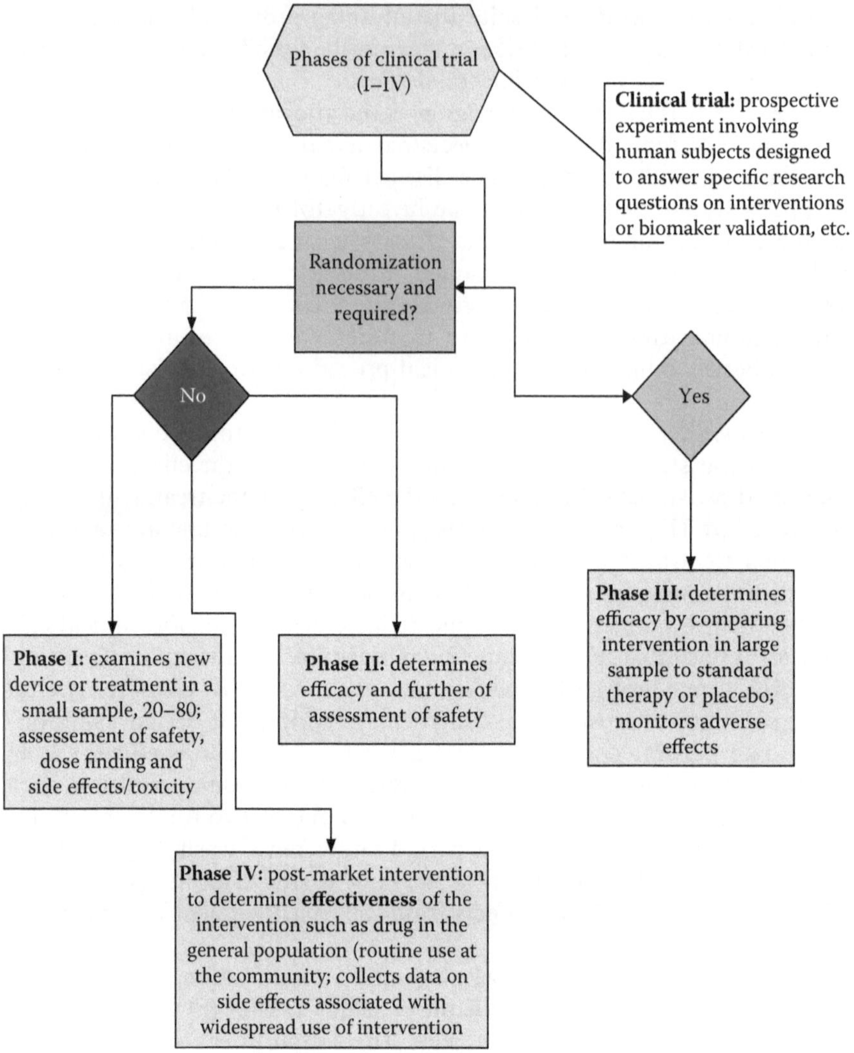

Figure 2.4 Phases of clinical trial illustrating randomized and nonrandomized phases of experiment.

2.5 Nonexperimental versus experimental design

Observational or nonexperimental studies are research designs in which investigators do not assign study subjects to the study groups/arms but passively observe events and determine the measures of association/magnitude of effect. The purpose is to draw inferences about possible causal relationships between exposure and some health outcome, condition, or disease.[3] These studies are broadly characterized as descriptive and analytic. The observational analytic designs so traditionally identified, but which remain inappropriately characterized (analytic designs have descriptive components as well as the description of incidence of disease over time), are cross-sectional, case–control, and cohort, and the several hybrids of these designs (nested case–control, case–cohort etc.). *Cohort studies* are observational or nonexperimental designs that commence with the identification of the exposure status of each subject and involve following the groups over time to determine the outcome in both the exposed and unexposed. Like most epidemiologic studies, cohort designs are intended to allow inferences about exposure influence on the occurrence of disease or outcome of interest.[5,6] While sampling (selection of study subjects) in *case–control* is based on the disease or health outcome, in cohort designs, sampling is performed without regard to the disease or health outcome but exposure status.[3] In comparison to *cross-sectional*, which is an "instant cohort" design, sampling (study population selection) is done without regard to exposure or disease status.[1] *Ecologic* studies are sometimes characterized as analytic because of their abilities to assess the effect of the exposure at the group level on the outcome, using the correlation coefficient. However, it is not uncommon to go through an introductory epidemiology text without finding mention of an ecologic design, or if it is discussed, it is classified as descriptive design. Therefore, the classification of epidemiologic designs into analytic and descriptive remains a meaningless distinction and should not be stressed (Table 2.1).

Table 2.1 Classical epidemiologic designs: experimental and nonexperimental (observational)

Design types and examples	*Description*
Experimental/clinical trial	Subjects are assigned to study arms by investigator—active manipulation of participants but not outcome. Used when feasible because of ethical considerations in examining the effects of screening, diagnosis, therapeutics, and preventive practices on health.
Nonexperimental design (a) Cohort design—commences with exposure status, uses follow-up, and determines the outcome. (b) Case–control—commences with disease and examines exposure distribution in cases and controls. (c) Cross-sectional—snapshot examination of exposure and outcome without follow-up. (d) Ecologic group-level analysis.	Does not involve subject allocation or assignment to the arms of the study. Used to assess the etiology, effects of treatment on disease, screening, diagnosis, and prevention. Classical examples are cohort, case–control, cross-sectional, and ecologic designs.

2.6 Measures of disease association or effect

Whatever methods or study design is used, the primary objective of a methodologist or clinical researcher is to obtain valid and reliable evidence from the data. This evidence primarily involves the measurement of disease or outcome/response effect. Common measures of disease effects are (a) relative risk (RR), risk ratio, or rate ratio (relative measures of comparison); (b) rate or risk difference (absolute measures of comparison); (c) population rate difference; (d) attributable proportion among the exposed; (e) attributable proportion among the total population exposed; and (f) correlation coefficient and coefficient of determination. While the relative measure of disease effect compares two measures of disease frequency, such as RR or odds ratio (OR), and quantifies the strength of the relationship or association between exposure (independent, explanatory, or predictor variable) and disease (outcome or response), the absolute measure of disease effect describes and quantifies the effect or impact of disease by comparing the difference between two measures of disease frequency, such as incidence rate or prevalence proportion.

The measure of disease occurrence quantifies both the crude and adjusted rates and the proportion of disease or outcome of interest in a specific patient or community-based population. In clinical research settings, patients usually consist of those who show improvement after a procedure or medication and those who do not. The proportion of those with improvement measures the occurrence of the outcome of interest and could be characterized as the prevalence of improvement (measured by those with improvement divided by the total number of all patients studied). In a prospective cohort design, it is possible to measure the incidence of a complication among patients who received surgery (number of new cases of complications/person-time). We can also compare the incidence of an outcome/disease in one patient population with another patient population, provided the two populations are standardized with respect to confounders, such as age and sex, which allows one to compare the age- or sex-adjusted rate, also called the standardized rate.

BOX 2.1 VALIDITY—SYSTEMATIC ERROR (BIAS) AND RANDOM ERROR (PRECISION)

The objective of a study, which is an exercise in measurement, is to obtain valid and precise estimates of the effect size or measure of disease occurrence.

- The value of the parameter is estimated with little error.
- Related to the handling of *systematic errors* or biases and *random error.*
- Involves the generalization of findings from the study to the relevant target or source population.

- Comprises *validity* and *precision.*
    - Validity refers to estimate or effect size that has little systematic error (biases).
    - There are two components of validity: internal and external.
- *Internal validity* refers to accuracy of the effect measure of the inferences drawn in relation to the source population.
    - Inference of the source population
    - A prerequisite for external validity*
    - Measures of internal validity are (a) confounding, (b) selection bias, and (c) information bias (measurement error)
- *External validity* refers to the accuracy of the effect measure of the inferences in relation to individuals outside the source population.
    - Involves representation of the study population to the general population.
    - Do factors that differentiate the larger or general population from the study population modify the effect or the measure of the effect in the study?
    - Involves combination of epidemiologic and other sources, for example, pathophysiology.
    - Related to criteria for causal inference.
- *Precision* refers to estimates or measures of effect or disease occurrence with little random error.

* J. A. Freiman et al. The importance of beta, the type II error and sample size in the design and interpretation of the randomized clinical trial, *N Engl J Med* 299 (1978):690–694.

2.7 Precision, random error, and bias

Random error refers to unsystematic errors that arise from an unforeseeable and unpredictable process, such as a mistake in assessing the exposure and disease, and sampling variability (unrepresentative sample or chance). This is the lack of random error. Precision, and hence reduction in random error, may be improved by (a) increasing the sample size, (b) repeating the measurement within a study, and (c) utilizing an efficient study design in order to maximize the amount of information obtained.

Precision (lack of random error) may be influenced by (a) sampling, (b) hypothesis testing and p values, (c) confidence intervals estimation, (d) random variable probability distribution, and (e) sample size and power estimation.[7] Systematic error may be present in a study despite the absence of or reduction in random error (the study may be precise but findings are inaccurate). *Interaction* is said to occur when the incidence rate of a disease or outcome in the presence of two or more risk factors differs from the incidence rate expected to result from their individual effect. This rate may be greater than what is expected (synergism) or less than what is expected (antagonism).[8] Like the effect measure modifier, interaction is said to occur if there is a difference in the strata-specific risk point estimate (RR, OR) on the basis of the third variable.

Internal validity (random error, bias, and confounding) refers to accurate measurement of study effects without bias—this bias presents threats to the internal validity of the study. The precision and accuracy of measurement are essential to study validity. While precision refers to the degree to which a variable has nearly the same value when measured several times, accuracy pertains to the degree to which a variable actually represents what it is supposed to represent or measure. Precision may be enhanced by (1) repetition, (2) refinement, (3) observer training and performance verification, (4) standardization, and (5) automation, which minimizes variability owing to observers. Accuracy may be improved by (1) specific markers and better instruments, (2) unobtrusive measurement, (3) blinding, and (4) instrument calibration.

Role of Random Error: Assuming a random sample was taken from the population studied, is this sample representative of the population? Is the observed result influenced by sampling variability? Is there a recognizable source of error, such as the quality of questions, faulty instruments, and so on? Is the error due to chance, given no connection to a recognizable source or error? Random error can be minimized by (1) improving design, (2) enlarging sample size, and (3) increasing precision, as well as by using good quality control during study implementation.[9] It is important to note here that the sample studied is a random sample and that it is meaningless to apply statistical significance to the result designs that do not utilize random samples.[10]

Null Hypothesis and Types of Errors: The null hypothesis states that there is no association between the exposure and the disease variables, which, in most instances, translates to the statement that the ratio measure of association = 1.0 (null), with the alternate hypothesis stated to contradict the null (one-tail or two-tail)—that the measure of association is not equal to 1.0. The null hypothesis implies that the statistics (mean, OR, and RR) being compared are the results of random sampling from the same population and that any difference in OR, RR, or the mean between them is attributed to chance. There are two types or errors that are associated with hypothesis testing: (1) type I (rejecting the null hypothesis when it is in fact true) and (2) type II (failing to reject the null hypothesis when it is in fact false).[11]

Significance Level (Alpha): The test statistics that depend on the design as well as the measure of the outcome and independent variables yield a p value. The significance level or α is traditionally set at 5% (0.05), which means that if the null hypothesis is true, we are willing to limit type I error to this set value.[2] The p value (significance level) is the probability of obtaining the observed result and more extreme results by chance alone, given that the null hypothesis is true. The significance level is arbitrary cutoff at 5% (0.05). A $p < 0.05$ is considered statistically significant, implying that the null hypothesis of no association should be rejected in favor of the alternate hypothesis. Simply,

Table 2.2 Hypothesis testing and type I error

	No association	*Association*
No association	Correct	Type II error
Association	Type I error*	Correct

*p value is the probability of type I error. Because samples come from the population, the p value plays a role in inferential statistics by allowing conclusions to be drawn regarding the population or the universe of subjects. Since population parameters remain unknown but could be estimated from the sample, the p value reflects the size of the study, implying how representative the sample is with respect to the universe or population of subjects upon which the sample was drawn.

this is indicative of the fact that random error is an unlikely explanation of the observed result or point estimate (statistically significant). With $p > 0.05$, the null hypothesis should not be rejected, which implies that the observed result may be explained by random error or sampling variability (statistically insignificant) (Table 2.2).[2]

2.8 Confounding, covariates, effect measure modifier, interaction

One of the issues in validation of epidemiological research is to assess whether associations between exposure and disease derived from observational epidemiological studies are of a causal nature or not (due to systematic error, random error, or confounding). Confounding refers to the influence or effect of an extraneous factor(s) on the relationship or associations between the exposure and the outcome of interest. Observational studies are potentially subject to the effects of extraneous factors, which may distort the findings of these studies. To be a confounding, the extraneous variables must be (1) a risk factor for the disease being studied and (2) associated with the exposure being studied but is not a consequence of exposure.

BOX 2.2 CONFOUNDING—ELEMENTS AND CHARACTERISTICS

A confounder is an agent or extraneous factor that accounts for differences in disease occurrence or frequency or the measure of the effect between the exposed and unexposed.

- Predicts disease frequency in the unexposed or referent population. For example, in the association between oral cancer and alcohol consumption, smoking is considered confounding if it is associated with both oral cancer and alcohol consumption.
  - A confounder is not qualified by this association only.

    - To qualify as a confounder, smoking must be associated with the occurrence of oral cancer in the unexposed or referent group, apart from its association with alcohol consumption.
    - Also, smoking must be associated with oral cancer among nonalcohol consumers.
- If the effect of alcohol consumption is mediated through the effect of smoking, then it is not a confounder, regardless of whether there is an effect of exposure (alcohol consumption) on oral cancer (outcome or disease).
- Any variable that represents a step in the pathway between the exposure and disease does not represent a confounder, but could be termed an intermediate variate.

Alcohol consumption → Smoking → Oral cancer

- Surrogate confounders refer to factors associated with confounders. For example, chronologic age and aging, chronologic age is a surrogate confounder (K. Rothmans et al., p. 130).
    - Features of a confounder—It (a) must be an extraneous risk factor for disease, (b) must be associated with the exposure in the source population or the population at risk from which the case is derived, and (c) must not be affected by the exposure or disease, implying that it cannot be an intermediate in the causal pathway between the disease and exposure.

Effect measure modifier or effect modification (heterogeneity of effect) refers to the strength of association between exposure and the disease that differs per level of another variable (effect modifier). For example, age is a modifier in the association between ethnicity and hypertension. Differences are not observed between black and white men under the age of 35 with respect to hypertension incidence. After age 35, the incidence tends to be two to three times higher in blacks relative to whites of the same age. Biologically, an effect measure modifier is the third variable that is not a confounding but enters into a causal pathway between the exposure and the disease of interest.[13] For example, the relationship between lung cancer and cigarette smoking is modified by asbestos, because asbestos exposure has been known to increase the risk of dying by 92 times among smokers, whereas the risk of dying from lung cancer among those exposed to asbestos only is 10-fold. Another example is the modifying effect of cigarette smoking and obesity on the association between oral contraceptives and myocardial infarction in women. The effect measure modifier and confounding have similarities. Both confounding and effect measure modifiers involve a third variable as well as that assessed or evaluated by performing stratified analysis.[14] Effect measure modifier differs from confounding. In confounding, one is interested in knowing whether the crude measure of association (unadjusted point estimate) changes (distorted) and whether the stratum-specific and adjusted summary estimate differ from the crude or unadjusted estimate. In effect measure modification, one is interested in finding out if the association differs per the third variable (the difference in stratum-specific estimate from one another). This concept, which is not very well understood among researchers in the healthcare field, is covered in detail in the *Applied Epidemiologic Principles and Concepts* by Holmes, L. Jr. and *Modern Epidemiology* by Rothman, K. et al.

2.9 Summary

Research design transcends analysis, since no matter how sophisticated a statistical tool used is, the error of design and sampling remains, rendering the inference invalid. Study designs in biomedical and clinical research are experimental and nonexperimental. Often, the selection of one design over the other depends on multiple factors, some of which include the particular research question to be answered, feasibility, expenses, and the availability of subjects for a given design.

Subject selection is fundamental to how the inference from the study will be used. A well-designed study must clearly define the targeted population in order to apply the results of the study appropriately. Clinical/biomedical research designs are typically classified into (a) nonexperimental and (b) experimental. The fundamental difference between the two designs is the allocation of subjects to the study arms or subject manipulation. While nonexperimental designs do not employ subject allocation by the investigator, subject allocation is the hallmark of experimental design in humans; it is also known as a clinical trial. Regardless of the design used, both studies involve the observation of the outcomes of interest, hence the misnomer in characterizing nonexperimental design as observational.

Nonexperimental designs that are commonly used in clinical and biomedical research include (a) cross-sectional; (b) case–control, with cases being the basis of the design; and (c) cohort design, conducted on the basis of exposure. There are several hybrids of these designs, including case–cohort, case crossover, nested case–control, and so on.

While preference has been for prospective designs, since such designs are able to establish temporal sequence, a well-designed retrospective study can generate standard and valid evidence. Therefore, the preference of one design over the other should be based on the research question, availability of study subjects, resources, and sampling feasibility.

Clinical research involves humans and hence the potential for the influence of other factors in the results of experiments or nonexperimental studies. The interpretation of such designs depends on the ability to disentangle confounding, random error, and bias from the findings, as well as being able to address interaction and effect modifier. While the appropriate analytic tool is fundamental to discovery, the study could be driven by confounding and bias in the midst of statistically significant results.

Finally, whatever design applied in the conduct of biomedical and clinical research, caution should be exercised in the interpretation of the results, noting clearly that (1) no design no matter how sophisticated is immune from observational and measurement errors, (2) no design explains everything, and (3) all designs are subject to limitations, and hence some degree of uncertainties or chance in the application of the results.

Questions for discussion

1 Read the study report by Holmes et al. (2007) on androgen-deprivation therapy and the prolongation of survival of older men diagnosed and treated for locoregional prostate cancer. Comment on the research design, hypothesis, statistical methods, and conclusions. Is this a reliable inference? Why and why not?

2 Suppose you are conducting a study on the incidence of asthma among children (up to 4 years of age) exposed to maternal cigarette smoking, and a similar study is conducted in a different center with children (from 12 to 21 years old). (a) What is the measure of effect of maternal smoking? (b) What is the problem in comparing these two incidence rates? (c) How will you perform a valid comparisons in this case?

3 One way to measure the effect of disease is by RR or OR. What is the distinction between these two measures? Comment on the advantage of one over the other in determining the direct association between exposure and disease.

4 In a hypothetical study of the relationship between polycystic ovarian syndrome (POS) and endometrial carcinoma, 80 out of 280 with POS had developed endometrial carcinoma, compared with 600 out of 4000 control women, who had endometrial carcinoma at some time in their lives. (a) Compute the OR in favor of never having been diagnosed with POS for women with endometrial carcinoma versus the control group. (b) What is the 95% CI for this association? (c) What can be concluded for these data? (d) Is there an association between POS and endometrial cancer based on these data?

5 Suppose you are appointed as the director of a clinical taskforce to establish the guidelines for the assessment and treatment of avascular necrosis associated with sickle cell disease, and you intend to base this guideline on the meta-analysis or systematic quantitative review. (a) What will be your inclusion and exclusion criteria? (b) What method of meta-analysis will you employ if the studies indicate heterogeneity, and why? (c) What are the limitations of this approach in establishing clinical guidelines?

6 A study was conducted to examine the role of paternal exposure to cigarette smoking and asthma in children. The result was found to be consistent with a causal relationship. (a) If genetic predisposition was also

a likely explanation, can we affirm the conclusion regarding a causal relationship? (b) In terms of internal validity and causation, comment on the (i) consistency of this study with other evidence, (ii) specificity, (iii) biologic plausibility, and (iv) coherency of the effect with the distribution of the exposure and the outcome.

7 Comment on the assessment of random error, bias, and confounding in the establishment of study validity. (a) How relevant is the assessment of bias and confounding if the result of a study is statistically insignificant? (b) What is the significance of probability value in the interpretation of study findings if the sample studied was not a random sample?

References

1. S. Piantadosi, *Clinical Trials*, 2nd ed. (Hoboken, New Jersey: Wiley-Interscience, 2005); L. M. Friedman et al., *Fundamentals of Clinical Trials*, 3rd ed. (New York: Springer-Verlag, 1998).
2. B. W. Brown, The cross-over experiment for clinical trials, *Biometrics* 36 (1980):69–79.
3. S. Piantadosi, *Clinical Trials*, 2nd ed. (Hoboken, New Jersey: Wiley-Interscience, 2005).
4. S. Piantadosi, *Clinical Trials*, 2nd ed. (Hoboken, New Jersey: Wiley-Interscience, 2005); L. M. Friedman et al., *Fundamentals of Clinical Trials*, 3rd ed. (New York: Springer-Verlag, 1998); B. W. Brown, The cross-over experiment for clinical trials, *Biometrics* 36 (1980):69–79.
5. L. Holmes Jr., W. Chan, Z. Jiang, X. L. Du, Effectiveness of androgen deprivation therapy in prolonging survival of older men with locoregional prostate cancer, *J. Prostate Cancer*, Prostatic Dis. 10 no. 4(2007):388–395.
6. J. L. Fleiss, *The Design of Clinical Experiments* (New York: Wiley, 1986).
7. M. Elwood, *Critical Appraisal of Epidemiological Studies in Clinical Trials*, 2nd ed. (New York: Oxford University Press, 2003).
8. J. E. Johansson, H. O. Adami, S. O. Anderson et al., High 10-year survival rate in patients with early, untreated prostatic cancer, *JAMA* 267 (1992):216–219.
9. R. S. Greenberg et al., *Medical Epidemiology*, 4th ed. (New York: Lange, 2005).
10. D. L. Sackett, W. S. Richardson, W. Rosenberg, and R. B. Haynes, *Evidence-Based Medicine: How to Practice and Teach Evidence-Based Medicine*, 2nd ed. (Edinburg: Churchill Livingstone, 2000).
11. M. Szklo and J. Nieto J. *Epidemiology: Beyond the Basics* (Sudbury, MA: Jones & Bartlett, 2003); D. A. Savitz, *Interpreting Epidemiologic Evidence* (New York: Oxford University Press, 2003).
12. B. W. Brown, The cross-over experiment for clinical trials, *Biometrics* 36 (1980):69–79; M. Szklo and J. Nieto J. *Epidemiology: Beyond the Basics* (Sudbury, MA: Jones & Bartlett, 2003); D. A. Savitz, *Interpreting Epidemiologic Evidence* (New York: Oxford University Press, 2003).
13. L. M. Friedman et al., *Fundamentals of Clinical Trials*, 3rd ed. (New York: Springer-Verlag, 1998).
14. S. Piantadosi, *Clinical Trials*, 2nd ed. (Hoboken, New Jersey: Wiley-Interscience, 2005); B. W. Brown, The cross-over experiment for clinical trials, *Biometrics* 36 (1980):69–79.

3 Population, sample, probability, and biostatistical reasoning

3.1 Introduction

Biostatistical inference is about the sample; the population parameters, like the mean, remain estimates, implying the uncertainty of absolute population parameters. All biomedical and clinical inferences about samples studied carry some uncertainties, requiring caution in the interpretation of findings for application to improvement of care or suggestions of diagnostic and screening guidelines. A parameter in biostatistics is a number that describes the population, while the population is the entire group of individuals or animals about which we require information or data. Ideally, the parameter is a fixed number, but in reality, this value remains unknown. Since the parameter from the population is unknown, statistics is used to describe the sample. The sample is a part of the population from which researchers obtain data, which they used to draw inferences or conclusions about the population. While the value of the statistic is known, this value is not fixed and can change from sample to sample. Based on this sample-to-sample variability, all findings have underlying uncertainties, and population parameters remain unknown, implicative of extreme caution in the interpretation and application of study findings in the improvement and provision of quality medical and psychosocial care to our patients.[1]

Sample design is the technique used to select the sample from the population and is essential to the validity of study inference. From poor sample design follows invalid and misleading inference from the data.

What is biostatistical reasoning? Inference about the sample studied in terms of the magnitude of difference in treatment is based on biostatistical techniques. For example, the length of hospital stay following spinal fusion for curve deformities in cerebral palsy has financial consequences. Orthopedic surgeons should be involved in logical and educated discussions on design process and biostatistical models that will enable the quality and internal as well as external validity of evidence to be assessed in reducing the length of stay without adversely affecting patient recovery. Biostatistical reasoning thus involves the assessment of the quality of evidence by considering the sampling design and the analysis technique or model used to identify the risk factors to a disease, supporting or negating the procedure or treatment studied. Such reasoning leads to a design sample that reflects a representative sample in order to test hypotheses that will enable one to generalize the observed findings to the population of interest, including those individuals with the disease who were not studied in the sample. Statistical inference is based on how reliable or trustworthy a procedure is, and what the outcome or observation will be if the procedure is repeated many times.[1]

To critically appraise scientific literature, clinicians and biomedical researchers are expected to be able to understand and examine statistical techniques used to generate the evidence as well as the design and the protocol used in the study implementation. Since statistical methods have been used incorrectly and continue to be erroneously implemented in scientific and medical literature, we attempt in this chapter to explain the flaws in the use of some of the most commonly abused tests, namely, the chi-square and *t* test. This chapter presents the biostatistical notion of populations, samples, sampling distribution and probability, bias, and variability. In addition, an attempt is made to expose the flaws in analysis and interpretation of biomedical, translational, and clinical research data as biostatistical reasoning.

3.2 Populations

Biostatistics is concerned with health populations from basic sciences (bench) via the patients (clinical science) to the community (population science and public health). The population of interest to biostatistics include humans and other animals as well as the environments associated with these species.[2] Population could also refer to events, procedures, or observations. Within this broad context, population refers to the aggregate of species, objects, cases, and so on.

Since biostatistics is not concerned with studying the entire population or the targeted population of interest, such as US males with prostatic adenocarcinoma, but a sample of such a population, knowledge of the population from which the sample was obtained is extremely important for a valid inference to be drawn. Consider a study on the effectiveness of androgen deprivation therapy in prolonging the survival of older US males with locoregional prostate cancer. The population of US males with CaP should be clearly defined. For example, not all US males with CaP reside in the United States, and the racial/ethnic, genetic, cultural, and social backgrounds of those who reside in the United States may differ substantially. In addition, the Gleason score, tumor stage, state or residence at the time diagnosis, age at diagnosis, PSA level, and so on, may also vary across the population of US males.

While the true population parameters, such as mean and standard deviation, remain unknown, since it may not be convenient to study the entire population, samples are normally drawn.[2,3] These samples are expected to be representative of the population of interest in order to allow accurate and true inferences to be drawn on the population.

The population mean (μ) and standard deviation (σ) differ from those of the sample, but the more representative the sample, the closer the sample mean and SD are to the population parameter. It is very important that the population be clearly characterized before the drawing of the sample. For example, the population of US males with CaP in the hypothetical study above should be described as "all men with locoregional prostate cancer, all patients aged sixty-five and older in the SEER database from 1993 to 2012."

3.3 Sample and sampling strategies

While adequate statistical analysis of the sample is important for the accuracy of inference, obtaining a representative sample implying a satisfactory sample is more important. Since samples are drawn from the population, populations must be clearly defined and characterized before the application of any sampling technique. We must stress an important aspect of a sample, which is the nonzero chance (*known probability*) of individuals, patients, eligible participants, or subjects being included in the study. Simply, each individual should have an equal and a known probability of being selected into the study.

Sample selection involves the concept of *independence*. The selection of one subject from the population should not affect the chance of other eligible participants being selected into the study sample. The requirement of independence in sampling is ensured by the process in which chance determines selectability. For example, in a study to assess the effect of medication adherence in pediatric asthma, if there are 3000 children with asthma, and the appropriate sample size is 372 (medication adherence) and 372 (nonadherence), the selection of these subjects must be achieved via a "chance process" such as coin spinning or random numbers table. The subjects selected in this exercise are termed a *random sample* and the variables collected from this sample are the *random variable*.

Earlier in the chapter, we observed that obtaining a representative sample from a population of interest into a study sample is an extremely important step in statistical analysis, since the end point of hypothesis testing is to generalize the findings to the targeted population based on the sample. Sampling selection should be representative for such generalization to be valid and reliable. For instance, epidemiologic data have indicated an inverse dose–response in the association between educational status and diabetes mellitus (DM) prevalence, implying higher prevalence of DM among those without high school education. In effect, a sample to be utilized in estimating the prevalence of DM in any population must be selected to reflect the educational status of that population. The inability to do so will result in underestimation or overestimation of DM prevalence in the targeted population.

The sampling technique identifies two types of sampling, namely, probability and nonprobability. The probability sampling, as observed previously, involves each or every member of the population to have a known probability of being selected into the sample, whereas in a nonprobability sampling, each member of the population is selected without the application of probability. Below are examples of probability sampling.

Simple Random Sampling (SRS)

This technique involves the identification of a sampling frame implying the complete list of all the population and assignment of a unique identification number, and the sample is selected at random. With this sampling scheme, every element in the population has an equal chance or probability of being selected.

Systematic Random Sampling (SS)

Like simple random sampling, SS begins with sampling frame as well as the assignment of a unique identification number. Additionally, samples are selected at fixed intervals, with the interval between selections determined by the ratio of the population size to the sample size (N/n) termed sampling fraction. For example, if the population size is 100 (N) and the required sample size is 10 (n), then the sampling fraction is 100/10 = 10, implying the selection of every 10th individual or element into the sample. Is it possible to obtain a nonrepresentative sample from such technique? Suppose the 100 people in the population consist of heterogeneous groups (racial/ethnic minorities and whites), systematic random sampling may result in the undersampling of certain racial/ethnic group, implying nonrepresentative sample.

Stratified Sampling

This technique involves the creation of strata or blocks based on certain characteristics of the population (race/ethnicity) and applying the techniques above in SS or SRS and sampling within each strata. With this technique, adequate representation of individuals in each block or stratum is ensured. For example, if the racial/ethnic composition of pediatric patients seen at a pediatric hospital in New-State is n = 1000 Whites, n = 450 Blacks/AA, n = 100 Asians, n = 380 Hispanics/Latinos, the sampling of this population should follow this distribution for representative sample by race/ethnicity.

In contrast, nonprobability samples arise from the inability to obtain a sampling frame, implying an unknown probability of selecting an individual into the sample. Below is an example of nonprobability sampling.

Convenience Sampling

Involves the selection of individuals into the study based on the availability of study subjects, implying unknown probability and nonrepresentative sample.

Quota Sampling

Is a process that reflects the selection of samples based on a specific number. For example, if we intend to sample 100 pediatric cancer patients, and we are aware of the percentage distribution of the patients by age group (0–4 years, 25%; 5–9 years, 15%; 10–14 years, 25%; and 15–19 years, 35%), then the sample will comprise 25, 15, 25, and 35 in the age groups, respectively.

3.4 Biostatistical reasoning

The purpose of biostatistical reasoning is to ensure appropriate decision-making about hypothesized states of the patient population.[1] Conducting a study for application in improving health conditions, providing early diagnosis, screening for disease, or minimizing the complications and adverse events requires obtaining data toward the clinical or biomedical relevance of the study. This relevance is reflected by the measure of effect or association. But in generalizing the results so obtained, statistical inference must be drawn.[2,3] Simply, biostatistical reasoning implies the use of probability to determine whether or not the sample studied represents the population from which the sample is drawn.[4]

This reasoning is slightly different from statistical reasoning, which is the rejection of the null hypothesis and the inclination toward the alternative hypothesis, given the established significance level. We commonly misconceive a statistically significant finding to mean the effective or efficacious treatment. Such an assumption is very misleading and should be discouraged in scientific evidence discovery. While we wish to ensure that the result of our study is not due to chance or luck in the sample we studied, it is equally important to realize that if proper effort has been made in terms of inclusion criteria with respect to our sample (random or consecutive), the effect of treatment or association is measured by the point estimate, such as the odds ratio, risk ratio, proportion, percent, and so on.

In conducting a study, we recommend that researchers critically examine the measures of effect or association that are appropriate to the data. For example, if a study is conducted to determine the effect of inhaled corticosteroid in racial/ethnic disparities in pediatric asthma survival, the appropriate measure of effect is the hazard ratio (HR), a measure of effect that considers time in the computation of survival experience of the treated versus the untreated cohort. In contrast, if the data are not time-to-event, but case-comparison/control, the odds ratio (OR) remains a useful and efficient measure of effect. Since such point estimate may be misinterpreted, a distinction must be made between descriptive and inferential statistics in the interpretation and application of the point estimate in clinical and biomedical decision-making.

In presenting inferential results (study involving hypothesis testing), both the point estimate and the precision of the point estimate are expected to be reported. If the purpose of the study was to determine the effectiveness of a treatment modality or outcome, confidence intervals (CIs) should be used. This practice allows the quantification of point estimate and the appropriate measure of uncertainty or measurement error. For example, if a study was conducted to determine the effectiveness of pelvic osteotomy in normalizing the hip, and the outcome is the migration index (MI), the mean MI after 2 years of follow-up quantifies the point estimate, while 95% CI reflects the uncertainty. We can interpret this 95% CI as a 95% chance of the obtained mean, MI, being included in the interval. Since samples that we study are not unique, it is important to realize that samples from the same population will generate different estimates of the population parameters, as well as different 95% CIs.

3.5 Measures of central tendency and dispersion

We are always required to describe our sample before the testing of any hypothesis in an inferential study. Understanding of the sample used in a study must precede the measures of effects or association. Summarizing our data requires knowledge of appropriate summary statistics, implying measures of central tendency and dispersion or variability. A measure of central tendency is a single value that attempts to describe a set of data by identifying the central position within that set of data. For this reason, the measures of central tendency are also termed *measures of central location*, as well as *summary statistics* (Figure 3.1 and Table 3.1). In addition, before hypothesis

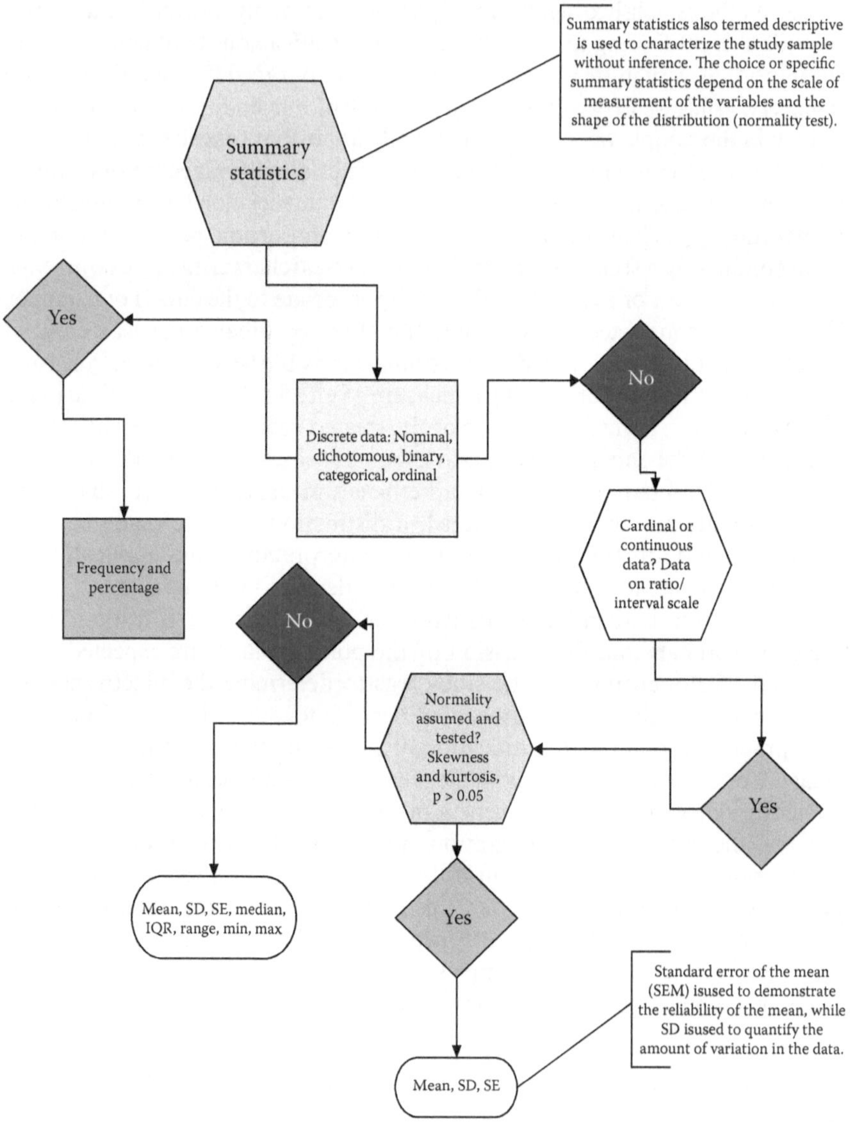

Figure 3.1 Summary statistics and measures of central tendency/location and dispersion.

Table 3.1 Choice of measures of central tendency or location

Scale of measurement of variable	*Measure of central tendency*	*Rationale*
Nominal	Mode	Variables, such as sex, with male = 1 and female = 2
Ordinal	Median/mean[a]	Variables, such as severity of illness (low, moderate, and severe)
Cardinal data—interval/ ratio (nonskewed)	Mean	Variables, such as systolic or diastolic BP and age—normal distribution (bell curve)
Cardinal data—interval/ ratio (skewed)	Median	Variables, such as systolic or diastolic BP and age that violate the normality assumption

[a] Ordinal data should be summarized with median and mean, which allows one to examine the proximity of the two parameters.

testing where the shape of distribution is assumed, a normality test is required, as are descriptive statistics. Box 3.1 illustrates such a practice from hypothetical data on the BMIs of children:

BOX 3.1 NORMALITY TEST TO EXAMINE THE NORMAL DISTRIBUTION OF BMI AND BMI% FROM A DATA SET WITH A SAMPLE OF 65,255 CHILDREN

```
Shapiro-Francia W' test for normal data

    Variable |   Obs        W'          V'           z       Prob > z
-------------+----------------------------------------------------------
         bmi |  65255    0.13984    2.8e+04     30.266      0.00001
       bmipc |  65241    0.91733    2730.033    23.352      0.00001

Note: the normal approximation to the sampling distribution of
W' is valid for 10 ≤ n ≤ 5000 under the log transformation.
```

What is skewness?

This refers to the variability of the data from the symmetry and implies the distributions below and higher than the mean. It is the measure of symmetry around the mean.

What is kurtosis?

This measures the peakness at the mean.

BOX 3.2 DESCRIPTIVE/SUMMARY STATISTICS OF BMI AND BMI PERCENT OF CHILDREN

```
tabstat bmi bmipc, stat (mean sd p50 iqr range min max n)
```

stats	bmi	bmipc
mean	19.19283	64.24659
sd	12.99647	29.16575
p50	17.46	70.66
iqr	5.049999	48.61
range	2131.16	100
min	1.92	0
max	2133.08	100
N	65255	65241

The above STATA output indicates that the data are nonnormal, requiring mean and SD, as well as median and IQR, to be used in summarizing the data, contrary to the mistaken practice of summarizing such data with median and IQR only.

How is the mean of a sample estimated? Consider a study conducted to examine the effect of age on systolic blood pressure (SBP). The ages of participants in years were 56.7, 45.9, 78.5, 46.8, 60.0, 89.2, 56.9, 50.0, 67.8, 48.6, 70, and 56.8, and the SBPs were 156, 148, 150, 160, 126, 144, 132, 160, 138, 148, 150, and 163. What is the mean age? What is the average SBP? What is the SD for these two variables, and how could this be interpreted? Is there a relationship between age and SBP?

The mean is the most commonly used measure of central tendency. We estimate the mean by summing all the ages of the participants and dividing it by the number of participants in the sample or sample size. We use the symbol μ for the mean of a population and sometimes the symbol for the mean of a sample. To calculate μ, we use the formula $\mu = \Sigma X/N$, where ΣX is the sum of all the ages in the population and N is the number of participants in the population. Similarly, the sample mean is the sum of all the values in the data set divided by the number of values (sample size) in the data set. Therefore, if there are n values in a data set and these values have $x_1, x_2, \ldots, x_n$, the sample mean is denoted by $\bar{x}$.

$$\bar{x} = \frac{(x_1 + x_2 + \cdots + x_n)}{n}$$

This can be further simplified as

$$\bar{x} = \frac{\sum x}{n}$$

3.5.1 Median

The median is the middle score for a set of data that has been arranged in order of magnitude. Consider the example with the SBP above: 126, 132, 138, 144, 148, 160, 148, 150, 150, 156, 160, and 163. Since these data have been ordered from lowest to highest, we estimate the median as the middle SBP for the set of SBP. The median is less affected by outliers and skewed data.

Box 3.3 presents the normality test for the SBP using STATA statistical software. The syntax for the normality test is as follows: `sktest var` x_a ... `var` x_z.

BOX 3.3A NORMALITY TEST UTILIZING SKEWNESS AND KURTOSIS (SK), SYSTOLIC BLOOD PRESSURE (SBP) OF 11 SUBJECTS

```
. sktest spb

               Skewness/Kurtosis tests for Normality

                                                     ------ joint ------
Variable |  Obs  Pr(Skewness)  Pr(Kurtosis)  adj chi2(2)    Prob>chi2
---------+-------------------------------------------------------------
     spb |   11     0.4585        0.9700         0.58          0.7499
```

BOX 3.3B NORMALITY TEST UTILIZING FRANCIA AND SHAPIRO'S METHOD, SBP OF 11 SUBJECTS

```
. sfrancia spb

                Shapiro-Francia W' test for normal data

Variable |    Obs       W'          V'        z          Prob>z
---------+------------------------------------------------------
     spb |     11    0.97046      0.524    -1.128       0.87027
```

The SBP showed normal distribution, which enables the selection of the mean as the best measure of central tendency. Since the null hypothesis is that data are normal, with $p = 0.7499$, we fail to reject the normal hypothesis.

BOX 3.4A EXPLORATORY STATISTICS, ILLUSTRATING THE CENTRAL TENDENCY AND THE SPREAD OF THE SBP DATA OF 10 SUBJECTS

```
. tabstat spb, stat (mean sd var p50 p75 p25 iqr range min max n)
```

variable	mean	sd	variance	p50	p75	p25	iqr	range	min	max	N
spb	146.8182	11.32094	128.1636	148	156	138	18	37	126	163	11

BOX 3.4B EXPLORATORY STATISTICS, ILLUSTRATING THE CENTRAL TENDENCY AND THE SPREAD OF THE SBP DATA OF 10 SUBJECTS (STANDARD ERROR OF THE SAMPLE MEAN INCLUDED)

```
. tabstat spb, stat (mean sd var sem p50 p75 p25 iqr range min max n)
```

variable	mean	sd	variance	se(mean)	p50	p75	p25	iqr	range	min	max	N
spb	146.8182	11.32094	128.1636	3.413391	148	156	138	18	37	126	163	11

Another sample of 31 patients was selected from the same population of men and women with hypertension, and the normality test was performed and the mean SBP was estimated. Box 3.5 presents the normality test and the measures of central tendency.

BOX 3.5A NORMALITY TEST, SK OF 31 SUBJECTS WITH SBP (HYPOTHETICAL DATA)

```
. sktest spb
```

Skewness/Kurtosis tests for Normality

Variable	Obs	Pr(Skewness)	Pr(Kurtosis)	——— joint ——— adj chi2(2)	Prob>chi2
spb	31	0.3117	0.5574	1.47	0.4801

.

Notes: The above normal distribution test indicates that the data are normal, given the null hypothesis that data are normal. With the significance level, 0.48, and the type I error tolerance of 0.05, there is no evidence against the null hypothesis, implying the acceptance of the null.

BOX 3.5B MEASURES OF CENTRAL TENDENCY OF 31 SUBJECTS WITH SBP (HYPOTHETICAL DATA)

```
. tabstat spb, stat (mean sd var sem p50 p75 p25 iqr range min max n)
```

variable	mean	sd	variance	se(mean)	p50	p75	p25	iqr	range	min	max	N
spb	145.871	10.61679	112.7161	1.906831	148	150	138	12	37	126	163	31

BOX 3.5C MEASURES OF CENTRAL TENDENCY OF 31 SUBJECTS WITH SBP BY RACE (SUBGROUP EXPLORATORY ANALYSIS)

```
. tabstat spb, stat (mean sd var sem p50 p75 p25 iqr range min max n) by ( race)
Summary for variables: spb

     by categories of: race
```

race	mean	sd	variance	se(mean)	p50	p75	p25	iqr	range	min	max	N
1	138	9.012811	81.23077	2.408775	138	148	132	16	24	126	150	14
2	152.3529	6.818552	46.49265	1.653742	150	156	148	8	25	138	163	17
Total	145.871	10.61679	112.7161	1.906831	148	150	138	12	37	126	163	31

Abbreviations: N = sample size, iqr = interquartile range, se (mean) = standard error of the mean, p50 = median, 1 = white, and 2 = black (race).

BOX 3.5D MEASURES OF CENTRAL TENDENCY OF 31 SUBJECTS WITH SBP BY SEX (SUBGROUP EXPLORATORY ANALYSIS)

```
. tabstat spb, stat (mean sd var sem p50 p75 p25 iqr range min max n) by ( Sex)

Summary for variables: spb
     by categories of: race
```

race	mean	sd	variance	se(mean)	p50	p75	p25	iqr	range	min	max	N
1	152.9231	8.30122	68.91026	2.302344	150	160	150	10	31	132	163	13
2	139.8824	8.644958	74.73529	2.09671	144	148	132	16	24	126	150	17
Total	145.5333	10.62766	112.9471	1.940336	148	150	138	12	37	126	163	30

Abbreviations: N = sample size, iqr = interquartile range, se (mean) = standard error of the mean, p50 = median, 1 = male, and 2 = female (sex).

3.5.2 Mode

The mode is the most frequent SBP in the example of hypothetical data used here. Using a histogram to present the data, the mode represents the highest frequency (Figure 3.2).

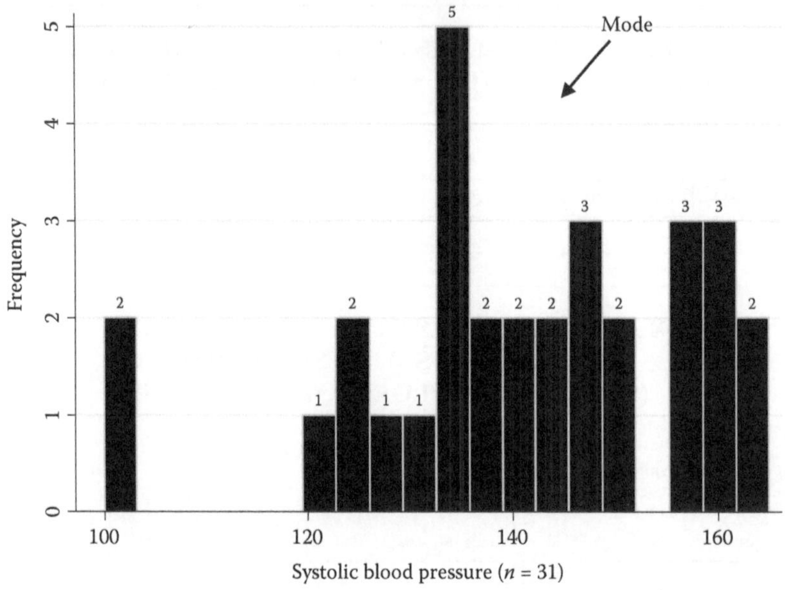

Figure 3.2 Histogram of 31 patients with SBP illustrating the mode.

Since the SBP data above are normally distributed from the two samples drawn from this hypothetical population, both the mean and median could be used as measures of central tendency. In general, given a symmetrical distribution, the mean, median, and mode are almost nearly equal. One would recommend the mean in this context as a better choice for the central tendency measure since it includes all the SBP values in its estimation or calculation. Consequently, any alteration in any of the SBP values will influence the mean but not the median or mode, implying the sensitivity of the mean to outliers.

3.5.3 Measures of dispersion

Measures of dispersion reflect a deviation of values from the measure of central tendency.[2] For example, if the SBP of a sample of African-American women were the same, there would be no need to estimate the sample mean. Since the SBPs of African-American women vary by age, family history, and so on, the extent to which they differ from each other is the dispersion of the distribution. There are several measures of dispersion, namely, range, variance, standard deviation, standard error of the mean, and so on.

3.5.4 Range

Range is the simplest measure of dispersion and is the difference between the highest and lowest SBP in the example above. As an interval, range could also represent the lowest and the highest SBP.

Vignette 3.1: Estimation of range as quantity and interval. A study was conducted to determine serum lipid concentration as a biomarker of higher BMI. The following data were available. The ages of the subjects are 10, 10, 11, 11, 11, 12, 12, 12, 12, 13, 13, 13, 13, 13, 14, 14, 14, 14, 14, 14, 15, 15, 15, 15, 15, 15, 15, 16, 16, 16, 16, 16, 16, 16, and 16. What is the mean age and the range of subjects? Estimate the range as quantity and interval. What is the median age and interquartile range?

BOX 3.6A VIGNETTE SOLUTION. SKEWNESS/ KURTOSIS TESTS FOR NORMALITY

				joint	
Variable	Obs	Pr(Skewness)	Pr(Kurtosis)	adj chi2(2)	Prob>chi2
sbp	35	0.3032	0.2779	2.41	**0.2995**
age	35	0.1926	0.1989	3.63	**0.1625**

BOX 3.6B EXPLORATORY (SUMMARY STATISTICS) ANALYSIS OF THE SBP AND AGE DISTRIBUTION BY THE TYPE OF ANTIHYPERTENSIVE TREATMENT (HTN-TX)

```
. tabstat SBP age, stat (mean sd var sem p50 iqr range min max n) by ( HNT_TX)

Summary statistics: mean, sd, variance, se(mean), p50, iqr, range, min, max, N
  by categories of: HNT_TX
```

HNT TX	SBP	age
1	113.0308	38.04615
	12.01688	6.627195
	144.4053	43.91971
	1. 49051	.8220024
	115	40
	20	9
	37	35
	98	30
	135	65
	65	65
2	143.413	49.06522
	11.9714	10.76084
	143.3145	115.7957
	1.765087	1.586599
	142.5	43
	15	16
	61	35
	98	30
	159	65
	46	46
Total	125.6216	42.61261
	19.20135	10.13201
	368.6919	102.6577
	1.822512	.961688
	132	41
	30	10
	61	35
	98	30
	159	65
	111	111

Abbreviations: 1 = Treatment with new agent and 2 = treatment with standard of care (old agent).

BOX 3.6C SUMMARY STATISTICS OF SBP BY HTN TREATMENT

```
. tabstat SBP , stat (mean sd var sem p50 iqr range min max n) by ( HNT_TX)

Summary for variables: SBP
     by categories of: HNT_TX
```

HNT_TX	mean	sd	variance	se(mean)	p50	iqr	range	min	max	N
1	113.0308	12.01688	144.4053	1.49051	115	20	37	98	135	65
2	143.413	11.9714	143.3145	1.765087	142.5	15	61	98	159	46
Total	125.6216	19.20135	368.6919	1.822512	132	30	61	98	159	111

BOX 3.6D EXPLORATORY ANALYSIS (SUMMARY STATISTICS) OF NEW AND STANDARD HTN TREATMENT BY SEX

```
. tabstat SBP if HNT_TX ==1, stat (mean sd var sem p50 iqr range min max n ) by (  Sex)

Summary for variables: SBP
     by categories of: Sex
```

Sex	mean	sd	variance	se(mean)	p50	iqr	range	min	max	N
1	116.125	7.825891	61.24457	1.597453	120	10	35	100	135	24
2	111.2195	13.66476	186.7256	2.134077	110	15	34	98	132	41
Total	113.0308	12.01688	144.4053	1.49051	115	20	37	98	135	65

```
. tabstat SBP if HNT_TX ==2, stat (mean sd var sem p50 iqr range min max n ) by ( Sex)

Summary for variables: SBP
     by categories of: Sex
```

Sex	mean	sd	variance	se(mean)	p50	iqr	range	min	max	N
1	148.4063	8.151229	66.44254	1.440947	145	19	19	140	159	32
2	132	11.661	136	3.116775	135	0	47	98	145	14
Total	143.413	11.9714	143.3145	1.765087	142.5	15	61	98	159	46

Abbreviations: Sex: 1 = male and 2 = female. HTN_TX: 1 = new agent and 2 = standard of care.

BOX 3.6E EXPLORATORY ANALYSIS (SUMMARY STATISTICS) OF NEW AND STANDARD HTN TREATMENT BY RACE

```
. tabstat SBP if HNT_TX ==1, stat (mean sd var sem p50 iqr range min max n ) by ( Race)
Summary for variables: SBP
     by categories of: Race
```

Race	mean	sd	variance	se(mean)	p50	iqr	range	min	max	N
1	11.8	11.53594	133.078	1.489284	110	20	34	98	132	60
2	127.8	7.224957	52.2	3.231099	132	12	15	120	135	5
Total	113.0308	12.01688	144.4053	1.49051	115	20	37	98	135	65

```
. tabstat SBP if HNT_TX ==2, stat (mean sd var sem p50 iqr range min max n ) by ( Race)

Summary for variables: SBP
     by categories of: Sex
```

Race	mean	sd	variance	se(mean)	p50	iqr	range	min	max	N
1	136.8333	24.90315	620.1667	10.16667	145	44	61	98	159	6
2	144.4	8.842786	78.19487	1.397167	140	10	24	135	159	40
Total	143.413	11.9714	1 43.3145	1.765087	142.5	15	61	98	159	46

The STATA output for the normality test for SBP and age indicate normally distributed data. The mean represents the best measure of the central tendency while the standard deviation reflects the values of individuals in the sample who vary from the mean. Box 3.7 presents the mean, median, range, and maximum and minimum values of age of the subjects in the hypothetical study.

BOX 3.7 RANGE OF SBP IN A SAMPLE OF 100 PATIENTS BY SEX, RACE, AND HTN TREATMENT

```
. tabstat SBP , stat (p50 iqr range min max n  )
```

variable	p50	iqr	range	min	max	N
SBP	132	30	61	98	159	111

```
. tabstat  SBP , stat (p50 iqr range min max n  ) by ( Sex)

Summary for variables: SBP
     by categories of: Sex
```

Sex	p50	iqr	range	min	max	N
1	140	25	59	100	159	56
2	115	32	47	98	145	55
Total	132	30	61	98	159	111

```
. tabstat SBP , stat (p50 iqr range min max n  ) by (  Race)

Summary for variables: SBP
     by categories of: Race

    Race |     p50     iqr     range       min       max       N
---------+------------------------------------------------------
       1 |   112.5      20        61        98       159      66
       2 |     140      10        39       120       159      45
---------+------------------------------------------------------
   Total |     132      30        61        98       159     111
----------------------------------------------------------------

. tabstat  SBP , stat (p50 iqr range min max n  ) by ( HNT_TX)

Summary for variables: SBP
     by categories of: HNT_TX

  HNT_TX |       p50     iqr     range       min       max       N
---------+--------------------------------------------------------
       1 |       115      20        37        98       135      65
       2 |     142.5      15        61        98       159      46
---------+--------------------------------------------------------
   Total |       132      30        61        98       159     111
------------------------------------------------------------------

.
```

Box 3.7 shows the SBP range as a single number of 111 subjects to be 61 (maximum SBP – minimum SBP) and as an interval to be from 98 (minimum) to 159 (maximum).

3.5.5 Quartiles and interquartile range and box plot

While percentiles in the hypothetical SBP data set describe the relative SBP along the distribution, quartile splits the SBP into fourths, so that an SBP falling in the first quartile lies within the lowest 25% of SBP values, while a score in the fourth quartile is higher than at least 75% of the SBP values in the data set.

A box plot graphically presents the SBP data with central location (median) and dispersion (quartiles) (Figures 3.3 through 3.7).

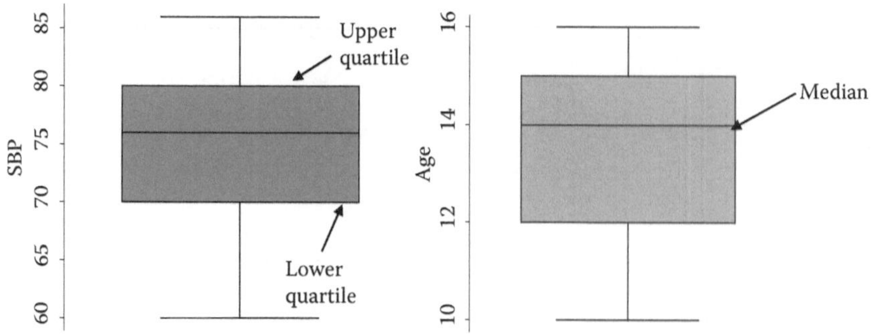

Figure 3.3 Box plots of SBP and age, respectively, illustrating the median (50th percentile), 25th percentile as the lower quartile, and the 75th percentile as upper quartile.

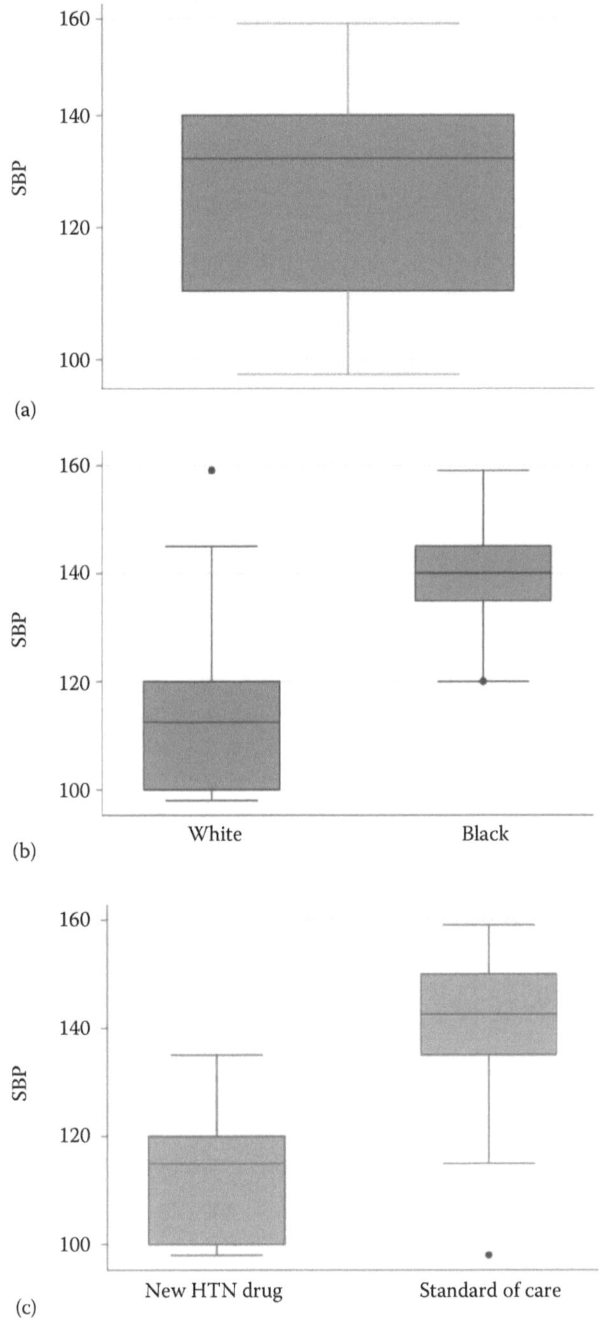

Figure 3.4 (a) Data visualization illustrating box plot of SBP in a sample of 100 patients. (b) Data visualization—SBP by race of patients on HNT treatment. (c) Data visualization—SBP by HNT treatment received.

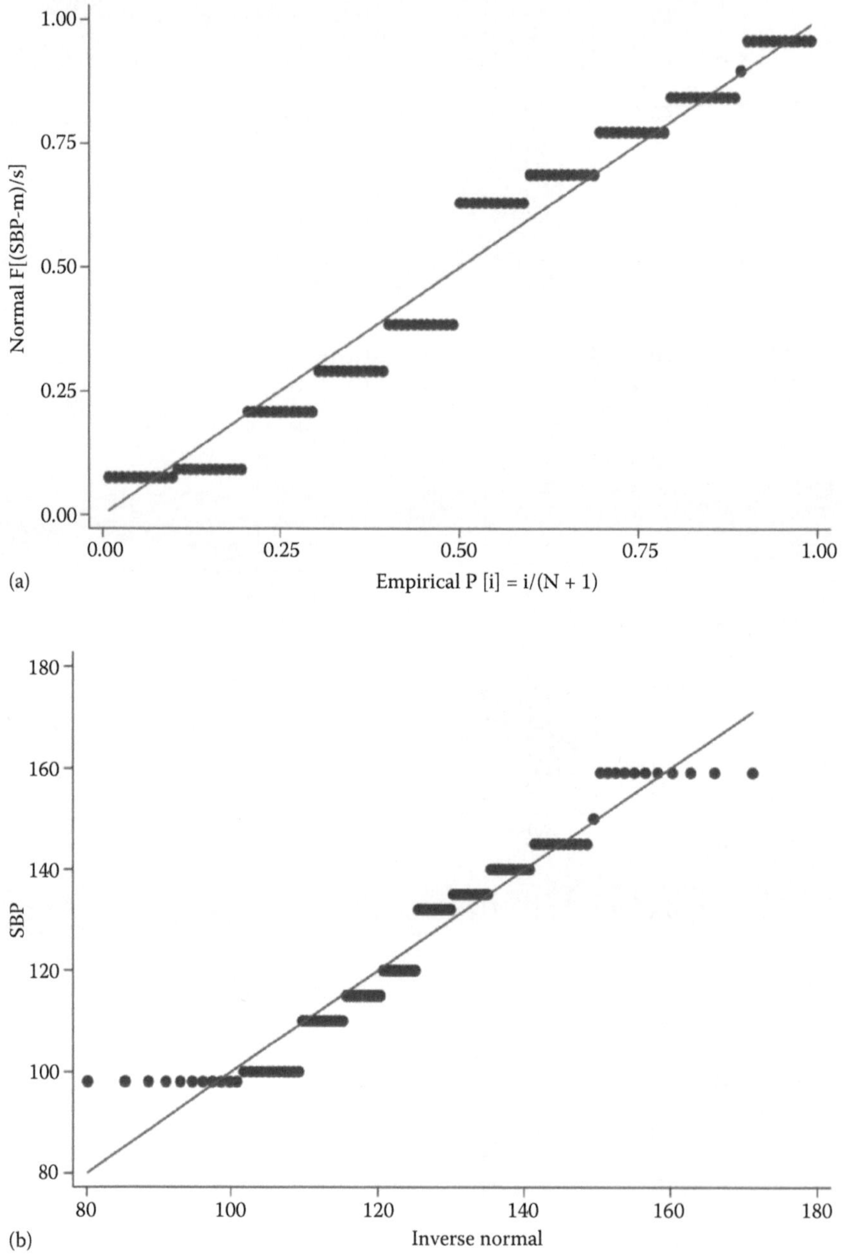

Figure 3.5 (a) Normal distribution of SBP. (b) Quantile normal distribution.

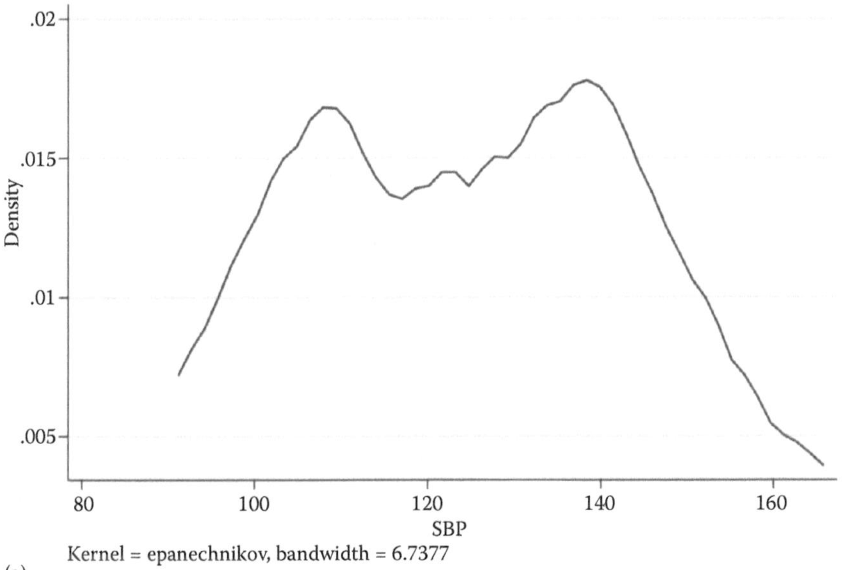

(a)

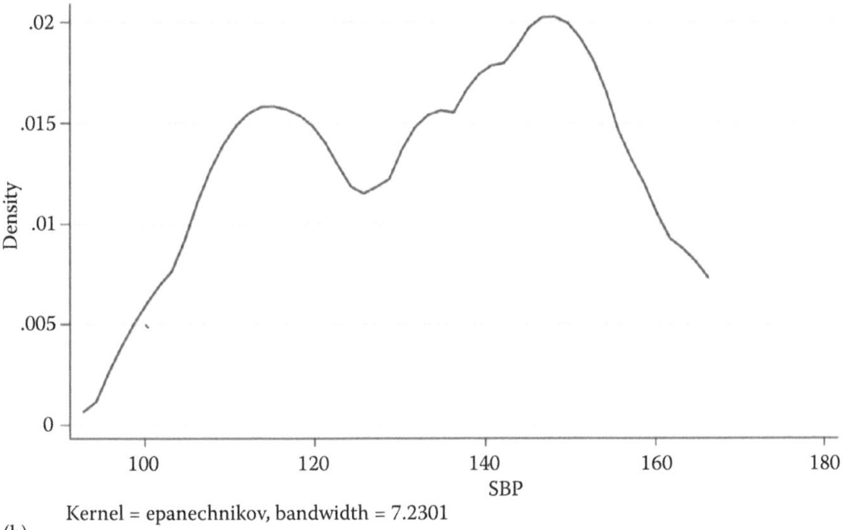

(b)

Figure 3.6 (a) Kernel density distribution, n = 100 (total sample). (b) Kernel density estimate (SBP distribution) in male (n = 56)—data skewed to the left.

(*Continued*)

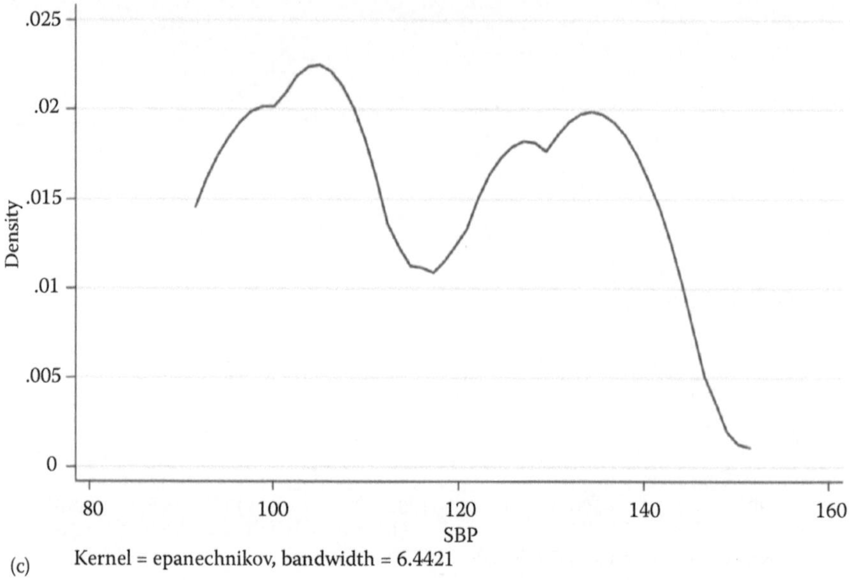

Figure 3.6 (Continued) (c) Kernel density estimate, female (n = 55)—data skewed to the right.

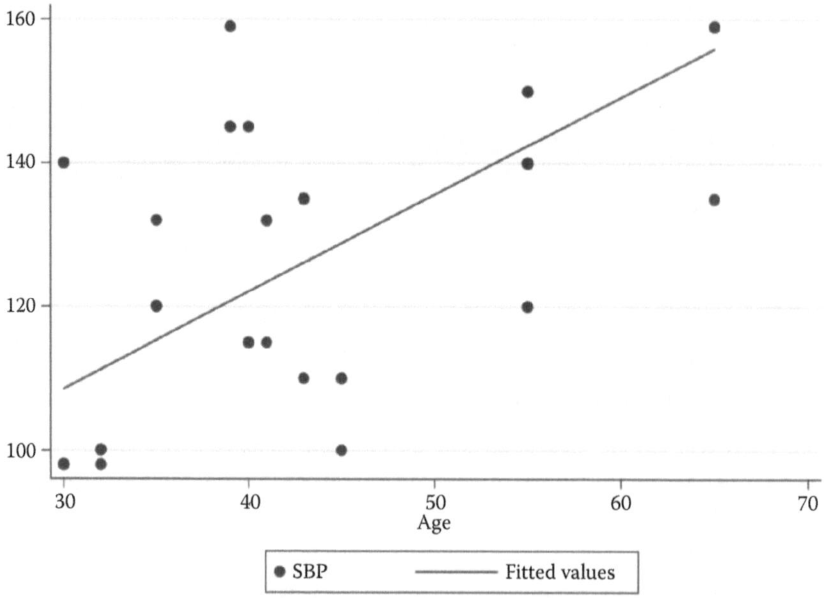

Figure 3.7 Scatter plot of SBP by age, using age to predict SBP.

Box 3.8 illustrates the first (p25) and third (p75) quartiles of the SBP. The quartiles are not as accurate as the variance or SD in describing the variability in the data since they do not have the mathematical properties of the SD or variance.

BOX 3.8 THE SBP QUARTILE, INTERQUARTILE, AND PERCENTILES BY SEX OF PATIENTS ($N = 100$)

```
. sum SBP, det

                             SBP
-------------------------------------------------------------
      Percentiles      Smallest
 1%           98             98
 5%           98             98
10%          100             98       Obs                 111
25%          110             98       Sum of Wgt.         111

50%          132                      Mean           125.6216
                        Largest       Std. Dev.      19.20135
75%          140            159
90%          150            159       Variance       368.6919
95%          159            159       Skewness       .0958709
99%          159            159       Kurtosis       1.895076

. sum SBP if Sex ==1, det

                             SBP
-------------------------------------------------------------
      Percentiles      Smallest
 1%          100            100
 5%          110            110
10%          110            110       Obs                  56
25%          120            110       Sum of Wgt.          56

50%          140                      Mean           134.5714
                        Largest       Std. Dev.      17.96953
75%          145            159
90%          159            159       Variance       322.9039
95%          159            159       Skewness       -.147815
99%          159            159       Kurtosis       1.716984

. sum SBP if Sex ==2, det

                             SBP
-------------------------------------------------------------
      Percentiles      Smallest
 1%           98             98
 5%           98             98
10%           98             98       Obs                  55
25%          100             98       Sum of Wgt.          55

50%          115                      Mean           116.5091
                        Largest       Std. Dev.      15.95349
75%          132            135
90%          135            135       Variance       254.5138
95%          135            140       Skewness       .0986213
99%          145            145       Kurtosis       1.381336

.
```

Abbreviation: Sex: 1 = male and 2 = female.

3.5.6 *Variance, standard deviation, and standard error of the mean (SEM)*

The variance reflects the average squared difference of the SBP above from the mean SBP of African-American women. Another commonly used measure of dispersion from the mean distribution is standard deviation. To estimate the variance of the SBP, the differences between each subject SBP and the mean is squared, since summing the differences directly without squaring will result in zero. The population variance, which is denoted by σ^2, is estimated by the following:

$$\sigma^2 = \sum_{i=1}^{N} \frac{(x_i - \mu)^2}{N}$$

while the sample variance (s^2) is estimated by the following:

$$s^2 = \sum_{i=1}^{n} \frac{(x_i - \bar{X})^2}{n}$$

The variance is the minimum sum of the squared differences of each SBP from *any* SBP number. Consequently, if we used any SBP other than the mean SBP as the value from which each SBP is subtracted, the resulting sum of squared differences would be greater.

The standard deviation (SD) is the square root of the variance. The population SD is designated by σ, while the sample SD is designated by s. The population SD is estimated by the following:

$$\sigma = \sqrt{\sum_{i=1}^{N} \frac{(x_i - \mu)^2}{N}}$$

while the sample SD is estimated by the following:

$$s \sqrt{\sum_{i=1}^{n} \frac{(x_i - \bar{X})^2}{n}}$$

where μ is the population mean, $\bar{X}$ is the sample mean, N is the population size, and n is the sample size.

3.5.7 *Standard error of the mean*

If not specified, the standard error often refers to standard error of the mean (SEM), but standard error of median or variance may also apply to SE. While SD and coefficient of variation are used to illustrate how much variation there is among individual observations, standard error or CI is used to demonstrate the reliability of the estimate of the mean. In reporting the amount of variation in the effect of a treatment, the SD becomes an appropriate measure of dispersion to use:

$$\text{SEM} = \frac{\sigma}{\sqrt{n}}$$

where σ is the SD and n is the sample size.

To illustrate the SEM, consider taking random samples from a population of 100 children with acute lymphocytic leukemia (ALL). The SEM simply reflects the deviation from the different sample means, while SD reflects the individual observations from the sample. If we take the mean age of a random sample of five children from this population, this mean may not reflect the population's parametric mean age of the children with ALL, but taking a sample of 30 ALL children may. However, as we increase the sample size, we are more likely to come close to the population mean age of the children with ALL, implying that the variability in the mean decreases with the increase in the sample size. The SEM can be used to describe the variability in the data if one is not interested in the amount of variation with respect to the effect of intervention or treatment.

A study (hypothetical) was conducted to examine elbow ligament thickness of 367 baseball players (population). If we take a random sample of 10 players, a sample of 40 players, and then 51 players, which of these means will be closer to the population parameter mean? Using STATA syntax for summary statistics (`sum var`) and confidence interval (`ci var`), the outputs shown in Box 3.9 were obtained:

BOX 3.9 SAMPLE MEAN, SEM, SE, AND SAMPLE SIZE

```
sum thick thick_01 thick_02 thick_03
```

Variable	Obs	Mean	Std. Dev.	Min	Max
thick	367	6.199728	1.650046	2.6	14.3
thick_01	51	6.303922	1.468055	3	9.3
thick_02	40	5.98	1.502852	3.1	9.3
thick_03	10	5.53	1.183263	3.1	7.1

```
ci thick thick_01 thick_02 thick_03
```

Variable	Obs	Mean	Std. Err.	[95% Conf.	Interval]
thick	367	6.199728	.0861317	6.030352	6.369103
thick_01	51	6.303922	.2055688	5.891025	6.716819
thick_02	40	5.98	.2376218	5.499365	6.460635
thick_03	10	5.53	.3741806	4.683545	6.376455

Box 3.9 illustrates SEM reduction with increasing sample size (thick represents the population: thick_01, the random sample with $n = 51$; thick_02, the random sample with $n = 40$; and thick_03, the random sample with $n = 10$). While SD fluctuates with sample size, it does not illustrate a dose–response effect as demonstrated by SEM.

3.6 Standardized distribution—*z* score statistic

In biomedical or clinical research, we may be interested in the top 20 biologic or specimen values in order to determine if our subjects will be classified as belonging to or not belonging to a certain treatment category. These answers may be complex, hence the utilization of probability distributions, such as a normal distribution (Figure 3.8). We assume that elbow ligament thickness in these players is normally distributed. With this assumption, we can use standard normal distribution and *z* scores to address such questions. Therefore, if a frequency distribution is normally distributed, we can determine the probability of a score occurring by standardizing the scores, such as for ligament thickness or hemoglobin level or test scores, by using the *z* score computation, which converts the group of data in the frequency distribution such that the mean = 0 and SD = 1. We express the *z* scores in terms of SDs and their means.

Mathematically, this appears as follows: standardized score (z) = $\chi - \mu/\sigma$, where μ is the mean (sample mean), χ is the score (individual score), and σ is the SD.

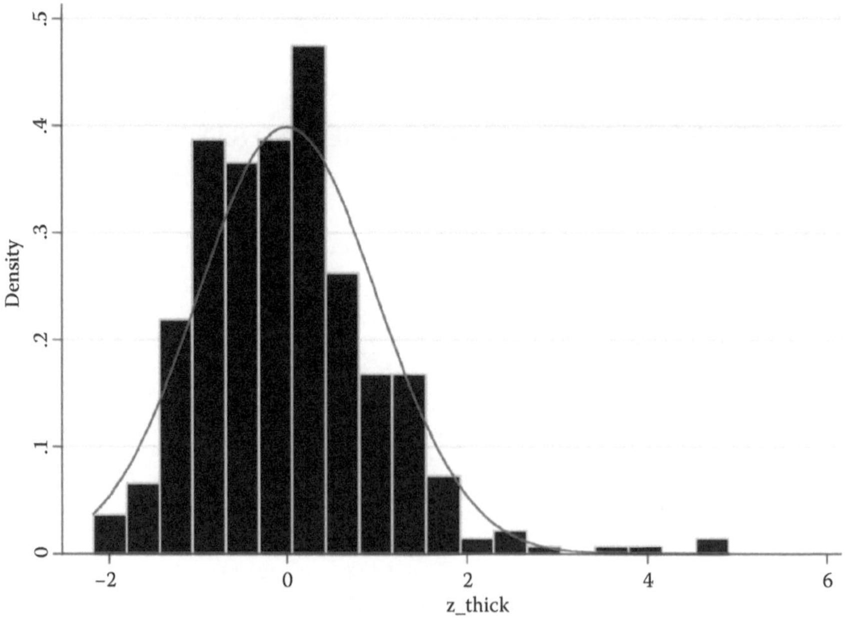

Figure 3.8 Normal distribution with mean (μ) = 0.

3.7 Basic probability notion

Statistics is about sample, and for a meaningful interpretation of statistical computation and the application in addressing health issues, a basic knowledge of probability is required.[5] Consider the chance of a normal or usual pregnancy resulting in a male child as 0.5 (50%) and that of not having a female child as 0.5 (50%). How do we compute this? Let us consider an example of 100 patients diagnosed with cystitis and prescribed erythromycin antibiotics (250 mg × 2 daily/7). If at the end of 2 weeks, 80 patients presented with no symptoms of cystitis; what is the probability that erythromycin is an effective antibiotics in treating cystitis?

We can compute the probability of an event occurring or success of erythromycin in treating cystitis as: Number of success/Overall or total number of trials (outcomes). Substituting: treated without symptoms (80)/All patients with cystitis (those without and with symptoms) (100). $P = 80/100 = 0.8$. The probability of failure (q) = $1 - P$. Substituting: $1 - 0.8 = 0.2$. Given the concept of probability, what are the odds of erythromycin producing a favorable outcome?

Odds or success = p/q, where p is the chance of an event occurring and q is the chance of the same event not occurring. Substituting, the success of erythromycin in treating cystitis is $0.8/0.2 = 4.0$, meaning that the odds of success is 4 to 1, while the odds of failure is 0.25 to 1. Simply, erythromycin, given these data, is more likely to yield a favorable compared to a non-favorable outcome.

Let us assume that early antibiotics used to treat cystitis had a success/cure or odds of 0.4 (p) and failure odds of 0.6 (q) in a comparable patient sample (age, sex, diagnosis, duration of illness, etc.) and sample size ($n = 100$). Since we are interested in the relative effectiveness of these two antibiotics, what is the crude odds ratio: odds ratio = odds of success in erythromycin antibiotic/odds of success in early antibiotic. Substituting: $0.8/0.4 = 2.0$, implying 2 to 1 success. How do we interpret this result? Simply, compared to early antibiotic, erythromycin antibiotic is two times as likely to relieve the symptoms of cystitis.

3.8 Simple and unconditional probability

Probability as observed earlier is a number that indicates the chance or the likelihood of an occurrence, and is expressed as a proportion ranging from 0 to 1, where 1 implies certainty and 0 implies no chance or likelihood of an event occurring. We can also express probability as a percentage. With respect to Table 3.2, what is the probability of selecting any cancer patient from this sample?

$$P(\text{characteristic}) = \frac{\text{Number of persons with characteristic } (\boldsymbol{n})}{\text{Total of population } (N)}$$

Table 3.2 Simple and unconditional probability estimate

	Race and ethnicity						
Cancer type	*White*	*Black/AA*	*Asian*	*American Indian/ Alaska Native*	*Hawaiian/ Pacific Islander*	*Multiracial*	*Total*
ALL	1000	400	100	60	70	200	1830
AML	400	180	30	10	15	120	755
Total	1400	580	130	70	85	320	2585

Abbreviations: AA, African-American; ALL, acute lymphocytic leukemia; AML, acute myeloid leukemia.

Substituting: 1/2585 = 0.0004 = 0.04%, implying < 1% chance of selecting any cancer patient.

Additionally, what is the probability of selecting a cancer patient that is white?

$$P(\text{white}) = \frac{\text{Number of white cancer patients}}{\text{Total population of cancer patients}}$$

Substituting: 1400/2585 = 0.54 = 54%, implying 54% chance of selecting a white patient with cancer.

Further, what is the probability of selecting a black patient with AML?

$$P(\text{black AML}) = \frac{\text{Number of blacks with AML}}{\text{Total population with AML}}$$

Substituting: 180/2585= 0.07 = 7%, implying a 7% chance of selecting a black cancer patient with AML in the sample.

The above examples reflect simple and unconditional probability estimation, given that the denominator reflects the total population, implying the chance of everyone in the population to be selected.

3.9 Conditional probability

Suppose we are interested in the subpopulation of patients with ALL, what is the probability of selecting an Asian who has ALL?

$$P(\text{Asian}|\text{ALL}) = \frac{\text{Number of cancer patients with characteristics (ALL)}}{\text{Total population } (N) - \text{ALL}}$$

Substituting: 100/1830 = 0.055 = 5.5%, implying 5.5% of AML among Asians in this sample.

3.10 Independence and conditional probability

An event is considered to be independent if the probability of one is not affected by the occurrence (P) or nonoccurrence ($1 - P$) of the other. Consider a diagnostic test for diabetes using percent A1C to examine independence probability. A1C also termed hemoglobin A1c, HbA1c, or glycohemoglobin test is used to determine blood sugar level for the diagnosis of diabetes. A normal A1C level is below 5.7%. An A1C level of 6.5% or higher on two separate occasions is indicative of DM, while A1C between 5.7% and 6.4% is considered pre-diabetic, suggestive of a high risk of DM (Table 3.3).

The probability that an individual has DM given he or she has a normal A1C is P(DM|normal A1C) = 10/60 = 0.167, while the probability that an individual has DM given he or she has an ACI between 5.7% and 6.5% is P(DM|A1C 5.7–6.5%) = 6/36 = 0.167, and the probability that an individual has DM given he or she has an A1C > 6.5% is P(DM|A1C > 6.5%) = 4/24 = 0.167. The probability that a subject had DM was 0.167, implying that the A1C test result does not affect the likelihood that an individual has DM in this sample. In this example, the probability that an individual has DM is independent of the A1C test result.

Consider these two events, A1C% test (A) and DM diagnosis (B). These two occurrences or events are said to be independent if P(A|B) = P(A) of if P(B|A) = P(B). Independence in probability could be verified by comparing a conditional with an unconditional probability. The equality of the conditional with unconditional is indicative of independence. Illustrating in the example above, P(A|B) = P(A1C < 5.7%|DM) = 10/20 = 0.50 and P(A) = P(A1C < 5.7) = 60/120 = 0.50. Additionally, independence can also be tested by examining whether P(B|A) = P(DM| < 5.7%) = 10/60 = 0.167 and P(B) = P(DM) = 20/120 = 0.167. Consequently, the probability of the patient having a diagnosis of DM given an A1C < 5.7% DM test, implying conditional probability, is the same as the overall probability of having DM diagnosis, implying an unconditional probability.

Table 3.3 Independence probability using A1C test result and DM diagnosis

A1C%	*DM*	*Non-DM*	*Total*
Normal (<5.7%)	10	50	60
Pre-diabetic (5.7%–6.5%)	6	30	36
Diabetic (>6.5%)	4	20	24
Total	20	100	120

3.11 Probability distribution

This refers to a listing of all the values the random variable can assume with their corresponding probabilities. There are several probability distributions, namely, binomial, Poisson, normal, and so on.

The binomial distribution model is an important probability model that is used when there are two possible outcomes (hence "binomial"). In a situation in which there were more than two distinct outcomes, a multinomial probability model might be appropriate, but here we focus on the situation in which the outcome is dichotomous.

For example, adults with allergies might report relief with medication or not, children with a bacterial infection might respond to antibiotic therapy or not, adults who suffer a myocardial infarction might survive the heart attack or not, and a medical device such as a coronary stent might be successfully implanted or not. These are just a few examples of applications or processes in which the outcome of interest has two possible values (i.e., it is dichotomous). The two outcomes are often labeled "success" and "failure," with success indicating the presence of the outcome of interest. Note, however, that for many medical and public health questions, the outcome or event of interest is the occurrence of disease, which is obviously not really a success. Nevertheless, this terminology is typically used when discussing the binomial distribution model. As a result, whenever using the binomial distribution, we must clearly specify which outcome is the "success" and which is the "failure."

The binomial distribution model allows us to compute the probability of observing a specified number of "successes" when the process is repeated a specific number of times (e.g., in a set of patients) and the outcome for a given patient is either a success or a failure.

$$\mu = np$$

$$\sigma = \sqrt{n(p)(1-p)}$$

3.12 Summary

Biostatistical reasoning reflects the degree to which evidence discovered from the observed data is generalizable across targeted populations. Being able to use appropriate test statistics or statistical techniques/procedures to make sense of the data collected during the course of our research is fundamental to evidence discovery. This ability depends on a careful understanding of the scale of measurement of our variables, especially the response variable, the sampling technique used, the type of study design—experimental or nonexperimental—and the power of the study. Where probability sampling was not applied or consecutive patient studies were conducted so as to reflect sample representativeness, it is not meaningful to quantify random error (p value) and estimate precision (CIs).

The fundamental thinking in inferential statistics is based on the assumption that observations represent random samples drawn from the population of patients, implying known and equal probability for all patients in the population to be included in our samples.[6] This is important in deciding the targeted population to which the study findings should apply, implying knowledge of the actual population the samples represent. The source of the sample is important for adequate generalization since in/outpatient subjects in a clinical investigation rarely represent a random sample of the population of patients with a given condition as a whole.

Measures of central tendency allow us to examine the location and the spread of our data. This exercise opens a window to the data besides the graphic presentation of data before the analysis. The mean remains the most commonly used measure of central tendency once data assume normality in terms of distribution, while the median is suitable in summarizing data that are skewed, since the median as a measure of central tendency is not subjected to outliers. The spread or dispersion of the data is commonly summarized with SD and SEM. However, care must be taken in the utilization of these two measures of dispersion.

Questions for discussion

1 If data are normally distributed, the mean and the median will be very close, and if data are not normally distributed, then both mean and median may provide useful information. Consider an ordered categorical variable on patient satisfaction rated as 1 = poor to 5 = excellent. What would be a preferred statistic for summarizing such patient satisfaction data?
2 SD is a measure of variability in variables with approximately symmetric distributions. Is range or interquartile range a better measure of variability for patients' ages?
3 Often, standard error is used to describe data, since standard error appears to be smaller relative to SD and thus indicative of a more precise study. (a) If the purpose is to describe the data and data are normal, is standard error a better measure of variability? (b) If the purpose is to describe the outcome of a study or the mean weight of children in an obesity clinic, is SD the best measure of variability of the data? (c) When should SD be used to describe variability in the data?
4 If the mean SBP of 100 women in a weight management clinic is 132 (SD=7.8) and that of 120 women in a hypertension clinic is 145 (SD=18.4), estimate the SEM in these two groups.
5 The urinary lead concentration (μmol/24 h) was obtained in two groups of children:

   Group A: 2.6, 3.4, 2.8, 1.9, 2.0, 3.9. 1.9, 2.1, 3.0, 1.7
   Group B: 2.7, 4.5, 2.6, 3.4, 3.8, 2.9, 1.6, 4.0, 3.5, 2.8

Table 3.4 Association between family history of breast cancer and breast cancer diagnosis

Family history of breast cancer	*Breast cancer*	*No breast cancer*	*Total*
Yes	491	368	859
No	152	5721	5873
Total	643	5089	6732

Using a statistical package of your choice, including STATA, estimate the mean difference in the urinary lead concentration. Is there a significant increase in concentration of urinary lead in group B?

6 Using Table 3.4, determine whether or not independent probability is involved in the family history of breast cancer and the prevalence of breast cancer.
   a Estimate the unconditional probability of breast cancer, which is simply the prevalence of breast cancer in this sample.
   b Estimate the conditional probability of breast cancer given the family history of breast cancer.
   c Compare the conditional and unconditional to determine the independent probability of these events.

Hints; *P*(breast cancer prevalence) = *P*(A) = Breast cancer prevalence/total sample while the unconditional probability of breast cancer prevalence given family history of breast cancer = *P*(A|B)= (Breast cancer prevalence|History of breast cancer).

References

1. M. Hardy and A. Bryman (Eds.), *Handbook of Data Analysis* (Thousand Oakes, CA: Sage, 2004).
2. B. Rosner, *Fundamentals of Biostatistics* (Belmont, CA: Thomson-Brooks/Cole, 2006).
3. R. L. Ott and W. Mendenhal, *Understanding Statistics* (Belmont, CA: Duxbury Press, 1994).
4. R. N. Forthofer and E. S. Lee, *Introduction to Biostatistics* (New York: Academic Press, 1995).
5. H. A. Kahn and C. T. Sempos, *Statistical Methods in Epidemiology* (Oxford: Oxford University Press, 1989).
6. J. Cohen, *Statistical Power Analysis for the Behavioral Sciences* (New Jersey: Lawrence Erlbaum Associates, 1988).

Section II

Biostatistical modeling

Evidence discovery requires assumptions and rationale around the data collected from research conduct or preexisting and secondary data. The reliability of evidence assumes an unbiased sample in order to ensure adequate generalizability.

The process of evidence discovery thus requires data processing, which is often ignored, data description via graphical presentation and summary statistics, and then hypotheses testing and interpretation. This section deals with biostatistical reasoning, categorical, and continuous data appraisal. The specific-hypothesis testing involves samples and relationships.

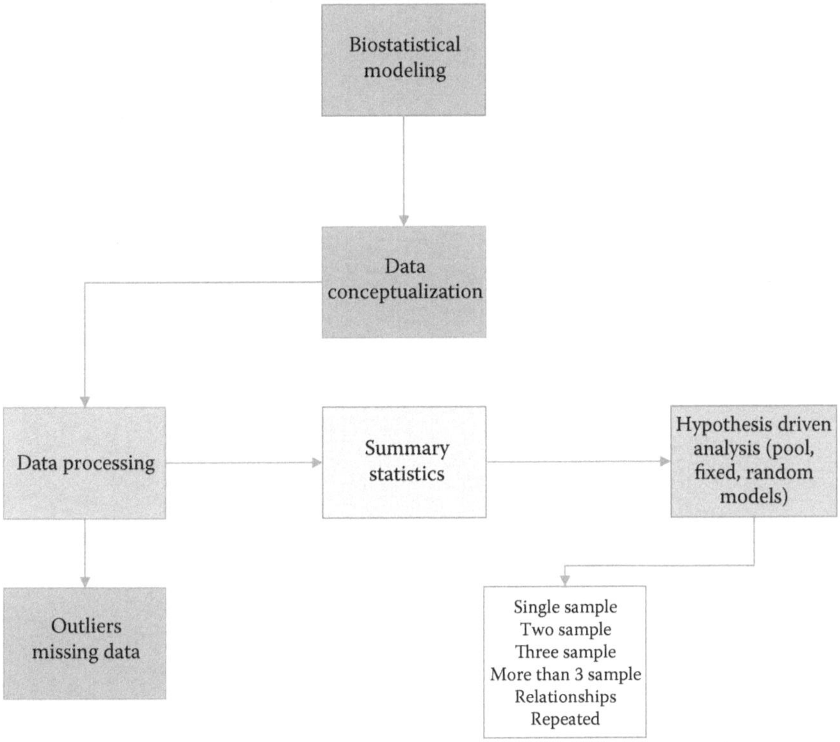

4 Statistical considerations in clinical research

4.1 Introduction

Conducting research centers on (a) conceptualization, (b) design process, and (c) statistical inference. Once the design is completed, the study is performed, and the data are collected, entered into the database, and edited, the next step is data analysis, which yields the study results. The initial step in the analysis, also termed *preanalysis screening*, is to obtain the summary statistics with frequency distribution (number and percentage) for discrete data and mean and standard deviation for continuous data. Therefore, the type of distribution or measurement scale (continuous, discrete) determines the nature of the descriptive summary or statistics.

In clinical research, we focus on a sample of patients and not the entire population of patients with a given condition. We use a random sample to ensure that every individual in the population has an equal and independent chance of being selected. Consider a study conducted to examine the association between residual postoperative Cobb angle and the prevalence of deep wound infection after posterior spine fusion among children with cerebral palsy. Of the 264 patients studied, 22 developed deep wound infection. The residual postoperative Cobb angle was compared between cases and noncases, and the difference in the mean Cobb angle was found. The next step was to determine whether the mean difference between the cases and noncases was due to chance alone. Since the sample studied was a random sample and the 264 patients represented the population of children with cerebral palsy, statistical significance must be considered using a probability model. The application of the probability model, which is indicative of how likely it is that we would obtain a certain mean difference in Cobb angle between cases and noncases in a sample of 264 patients if there were no real difference between the cases and noncases in the entire population of children with cerebral palsy who have undergone surgery for spinal deformity correction, reflects the notion of inferential statistics.

In the previous chapters (Section I), we presented data cleaning and editing, preanalysis screening, and hypothesis-specific test notions. These aspects of clinical research are required in the study protocol, and clinical investigators are required to develop and utilize a manual of procedures in addressing these issues. This chapter is concerned with the illustrative approach to understanding how sense is made from data through the steps outlined in various techniques of hypothesis testing. We attempt to present reliable and valid scientific research as that which applies appropriate statistical techniques in drawing evidence from the data. Statistics is presented as an informational science, with the purpose being to make sense of accurate data, since statistical methods, no matter how sophisticated, cannot generate valid and reliable evidence from an inaccurate measurement or poorly designed study.

BOX 4.1 NOTION OF STATISTICS

- Statistics is a highly developed information science.
- It is involved with the study of inferential processes, especially the planning and analysis of experiments, surveys or observational studies.[a]
- The study of how information should be employed to reflect on, and give guidance for action in a practical situation involving uncertainty.[b]
- A way of thinking or an approach to everyday problems that relies heavily on designed data production. It is essential in that its proper usability minimizes the chance of drawing incorrect conclusions from data.[c]

[a] V. Barnett, *Comparative Statistical Inference*, 2nd ed. (New York: Wiley, 1982).
[b] S. Stigler, *The History of Statistics* (Cambridge, MA: Belknap Press, 1986).
[c] S. Piantadosi, *Clinical Trials*, 2nd ed. (Hoboken, New Jersey: John Wiley & Sons, 2005).

The technique to be used in producing the result of a study or to test the proposed hypothesis depends on (a) design, (b) scales of measurement of the variables, (c) the assumption underlying the distribution of the data—parametric or nonparametric of distribution-free, (d) number in the comparison group, and (e) group independence. For example, using a retrospective cohort design, an investigator wanted to determine the outcome of cervical arthrodesis with instrumentation on pediatric patients with skeletal dysplasia (SKD), a heterogeneous disorder involving abnormality of skeletal development, growth, and degeneration. *What is the test statistic to examine the null hypothesis of no difference in the proportion of solid fusion comparing instrumented to non-instrumented patients?* To answer this question, the investigator needs to address the following issues:

a *What was the scale of measurement of the dependent or response variable?* The outcome of cervical arthrodesis was measured as the presence or absence of solid fusion as observed on x-ray imaging of SKD patients who underwent this procedure, where absence was coded as "0," and presence as "1."

b *What was the comparison or how many groups were being compared?* There were two comparison groups based on instrumentation, which was coded as "0" for absence of instrumentation and "1" for instrumentation.

c *What was the assumption underlying the data on response variable?* The response variable was measured on a binary scale and hence represents a proportion. Therefore, the proposed analysis must assume a nonparametric or distribution-free test.

d *Were the groups independent?* Simply, is the outcome or fusion obtained from a patient in the instrumented group dependent on that from a patient in the noninstrumented group? The groups were independent since the patients in the instrumented group were unrelated to the patients in the noninstrumented group, except for the disease of interest, SKD.

The approach to understanding hypothesis testing in clinical research is to attempt to answer the research questions. With the previous example, the investigator utilized chi-square statistics to examine the independence of the groups (instrumented versus noninstrumented) and binomial regression to predict the outcome of cervical arthrodesis in SKD, given instrumentation as the independent variable and solid fusion as the response variable. Are these two tests appropriate? Let us consider the adequacy of (a) chi-square and (b) binomial in answering the research questions or testing the null hypothesis of no difference (binomial regression) or dependence (chi-square).

4.1.1 Chi-square statistic

4.1.1.1 What is it?

This is the measure of how much the observed cell counts in a two-way table diverge from the expected cell count. It is easily described as a statistical technique used to test the null hypothesis of the equality of proportion, such as independence or no association between instrumented and noninstrumented patients with respect to certain study characteristics, such as age, sex, or type of medical insurance coverage. Simply, the chi-square tests the null hypothesis of no dependence or association between the row variable and the column variable by comparing the entire set of observed counts with the set of expected counts. Mathematically, it appears as follows: $\chi^2 = \Sigma$ (observed count − expected count)^1/expected count.

4.1.1.2 When is it used?

It is used to examine or test for independence or no association when variables are categorical or binary, and normality is not assumed (distribution-free data). Chi-square is appropriate in testing a null hypothesis of independence, or no association, when normality distribution cannot be assumed (nonparametric/distribution-free) and when variables are coded as categorical or binary. If the expected counts and observed counts are very different, a large value of chi-square will result. Therefore, large values of chi-square provide evidence against the null hypothesis.

4.1.2 *Binomial regression*

4.1.2.1 What is it?

Binomial regression is a test statistic based on the probability distribution that describes the number of successes "A" observed in independent trials or attempts (Bernoulli trial—named after the Swiss statistician, Jakob Bernoulli, who developed this distribution theory in the seventeenth century), each with the same probability of occurrence. For example, solid fusion based on x-ray imaging occurred as a binary event—presence (1 = Yes) or absence (0 = No)—and can be denoted as X and Y or A and B. Simply, the probability of X (fusion proportion) is denoted by π, or $P(X) = \pi$, and π remains the same each time fusion occurs or is observed, while the probability of fusion not occurring (Y) is denoted by $1 - \pi$, since Y occurs each time X does not occur. This distribution presents the probability that solid fusion occurs in a certain number of cervical arthrodesis performed for cervical stability on SKD pediatric patients with cervical instability. Therefore, since cervical arthrodesis is performed on different patients, implying the occurrence of cervical arthrodesis in *n* times, and the outcome (solid fusion) is independent from one arthrodesis performed to another, binomial regression computes the probability that solid fusion occurs exactly Z times (proportion of solid fusion in instrumented versus noninstrumented patients with risk ratio as the measure of effect or point estimate).

4.1.2.2 When is binomial regression used?

When the distribution follows Bernoulli's theory and the response or outcome variable is binary (fusion "1" and no fusion "0"); the independent variable is binary, discrete, or categorical or mixed (instrumentation "1" and noninstrumentation "0"); and the design is retrospective cohort, which allows for risk ratio as the measure of effect, binomial regression is used. The technique is also efficient in other observational designs.

4.1.2.3 Where is the binomial regression model used?

This test statistic is appropriate if the design of the study is retrospective cohort (Figure 4.1), which allows for the effect size to be presented as risk ratio, the outcome variable is measured on a binary scale (Yes = 1 and No = 0), with or without normality assumption (nonparametric or distribution-free),

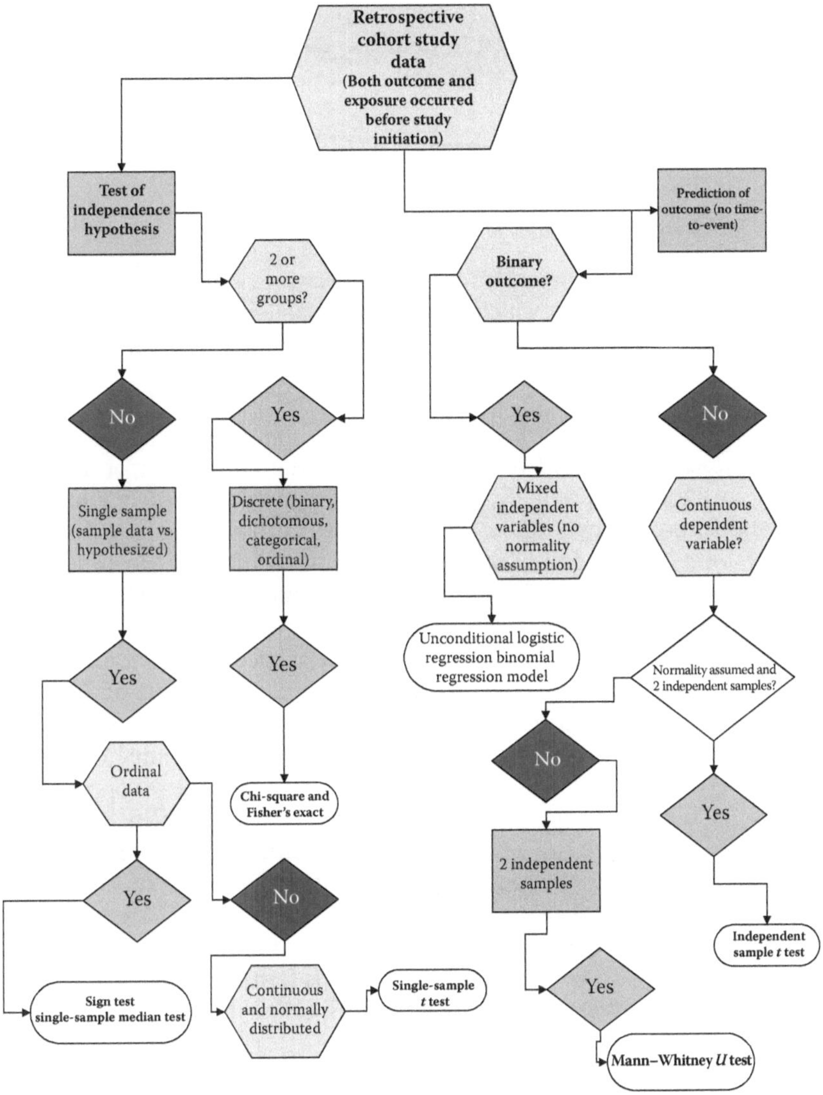

Figure 4.1 The use of statistical methods in a retrospective cohort study.

and the independent variables are measured in mixed scales (binary, discrete, categorical, or continuous). In addition, *how the test is used and interpreted* is essential to analysis, interpretation, and result presentation. These aspects are explained later in this chapter.

4.2 Types of variables

4.2.1 Random variables and probability distributions

Variable refers to a characteristic of interest in a study that has different values for different subjects (that which varies).[2] A variable is the measure of a single characteristic and is so termed because it varies or changes with subjects.

4.2.1.1 What is a random variable?

Clinical research involves the application of the conclusion of the study sample to the target population, implying the population of previous, current, and future patients. *Random variable* refers to a variable in a study in which subjects are randomly selected.[3] For example, if the subjects in a study to examine the survival of men treated for localized prostate cancer with radical prostatectomy represent a random sample selected from the larger population, then race and Gleason score are examples of random variables. Consider another example: investigators examined the effect of treatment on the racial variance in the survival of older women diagnosed with cervical cancer and treated for the disease; they selected a sample of subjects and observed the effect of treatment (less extensive surgery versus radical surgery) on the survival of these women. If a random variable is used in this sample, then inference can be drawn from the data, implying that the result of the study can be applied to all women, past, present, and future, who are diagnosed with cervical cancer and treated for the disease. Further, since the selected sample represents a population where all had equal probability or were equally likely to be selected, this sample is termed an unbiased sample, and *treatment* as a measure of survival is then called a random variable.[4]

4.3 Variables and sources of variation (variability)

There are attributes of variables, whether random or nonrandom. The common sources of variation are disease status, biologic differences, measurement conditions, measurement methods, measurement error, and random error. Statistical methods/tools are used to make sense of the variation in data. For example, if a random variable (treatment) used in a study and the observation in the sample are mutually independent (probability that an older woman selected is unaffected by the selection of another older woman in the sample), then the sample is said to be unbiased. Variability or chance is minimized, and the result is not due to chance (accurate) if an unbiased sample (equal probability of being selected from the target population into the sample) of independent observations is used in the study. Despite this, chance may influence the outcome of a study, resulting in the application of statistical technique to assess the effect of chance.

4.3.1 Types of variables in clinical research

Measurement scales or type of variable determines which statistical method is appropriate for a given set of data.[5] For example, if a variable, such as weight or blood pressure, is measured in a ratio scale, mean and standard deviation are appropriate measures of central tendency used to summarize the data. However, if the scale of measurement is ordinal, median and interquartile range become appropriate statistical methods for the summary, as well as frequency distribution (number and percentage).

4.3.1.1 What are the types of scales used in measuring variables?

Nominal (unordered) variables are those (naming or categorical) that have no measurement scales (e.g., skin color). The *binary* or *dichotomous variable* or observation is a nominal measure that has two outcomes (e.g., gender [male → 1, female → 2], survival [yes → 1, no → 0]). *Discrete variables* are binary and nominal, so termed because the categories are separate from each other (e.g., gender [male vs. female]). Ordinal *(ordered categories)* variables are those with underlying order to their values (e.g., fatigue scale [0–10], mild, moderate, severe). Continuous or dimensional variables are characteristics that are measured on a continuum (e.g., systolic blood pressure, diastolic blood pressure, height, weight, age, etc.). Compared with ordinal, nominal, or discrete data, continuous variables (interval and ratio) allow for more detailed information and inferences.

4.3.2 Additional terms explained

4.3.2.1 What is probability distribution?

Probability distribution is used to summarize values of random variables as a form of frequency distribution.

4.3.2.2 What are the types of probability distributions?

Binomial (yes and no) is a discrete probability distribution in which the associated random variable takes only integer values—0, 1, 2 … *n*. It provides the probability that a specified event or outcome occurs in a given number of independent trials. *Poisson* is a discrete distribution applicable, like binomials, when the outcome is the number of times an event occurs. *Normal (Gaussian) distribution (bell-shaped curve)* is a continuous probability distribution. This distribution takes any value; it is a smooth, bell-shaped curve, and it is symmetric about the mean of the distribution, symbolized by μ, and a standard deviation symbolized by σ.[6] *Standard normal (z) distribution* refers to the distribution with a mean of 0 and a standard deviation of 1.

$$Z \text{ or (Z-score, normal deviate, standard score or critical ratio)} = (\boldsymbol{X} - \mu)/\sigma$$[7]

4.4 Sampling, sample size, and power

Statistics deals with samples, and the main reason for research is to infer, or generalize, from a sample (sets of observations from one group of subjects) to a larger population (others who are similar to the subjects in the sample).[7] Statistics is the procedure by which some members of a given population are selected as representatives of the entire population.[8] The process of inference requires statistical methods based on probability. The probability of a given outcome is the number of times that outcome occurs divided by the total number of trials.

4.4.1 *What are the uses of probability?*

Probability is essential to research and is applied in (1) understanding and interpreting data; (2) indicating how much confidence there is in estimates, such as the means or relative risks; and (3) understanding the meaning of *p* values.[8]

4.4.2 *What are the types of probability rules?*

The following probability rules are commonly used:

a *Mutually exclusive events and the additional rule*: Two or more events are mutually exclusive if the occurrence of one precludes the occurrence of the others. The probability is found by adding the probabilities of two events—(addition rule) → $P(\text{A or B}) = P(\text{A}) + P(\text{B})$.[10]
b *Independent events and multiplication rule*: Two events are independent if the outcome of one event has no effect on the outcome of the second—(multiplication rule) → $P(\text{A and B}) = P(\text{A}) \times P(\text{B})$.[11]

4.4.3 *What is a population, and how does it differ from a sample?*

Population describes a large set or collection of items with common characteristics, whereas *sample* refers to the subset of the population, selected so as to be representative of the larger population.[12] For example, if researchers study

236 pediatric patients with cerebral palsy to determine the association between nutritional status and deep wound infection, the sample is 236 patients studied, while the population is the children with cerebral palsy. *Why use a sample? "Bigger is not always better."*

1 Samples are quick to study.
2 They are less expensive.
3 It is difficult or impossible to study the entire population.
4 The accuracy of result can be compared with the total population.
5 If properly selected, probability methods can be used to estimate the error in the resulting statistics, making a probability statement about the observations in the study.
6 Samples can be selected to reduce heterogeneity.[13]

4.4.4 What is a sampling technique?

This refers to the process of selecting subjects into the study to constitute study population. This procedure includes probability sampling, which ensures that a sample will lead to a reliable and valid inference, and nonprobability sampling (unknown probability of selection), which is deprived of the randomness needed to estimate sampling errors.

4.4.5 What are the types of probability sampling?

Probability sampling types include simple random sampling, in which every subject has an equal probability of being selected for the study; systematic sampling, in which every kth item is selected, where k is determined by the number of items in the sampling frame divided by the desired sample size; stratified sampling, in which the population is first divided into relevant strata or subgroups, and a random sample is then selected from each stratum or subgroup; and cluster sampling, in which the population is divided into clusters and a subset of the clusters is randomly selected.[14] *Sampling unit or element* refers to the subject under observation on which information is collected (e.g., women aged fifty-five or older undergoing mammography).

4.4.6 What is sampling fraction, frame, and scheme?

The *sampling fraction* refers to the ratio between sample size and population size (e.g., 100 out of 1000 or 10%). The *sampling frame* is the list of all sampling units from which a sample is drawn (e.g., list of women aged 55 or older undergoing mammography). The *sampling scheme* is the method of selecting sampling units from the sampling frame (e.g., random selection, convenience sample, etc.).

4.4.7 *How is sample or study size estimated?*

The sample or study size is always an estimation. The strategy used to estimate the sample size depends on the study design and the number of groups compared. Sample size is influenced by significance level, effect size, variability, and power. The following are the methods used to estimate sample size:

a Sample size estimation for descriptive survey—one proportion. This is the formula for one proportion:

$$n = z^2 \times (p \times q)/d^2$$

where n is the sample size, z is the alpha risk expressed in z score, p is the expected prevalence, $q = 1 - p$, and d is the desired/absolute precision.

b Sample size estimation—two proportions or groups. This is the formula for two proportions:

$$n = z_1 - \alpha/2[P_1(1 - P_1) + P_2(1 - P_2)]/d^2$$

where n is the sample size (each group), $z_1 - \alpha/2$ is the confidence interval, P_1 is the estimated proportion (larger), P_2 is the estimated proportion (smaller), and d is the desired precision.[15]

BOX 4.2 INFLUENCE ON CONFIDENCE INTERVAL (CI)

- The length of confidence interval is influenced by (a) sample size, (b) standard deviation (SD), and (c) type I error (α).
- Sample size—as sample size increases, the width of CI decreases (increased precision).
- Variability—as SD increases, the length of CI increases (decreased precision).
- Type I Error Tolerance—as the confidence desired increases, the length of the CI increases.

4.4.8 *What is statistical power?*

This is the probability that the test will reject a false null hypothesis. It refers to the probability that a study will not result in a type II error. The power computation depends on significance criterion (statistical stability) as well as the effect size or the size of the difference. The ability of a test to reject the null hypothesis when the alternative hypothesis is indeed true = $1 - \beta$.[16] Simply, the higher the power, the greater the chance of obtaining a statistically significant result when the null hypothesis is false (Table 4.1).

Table 4.1 Hypothesis testing and relationship between type I and type II errors

		Null hypothesis	
		False	True
Test results	Significant	Power	Type I error
	Nonsignificant	Type II error	

4.5 Research questions, hypothesis testing, and statistical inference

In Section I of this book, we explained research questions and hypotheses. However, to understand statistical inference, it is essential to repeat these concepts. Reading and interpreting scientific research requires understanding how research questions are formulated, how hypotheses are asserted, and how specific test statistics are selected to test the hypotheses.

Scientific finding, which commences with hypothesis testing and asserting an association, involves measurement of the magnitude of the outcome effect of interest by comparing outcome between groups with different exposure experience, or comparing pre- and posttreatment measures within subjects, as in repeated-measures design; measurement of variation among the observations of interest within exposure groups; measurement of the ratio of outcome effect to variation (e.g., confounding); elimination of alternative explanations (e.g., confounding, bias, random error or chance); and ascertainment of association.[17]

4.5.1 What is the research question?

Research question refers to a statement that identifies the phenomenon to be investigated (e.g., “Does coffee drinking result in pancreatic neoplasm?”). Research questions could involve one group of subjects who are measured on one or two occasions (e.g., mean milk consumption and bone density in women 45 years and older). Other examples of appropriate research questions are as follows:

1 Is the mean milk consumption of women 45 years and older different in our sample compared with the National Study on Nutrition sample? In other words, How confident are we that the observed mean milk consumption in our sample is X ounces per day?
2 Is the mean bone density (X) in the National Study on Nutrition of women 45 years and older significantly different from our sample?

4.5.2 What is the hypothesis?

The hypothesis tests or estimates the mean value of a numerical value (e.g., milk consumption, bone density). This hypothesis testing involves the examination of the mean in one group when the observations are normally distributed (e.g., bone density, milk consumption).

4.5.3 Which test is appropriate?

Earlier in this chapter, we used binomial regression as a statistical method to test hypotheses in a retrospective cohort study when proportion was involved. Here, we wish to examine hypothesis testing when the variable is continuous, such as bone density in a single or more than one group sample, implying single sample statistical inference. The appropriate test statistic in this context is the t test. The t distribution is appropriate in performing the test statistic and obtaining the confidence limits.[18] Simply stated, the single- or one-sample t test compares the mean of a single sample to a known population mean.[19] The purpose of this test (t) or Student's t test is to answer research questions about means. The formula for the t test is (statistic − hypothesized value)/estimated standard error of the statistic.[20] Mathematically, it appears as follows:

$$t = (X - \mu)/(\text{SD} / \sqrt{n}) = (X - \mu)/\text{SE}$$

where X is the observed or sample mean, μ is the hypothesized mean value of the population (true mean in the population), and SE is the standard error of the mean (X). Simply, mean (x) − constant (μ)/SD(x), where SD(x) is the sum $\{(x_i - \text{Mean}(x)\}^2/(n - 1)$.[21]

To find out whether the observed mean is "real" (i.e., the observed mean is different from the mean of the National Study of Nutrition [NSN], termed the *norm* or *population mean*) and not just a random occurrence, the following factors need to be considered: (1) the difference between the observed mean and the norm (NSN) or population mean, implying much larger or smaller—magnitude of the mean difference → greater difference; (2) the amount of variability among subjects, implying less variation—smaller standard deviation in the sample (i.e., homogeneous sample and relatively precise method of measurement); and (3) the number of subjects in the study, implying a larger rather than smaller sample.

Vignette 4.1: Consider a study conducted to compare the mean vitamin C intake among eighth-grade schoolchildren at New School, Texas, with the population mean (Texas Study of Nutrition, or TSN). If the investigator found a greater standard deviation (SD), what is the probable explanation?

Solution: If the SD is greater in the sample studied (eighth-grade children at New School), it is likely that (1) vitamin C intake varies widely from one child to another or (2) a biased or crude measurement device is used to ascertain the vitamin C intake (improper, imprecise, or crude measure).

Assumptions: The following assumptions are necessary before the use of the *t* test: (a) normal distribution; (b) if normality is not assumed, observations should be more than 30 subjects; thus, observation becomes normally distributed above this number regardless of the distribution of original observations (central limit theorem); and (c) even with violation of normal distribution, a *t* test could still be performed since it is robust for nonnormal data, implying the drawing of a proper conclusion even when the assumptions are not met, including normality.

Interpretation: The null hypothesis assumes the equality of means; a significant result at significant level (<0.05) is indicative of the significant difference between the sample mean (X) and the population mean (μ). A nonsignificant mean difference implies that the difference may be due to random error or chance, given the significance level ($p > 0.05$); it does not mean that the two means are equal.[22] Simply, it is not possible to be confident about accepting the observed difference because this might be due to random occurrence.

4.5.4 *What are the types of* t *test?*

There are several types of test, and these tests are used depending on the number of groups compared and whether or not one is examining a single subject with repeated measures as in pre- and posttreatment mean blood pressure for a single treatment group. The following are examples of *t* test:

a *One-sample t test*, which compares the sample mean to the population mean.

b *An independent samples t test*, which compares the means of two samples. The following assumptions apply to independent or two-sample *t* tests: (1) two groups being compared should be independent of each other, (2) the scores should be normally distributed, (3) dependency must be measured on an interval or ratio scale, and (4) the independent sample should have only two discrete levels.

c *A paired samples t test, also called a dependent t test or t test for correlated data,* compares the means of two scores from related samples. The assumptions of this test are (1) both variables (pre- and posttest) are at interval or ratio scales; (2) both are normally distributed; (3) both are measured with the same scale; and (4) if different scales are involved, the scores should be converted to *z* scores before *t*-test analysis.

The difference between *t* and *z* is very small when $n > 30$ subjects. Clearly, as sample size increases, degree of freedom (df) increases, and the *t* distribution becomes almost the same as *z* (Table 4.2). With $n > 30$, either of the two distributions can be used in hypothesis testing.

Table 4.2 Comparison between standard normal distribution (Z score) and *t* distribution

Test	*Description*
z score	Symmetric with mean of 0 and SE = 1.0 Narrower and lower in tails compared to *t* distribution. Why? Smaller SE.
t distribution	Symmetric with mean of 0 and SE > 1.0 Degree of freedom (df) is $n - 1$. Wider and higher in tails compared to *z*. Why? Larger SD.

4.5.5 Other test statistics

The nonparametric analog to the above tests used to examine the mean differences include (a) the Wilcoxon signed-rank test for paired *t* test and (b) the Wilcoxon rank-sum test for independent sample *t* tests. These nonparametric tests examine the median difference in ranked or distribution-free data.

Because using a *t* test involves a normal distribution and equal variance, a nonparametric alternative test statistic for evaluating mean differences when these assumptions are not met is the Wilcoxon test (Mann–Whitney test), which is adequate for paired design as well as an independent sample *t* test.

4.5.6 Hypothesis testing about the proportion is performed using the z distribution

This process involves a research question. For example, is there a significant difference in the observed proportion (0.20) of children with moderate to high physical activity in a sample, compared with the population proportion of 0.40? Comparing two independent proportions involves the use of a *z* test, while comparing frequencies of proportion in two groups can be achieved with the chi-square test of independence. Like the *t* test, it is *z* approximation (approximate test). It is based on a null hypothesis of no difference/relationship/association or dependency.

4.5.7 Nonparametric procedure

The nonparametric procedures are used when the distribution-free assumption is applied to the data and research questions fit such a procedure.

4.5.8 What are possible research questions?

The examples of research questions that justify the use of a nonparametric test are as follows: (1) Is there a difference in the proportion of older men treated for prostate problems who received hormonal therapy relative to those who did not receive hormonal therapy? (2) Is there an association or relationship between autoimmune disorder and race in women?

4.5.9 What are the hypotheses?

The hypothesis in this context tests the equality of these two proportions. The null hypothesis for dependency is that there are no racial differences among women with autoimmune disorders or, simply, women with autoimmune disorders do not differ by race. This hypothesis could be tested using chi-square. Mathematically, it appears as follows:

$$\chi^2 = (0 - E)^2 / E$$

where O is the observed frequency, E is the expected frequency → $\chi^2_{(df)} = \Sigma$ (observed frequency − expected frequency)/expected frequency.[23] If no relationship exists, the observed frequencies will be very close to the expected frequency, thus rendering the chi-square value small. If more than 20% of the expected, not the observed, frequency is <5 → Fisher's exact test, [24] and if the expected cell count is <2.0, Fisher's exact should be used, since the smaller the denominator, the higher the likelihood of a higher chi-square value, resulting in a lower significance level. *Chi-square assumption*: Statisticians vary with respect to the chi-square assumptions. However, these assumptions have commonly been used: (1) The expected frequency for each category should not be less than 2. (2) No more than 20% of the categories should have expected frequencies of <5. *Test statistic*: chi-square test of independence. *Interpretation*: A significant chi-square test implies that two variables are not independent, meaning that there is an association between the two variables, whereas a nonsignificant result indicates that the variables do not differ significantly.[25]

Vignette 4.2: Consider a study conducted to assess the relationship between sex and cardiomyopathies among US residents. If the investigators found that cardiomyopathies were 68% among men and 40% in women, and the significance level was <0.05, with a $\chi^2 = 27.32$, and df = 1, would you consider this finding to indicate that men are significantly more likely to have cardiomyopathies relative to women?

Solution: With the chi-square value (27.32), which is large, given 1 degree of freedom (3.84 critical value), and the p value, <0.05, there is a significant association between sex and cardiomyopathies, leading to the rejection of the null hypothesis of independence or no association. Therefore, the conclusion drawn is accurate: men are more likely to have cardiomyopathies compared with women, based on the proportion in the result of the investigation.

4.5.10 *What is analysis of variance?*

Whereas the t test compares means in two groups, the analysis of variance (ANOVA) is used to compare means in two or more groups. ANOVA is also termed *univariate* or *one-way ANOVA*. *Assumptions*: (1) group independence; (2) one independent variable (if more than one independent variable → factorial ANOVA [two-way ANOVA]); (3) dependent variable is at interval or ratio levels and is *normally distributed* → *parametric procedure*; (4) equality of variance is the same in each group (homogeneity of variance); and (5) observations are obtained from a random sample.[26] The test statistic for ANOVA (F test) is not influenced by moderate departure from the assumption of normality, especially with a large number of observations—*robust*.

4.5.11 *What is the nonparametric alternative?*

In skewed observations, Kruskal–Wallis test (nonparametric procedure) is an alternative to ANOVA. Similarly, as discussed above, serious violation of independent t-test assumptions requires the use of the Wilcoxon rank-sum test (nonparametric procedure). When the one-way ANOVA for repeated measures is not feasible because of an assumptions violation, the Friedman test, which is a nonparametric procedure,[27] is recommended.

4.5.12 *What is the hypothesis testing in one-way between-subject ANOVA?*

The null hypothesis is that the two variances are equal (i.e., the variation among means is not much greater than the variation among individual observations within any given group).[28] *Interpretation*: The F value, degrees of freedom, and the significance level are necessary for the conclusion to be drawn on the significant mean differences between the groups.[29]

4.5.13 *What is the test statistic and assumptions for one-way between-subjects ANOVA?*

The F test for two variances is the test statistic for ANOVA. This is the ratio of the variance among means to the variance among subjects within each group.[30] The F ratio under certain conditions corresponds to F distribution. This reflects the between-group variability, implying both sampling error and the effect of the independent variable. However, the within-group variability merely reflects the sampling error. The ratio of the two sources of variability in ANOVA, which is the variance ratio, can be computed by between-group variability/within-group variability = sampling error + effect of the independent variable/sampling error. The F test for one-way ANOVA is appropriate when (a) the dependent variable is quantitative and measured on an interval/ratio scale, (b) samples are independent and randomly selected, (c) data are normally distributed, and (d) there is homogeneous variance. The assumptions b to c are met if the sampling distribution of the *F* ratio is distributed in accordance with the relevant *F* distribution.

4.5.14 *What is ANCOVA?*

Comparison of means in three or more groups with a covariate that is confounding involves the use of covariates (ANCOVA). ANCOVA serves as a method of controlling for confounding.[3]

4.5.15 *What are the analysis techniques used in the analysis of clinical research data?*

Various test statistics are available for analyzing the relationship between two or more variables. The selection of a test or statistic (e.g., *t* test [testing for statistical significance]) depends on (1) the scale of the measurement of the dependent and independent variables, parametric (continuous scale data), or nonparametric (nominal/discrete scale data) distribution; (2) the type of design (before and after comparison); and (3) the sampling procedure (random sampling), among other factors.[32] The following are selective examples of statistical techniques:

a *Bivariable* or *univariable* analysis refers to the analysis of the relationship between *one* independent (X) and *one* dependent variable (Y). For example, if an investigator decides to examine the relationship between height and weight of 100 high school children, she or he may wish to determine if weight (Y) depends on height (X).[33]

b *Multivariable analysis* refers to the analysis between a single dependent variable and more than one independent variable (e.g., a study to determine the impact of race and gender in the development of colorectal cancer). The independent variables are age (X_1) and race (X_2), while the dependent variable is colorectal cancer (Y).

c *Multivariate analysis* is the technique that involves more than one dependent and more than a single independent variable. This term is *not* interchangeable with multivariable analysis, and it is often used incorrectly.

d *Correlation analysis* is used to measure the change in two variables. However, unlike linear regression, which is discussed below, neither of the variables are considered dependent variables. This technique allows for the determination of the strength of the relationship between the two variables and does not assume causality or the prediction of the response variable by the independent variable (Table 4.3). For example, investigators examined the correlation between pedobarographic and radiographic measures of surgically treated clubfoot and obtained the correlation coefficient that allowed them to conclude that there was a moderate direct correlation between heel rise and some radiographic measure of clubfoot.

Table 4.3 Analysis of research questions about relationships among variables: correlation

Statistical method	*Variable*	*Assumption*	*Statistic*
Correlation: Pearson	Dependent (outcome, response) and independent (predictors, explanatory) must be measured in continuous scale	1 Random sample 2 Bivariate normal distribution	Pearson product moment correlation coefficient (*r*)
Correlation: Spearman's rho/ Kendall's tau	1 Numerical variables that are not normally distributed 2 Ordinal variables	1 Rank order data 2 Ordinal data, or interval or ratio 3 Nonparametric data	Spearman's rho or rank correlation (*r*)

Note: Bivariate implies normal distribution for the two variables (*X* and *Y*) in the correlation coefficient.

In this analysis, the intent of the researcher was not to establish a causal association but to determine the strength of the relationship. The results were present as Pearson correlation and Spearman rank correlation coefficients. The Pearson product moment correlation coefficient is used to assess the strength of the relationship between two variables when these variables are normally distributed. If either of the two variables is not normally distributed, Pearson correlation is considered inappropriate.[34]

4.5.16 *What is a nonparametric alternative to Pearson correlation?*

If either of the variables is distribution-free, then the alternate approaches are (1) both variables should be transformed to achieve near-normal distribution and (2) the Spearman rank correlation coefficient, which is a nonparametric test, should be used if any of the variables is not normally distributed, meaning when the p value is <0.05. Please note that the null hypothesis for the test of normality is that the data are normal. Thus, when $p < 0.05$, we reject the null hypothesis and tend to the alternative hypothesis that the data are not normally distributed.

4.5.17 *How is the result of correlation analysis interpreted?*

The measure of effect or relationship in correlation analysis is correlation coefficient (r). What is the *interpretation of r?* (1) Correlation coefficient is between -1.0 and $+1.0$, with r close to 0.0 considered to be a weak relationship; (2) 1.0 or -1.0 = perfect relationship; (3) >0.7 = strong correlation; (4) 0.4 to 0.7 =

moderate correlation; (5) <0.4 = weak correlation.[35] A significant correlation at the 0.05 significance level implies that the observed r is different from zero.

4.5.18 What is linear regression analysis?

Linear regression, also called *least squares regression*, refers to a regression method that is based on the least squares method. This is an analytic technique used to predict the value of one characteristic or variable (Y) from knowledge of the other (X). The regression equation is given as follows:

$$\hat{Y} = \beta_0 + \beta_1 \boldsymbol{X} + \varepsilon$$

It is called *linear* because this method, unlike correlation, measures only a straight line or linear relationship between two variables (simple linear regression). The least squares method minimizes the differences between the actual value of Y and the predicted value of Y, $\{\Sigma(Y - \hat{Y})^2\}$, which is measured by the error term ε $(Y - \hat{Y})$ in the regression equation above.[36] In *simple linear regression*, only a single independent or explanatory variable (X) is used to predict the outcome (Y).

4.5.19 What is multiple or multivariable linear regression?

Multiple or multivariable linear regression refers to a regression technique that, like the simple linear regression, is based on the least squares method, where more than one independent variable is included in the prediction equation. Mathematically, it appears as follows:

$$\hat{Y} = \beta_0 + \beta_1 X_1 + \beta_2 X_2 \ldots \beta_i X_i$$

with β_0 and β_1 … β_i as the regression parameters.

4.5.20 How are the results of linear regressions interpreted?

The *simple linear regression* equation is given by $\hat{Y} = \beta_0 + \beta_1 X + \varepsilon$, where β_1 is the slope or the regression coefficient, β_0 is the intercept of the regression line (β_1 and β_0 are the parameters), and ε is the error term, which is the distance the actual value of Y departs from the regression line. The *R square (R^2)* in the linear regression model output is the coefficient of determination that measures the proportion of the variance of the dependent variable (Y) that can be explained by the variation in the independent variable (X). *The standard error of estimate* (model output) measures the dispersion for the prediction equation. *Test statistics*: (1) ANOVA in the model uses F statistic to determine the statistical significance of the regression equation, and (2) the t statistic tests whether or not the regression coefficient is statistically significant (Table 4.4).[37]

Table 4.4 Analysis of research questions about relationships among variables: linear regression

Statistical method	*Variable*	*Assumption*	*Statistic*
Simple linear regression (SLR)	1 Response is measured in continuous scale 2 Independent may be in continuous or binary scale	1 Both variables are interval or ratio scaled 2 Dependent (*Y*) must be normally distributed along the predicted line (homogeneity) 3 Relationship is linear	Regression statistic: (1) *t* statistic (2) *F* statistic
Multiple linear regression (MLR)	Same as SLR; more than single independent variables	Same as SLR; variables are also related to each other linearly	Same as SLR

Note: Perform the statistical test to determine the likelihood of any observed relationship between *X* and *Y* variables.

4.5.21 *What are other types of regressions?*

Examples of regressions include (a) *polynomial regression*, which refers to multiple or multivariable regression, in which each term in the equation is a power of *X*;[38] (b) *discriminant analysis*, which predicts group membership with only two groups and uses continuous independent variables only; (c) *log-linear analysis*, which focuses on the analysis of the conditional relationship of two or more categorical values (unlike logistic regression, the dependent variable is categorical and the link function is the log [log of the dependent variable], not logit, and the predictions are estimates of the cell counts in a contingency table, not the logit of the dependent variable, *y*);[39] and (d) *logistic regression (LR)*.

4.5.22 *What is logistic regression?*

Logistic regression is a form of regression analysis (logit transformation) in which the outcome is binary and the independent variables could be measured in mixed scales (categorical, binary, mixed continuous, and categorical).[40] Logit transformation (logit p) for the binary outcome or dependent variable is denoted by $\ln[p/(1-p)]$, where the logit transformation takes any value from minus infinity to plus infinity.[41] This method calculates the probability of success over the probability of failure, thus presenting the odds ratio as the final result (e.g., logistic regression [LR] is used in determining the probability of developing prostate cancer, given exposure to organophosphates [pesticides] after adjusting for other known and postulated risk factors). It is classified under the generalized linear model (GLM). Further, the dependent variable can have more than two levels (e.g., multinomial and polytomous logistic regression). Like SLR or MLR, logistic regression is a predictive model and is used to predict the outcome or dependent variable on the basis of continuous and/or binary/categorical independent or predictor/explanatory variables, as well as to determine the percent variance of the dependent variable that is explained by the independents, rank the relative importance of independents, assess the interaction effects, and control for confounding in the multivariable LR. This method uses maximum likelihood estimation after transforming the dependent variable into a logit, implying obtaining the natural log of the odds of the outcome or dependent variable occurring or not occurring—that is, the probability of the outcome occurring. The goal of this method is to correctly predict the outcome of the individual cases using the most parsimonious model. Unlike the SLR, the relationship between the predictor and the response variables is not a linear function but a logit transformation of the outcome variable. The changes in the log odds of the outcome are estimated and not the changes in the dependent or outcome variable itself. Mathematically, it appears as follows:

$$\theta = e(\alpha + \beta_1 X_1 + \beta_2 X_2 \ldots \beta_i X_i) / 1 + e(\alpha + \beta_1 X_1 + \beta_2 X_2 \ldots \beta_i X_i)$$

where α is the constant of the equation and β is the coefficient of the predictor or independent variables in the equation.[42] Given the probability of success (p) of a binary outcome variable (y), the logistic regression model is Logit(p) = $\ln(p/1 - p)$ = alpha + beta$_1$ X_1 + beta$_2 X_2$ ...beta$_k X_k$. Likewise, solving for $\boldsymbol{p} = \boldsymbol{e}(\alpha + \beta_1 \boldsymbol{X}_1 + \beta_2 \boldsymbol{X}_2 \ldots \beta_k \boldsymbol{X}_k) / 1 + \boldsymbol{e}(\alpha + \beta_1 \boldsymbol{X}_1 + \beta_2 \boldsymbol{X}_2 \ldots \beta_k \boldsymbol{X}_k)$.[43] The occurrence of outcome in this equation is an exponential function of the independent variables: $Px = 1/\{1 + \exp[-(b_0 + b_1x_1 + b_2x_2 + b_3x_3 + b_4x_4 \ldots b_ix_i)]\}$, where b_0 is the intercept (constant), b_1, b_2, b_3, b_4 ... b_i are the regression coefficient, while exp represents the base of the natural logarithm (2.718).[44] Mathematically, the odds ratio in LR can be computed from the coefficient of regression:

$$\beta \rightarrow \text{OR} = e^{\beta}$$

where exp = 2.718. The Wald statistic tests the statistical significance of the individual independent variable [each coefficient (β)]. The Wald test is a squared z test with chi-square distribution: $z = \beta/\text{SE}$ [coefficient (β)/standard error (SE)]. This is the squared ratio of the unstandardized logit coefficient to its standard error.

4.5.23 What is the interpretation of the Wald test in logistic regression?

Some statisticians have suggested that large logit increases standard errors, lowering the Wald statistic, thus leading to a type II error implying a false negative, assuming that the effect is not significant, which indeed it is (rejecting the alternate hypothesis of difference).

4.5.24 What is model and model testing?

Model testing (appropriateness of the model): Goodness of fit (Hosmer–Lemeshow), which is a chi-square statistic with a desirable outcome of nonsignificance, indicates that the model prediction does not significantly differ from the observed.[45] *Model testing (backward stepwise elimination)*: Likelihood-ratio test (LRT) uses the ratio of the maximized value of the likelihood function of the full model (L_1) over the maximized value of the likelihood function for the simpler model, such as the model without predictors and or interaction (L_0). Mathematically, $\text{LRT} = -2\log(L_0/L_1) = -2\{\log(L_0) - \log(L_1)\} = -2(L_0 - L_1)$.[46] The reduced model could be a baseline model or initial model with constant only; thus, it is termed a null model. The full model then becomes the model with the predictors. A likelihood ratio test can then test the difference between the initial or null model, model with constant only, and the model with the coefficients from the predictors. The model is significant at $p < 0.05$, indicating that the fitted model is significantly different from the null model or model chi-square test, as it is termed. This model does not ensure that every independent variable in the model is significant. The "Best model"—the final model—implies that adding another variable would not improve the model significantly (e.g., model with and without interaction).

4.5.25 Interpretation of logistic regression result ($OR = e^{\beta}$)

The odds in favor of success for a subject (A) (exposure = 1) are given by $\text{OR}_A = P_A/(1 - P_A)$, and the odds in favor of success for a subject (B) (exposure = 0) is given by $\text{OR}_B = P_B/(1 - P_B)$. The odds ratio is then $(\text{OR}) = \text{OR}_A/\text{OR}_B$. The odds ratio relates a disease or outcome to the *i*th exposure for two hypothetical subjects A and B, where A is exposed and B is not. In the multivariable regression, this odds ratio relates disease to the *i*th exposure variable, controlling for the levels of all other exposure variables in the regression equation (Table 4.5).

4.5.26 Other types of GLMs (counts data)

Included in GLM are (a) Poisson regression, (b) negative binomial regression, and (c) zero-inflated regression. These methods are appropriate for the analysis of count data that are (1) highly nonnormally distributed and (2) not well estimated by ordinary least squares (OLS) regression (Table 4.6).

Table 4.5 Analysis of research questions about relationships among variables: logistic regression

Statistical method[a]	*Variable*	*Assumption*	*Statistic*
Logistic regression: unconditional (ULR)	*Outcome* is binary *Independent* variables are categorical and continuous (mixed)	Does not assume linear relationship Outcome need not be normally distributed Outcome need not be homoscedastic for level of predictors No normally distributed error term	Wald statistic (β) Hosmer–Lemeshow (χ^2) (goodness of fit) Likelihood ratio test (overall model)
Logistic regression: conditional	Same as ULR; matched pairs (1 − 1 or 1 − K)[a]	Same as ULR	Same as ULR

[a] Matching tends to increase the degrees of freedom relative to the cases. A better approach to the analysis is conditional logistic regression, which maximizes the likelihood estimate in logistic regression.

Table 4.6 Statistical methods involving counts data

Statistical method	*Description and applications*
Poisson regression	To model the number of occurrences of an event of interest or the rate of occurrence of an event of interest, as a function of some independent variables. Efficient when the dependent variable is a count variable—with same length of observation time (e.g., number of days absent from work). Incidence rate ratio is the point estimate.
Negative binomial regression	Used to estimate count models when the Poisson model is inappropriate because of overdispersion (which is most of the time). In Poisson distribution, the mean and variance are equal; thus, when the variance is greater than the mean, the distribution is said to display overdispersion; if lower than the mean, it is underdispersion. When there is overdispersion, the Poisson estimates are inefficient with standard errors biased downward, yielding spuriously large z values. Efficient for dispersed count data, as an extension of generalized Poisson regression.
Zero-inflated Poisson (ZIP) regression model	Extension of generalized Poisson regression with count data having extra zeros. ZIP is useful to analyze such data. Efficient where overdispersion is assumed to be caused by an excessive number of zeros.

4.6 Summary

Conducting clinical research involves conceptualization, design, and statistical inference. Practically, a clinical research is conducted to improve care and provide guidelines for the screening, diagnosis, and treatment of future patients. Therefore, the inference drawn from such studies must be supported by biologic, clinical, and statistical evidence in terms of reliability and validity.

Previous chapters presented research conceptualization and design. This chapter introduces the statistical inference component of research conduct, with statistical consideration in research as its main focus. Statistical consideration in clinical research revolves around sample and the generalization of findings from the sample to the population of interest, termed targeted population. The method used in obtaining the sample is significant to this process of generalizability and requires a probability sample or representative sample, also termed a *random sample*. When the sample is random, we ensure that the variable from such a sample is representative of the population of interest and hence the possibility of applying inferential statistics or probability value in interpreting the statistical significance of the findings. However, it is not uncommon in clinical research and in epidemiologic studies to use nonrandom samples and still apply statistical significance in the interpretation of the results, which is meaningless and valueless to the statistical notion of p value or inference from the sample.

The statistical inference notion of research conduct involves hypothesis testing. Statistical inference involves the generalization of the findings beyond the sample. Hypothesis testing is dependent on the nature of the design and the scales of measurement of the main or independent and response variables. This selection (appropriate test statistic) is important in the understanding of the results and the interpretation of the data. These test statistics include (a) single-sample t test, (b) z test, (c) independent sample t test, (d) paired t test, (e) binomial regression, (f) logistic regression, (g) linear regression, (h) Poisson regression, (i) ANOVA, (j) correlation analysis, and (k) analysis of covariance (ANCOVA).

Essential to clinical research is the use of t test and ANOVA (which are so commonly applied because of the continuous scale encountered in the measurement of most laboratories) and radiographic and clinical variables. The t test and ANOVA assume normality as well as equality of variance, random sample, and independent sample except paired t test, single-sample t test, and repeated-measure ANOVA (there is no between-subject variability). In clinical, epidemiologic, or public health research, the application of logistic regression is very common and is due to the nature of public health data—presence or absence of outcome/disease. The selection of this statistical technique involves the dependent variable that is measured on a binary scale, while the independent variable can be measured on binary, discrete, continuous, or categorical scales. This technique belongs to a GLM group and is distribution-free (Figure 4.2).

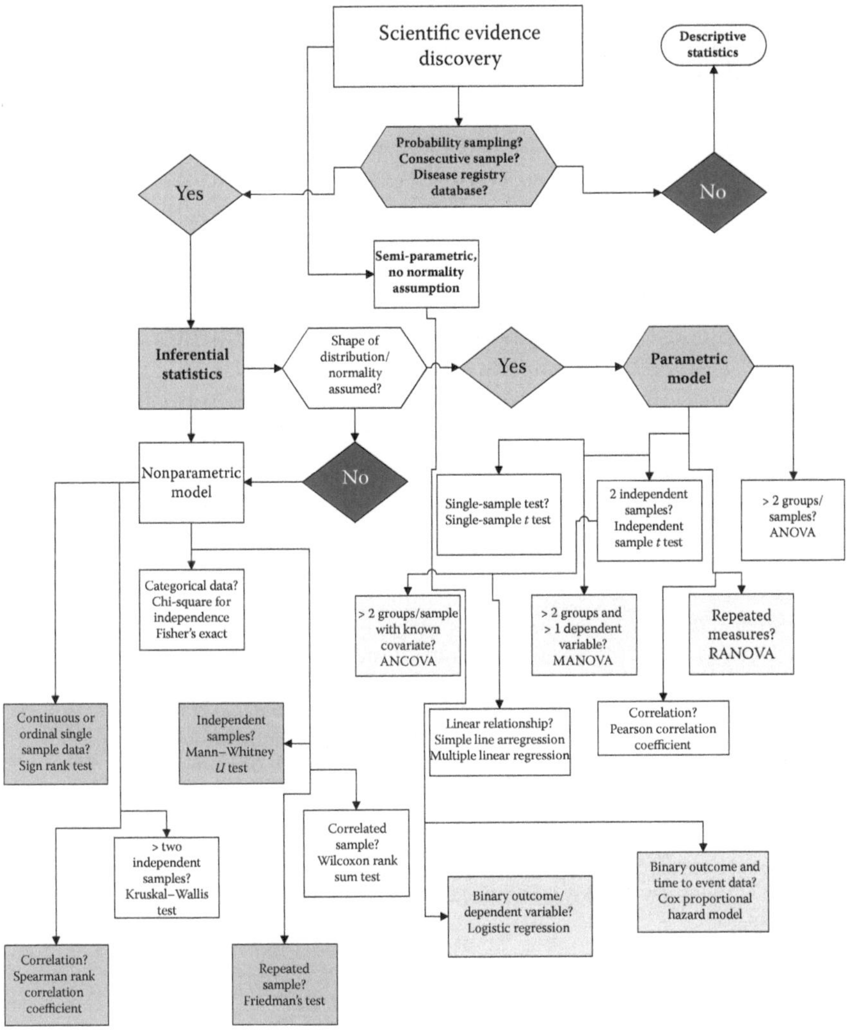

Figure 4.2 Selection of test statistic.

Questions for discussion

1 Suppose you are a principal investigator in a study intended to assess the relationship between radiographic and pedobarographic measure of surgically treated clubfoot. (a) How would you state the hypothesis? (b) What is the statistical technique to be used in testing the hypothesis? (c) What is the measure of the parameter? (d) What is the interpretation of the statistically significant finding? (e) If the correlation coefficient is 0.5, and the *p* value is 0.67, what can be concluded from the data on the

relationship between right heel impulse and right lateral calcaneal pitch angle? (f) If one of the variables is not normally distributed, what alternative test would you use to present your data?

2 Briefly discuss the difference between simple linear regression and correlation coefficient. (a) What is the interpretation of statistically significant finding in (i) simple linear regression and (ii) the Spearman rank correlation coefficient? (b) When is multiple linear regression a preferred statistical method?

3 Generate data on 100 patients with sepsis. The variables to be considered should include race, temperature, type of infection, sepsis, sex, age, length of hospitalization and comorbidity. Using this hypothetical data set, construct a box plot of temperature by sepsis. Chi-square is a standard distribution, with positive values where low values are consistent with null hypothesis while high values produce evidence to reject or disprove the null hypothesis. Thus, when χ^2_n is large, the null is rejected. Using these hypothetical data, examine the association between race and sepsis.

References

1. S. Stigler, *The History of Statistics* (Cambridge, MA: Belknap Press, 1986).
2. B. Dawson-Saunders and R. G. Trap, *Basic and Clinical Biostatistics*, 2nd ed. (Norwalk, CT: Appleton & Lange, 1994).
3. B. Dawson-Saunders and R. G. Trap, *Basic and Clinical Biostatistics*, 2nd ed. (Norwalk, CT: Appleton & Lange, 1994); W. D. Dupont, *Statistical Modeling for Biomedical Researchers* (Cambridge, UK: Cambridge University Press, 2003).
4. W. D. Dupont, *Statistical Modeling for Biomedical Researchers* (Cambridge, UK: Cambridge University Press, 2003).
5. B. C. Cronk, *How to Use SPSS: A Step-by-Step Guide to Analysis and Interpretation*, 3rd ed. (Glendale, CA: Pyrczak Publishing, 2004).
6. T. D. V. Swinscow and M. J. Campbell, *Statistics at Square One*, 10th ed. (Spain: BMJ Books, 2002).
7. B. Dawson-Saunders and R. G. Trap, *Basic and Clinical Biostatistics*, 2nd ed. (Norwalk, CT: Appleton & Lange, 1994); T. D. V. Swinscow and M. J. Campbell, *Statistics at Square One*, 10th ed. (Spain: BMJ Books, 2002); D. A. Freedman et al., *Statistics*, 4th ed. (New York: Norton, 2007); S. Greenland, Power, sample size, and smallest detectable effect determination for multivariate studies, *Stat Med* 4 (1985):117–127; J. M. Hoening et al., The abuse of power: The pervasive fallacy of power calculations for data analysis, *Am Stat* 55 (2001):19–24; D. Moher et al., Statistical power, sample size, and their reporting in randomized controlled trials, *JAMA* 272 (1994):122–124.
8. B. Dawson-Saunders and R. G. Trap, *Basic and Clinical Biostatistics*, 2nd ed. (Norwalk, CT: Appleton & Lange, 1994); T. D. V. Swinscow and M. J. Campbell, *Statistics at Square One*, 10th ed. (Spain: BMJ Books, 2002).
9. B. Dawson-Saunders and R. G. Trap, *Basic and Clinical Biostatistics*, 2nd ed. (Norwalk, CT: Appleton & Lange, 1994); T. D. V. Swinscow and M. J. Campbell, *Statistics at Square One*, 10th ed. (Spain: BMJ Books, 2002); D. L. Katz, *Clinical Epidemiology & Evidence-Based Medicine: Fundamental Principles of Clinical Reasoning & Research.* (Thousand Oaks, CA: Sage, 2001); D. G. Altman, *Practical Statistics for Medical Research* (London: Chapman & Hall, 1991); P. Armitage

and G. Berry, *Statistical Methods in Medical Research*, 3rd ed. (Oxford, UK: Blackwell Scientific Publishing, 1994); B. Rosner, *Fundamentals of Biostatistics*, 5th ed. (Duxbury Press, CA: 2000); J. A. Freiman et al., The importance of beta, the type II error and sample size in the design and interpretation of the randomized clinical trial, *N Engl J Med* 299 (1978):690–694; J. F. Jekel, L. Katz, and J. G. Elmore, *Epidemiology, Biostatistics, and Preventive Medicine* (Philadelphia: Saunders, 2001).

10. B. Dawson-Saunders and R. G. Trap, *Basic and Clinical Biostatistics*, 2nd ed. (Norwalk, CT: Appleton & Lange, 1994); D. L. Katz, *Clinical Epidemiology & Evidence-Based Medicine: Fundamental Principles of Clinical Reasoning & Research* (Thousand Oaks, CA: Sage, 2001).
11. B. Dawson-Saunders and R. G. Trap, *Basic and Clinical Biostatistics*, 2nd ed. (Norwalk, CT: Appleton & Lange, 1994); T. D. V. Swinscow and M. J. Campbell, *Statistics at Square One*, 10th ed. (Spain: BMJ Books, 2002); D. L. Katz, *Clinical Epidemiology & Evidence-Based Medicine: Fundamental Principles of Clinical Reasoning & Research.* (Thousand Oaks, CA: Sage, 2001); D. G. Altman, *Practical Statistics for Medical Research* (London: Chapman & Hall, 1991); P. Armitage and G. Berry, *Statistical Methods in Medical Research*, 3rd ed. (Oxford, UK: Blackwell Scientific Publishing, 1994); B. Rosner, *Fundamentals of Biostatistics*, 5th ed. (Duxbury Press, CA: 2000); J. A. Freiman et al., The importance of beta, the type II error and sample size in the design and interpretation of the randomized clinical trial, *N Engl J Med* 299 (1978):690–694; J. F. Jekel, L. Katz, and J. G. Elmore, *Epidemiology, Biostatistics, and Preventive Medicine* (Philadelphia: Saunders, 2001).
12. T. D. V. Swinscow and M. J. Campbell, *Statistics at Square One*, 10th ed. (Spain: BMJ Books, 2002).
13. T. D. V. Swinscow and M. J. Campbell, *Statistics at Square One*, 10th ed. (Spain: BMJ Books, 2002).
14. P. Armitage and G. Berry, *Statistical Methods in Medical Research*, 3rd ed. (Oxford, UK: Blackwell Scientific Publishing, 1994); B. Rosner, *Fundamentals of Biostatistics*, 5th ed. (Duxbury Press, CA: 2000); J. F. Jekel, L. Katz, and J. G. Elmore, *Epidemiology, Biostatistics, and Preventive Medicine* (Philadelphia: Saunders, 2001).
15. B. Dawson-Saunders and R. G. Trap, *Basic and Clinical Biostatistics*, 2nd ed. (Norwalk, CT: Appleton & Lange, 1994); B. Rosner, *Fundamentals of Biostatistics*, 5th ed. (Duxbury Press, CA: 2000); J. A. Freiman et al., The importance of beta, the type II error and sample size in the design and interpretation of the randomized clinical trial, *N Engl J Med* 299 (1978):690–694; J. F. Jekel, L. Katz, and J. G. Elmore, *Epidemiology, Biostatistics, and Preventive Medicine* (Philadelphia: Saunders, 2001); H. A. Khan and C. T. Sempos, *Statistical Methods in Epidemiology* (New York: Oxford University Press, 1989).
16. J. A. Freiman et al., The importance of beta, the type II error and sample size in the design and interpretation of the randomized clinical trial, *N Engl J Med* 299 (1978):690–694; J. F. Jekel, L. Katz, and J. G. Elmore, *Epidemiology, Biostatistics, and Preventive Medicine* (Philadelphia: Saunders, 2001); H. A. Khan and C. T. Sempos, *Statistical Methods in Epidemiology* (New York: Oxford University Press, 1989).
17. B. Dawson-Saunders and R. G. Trap, *Basic and Clinical Biostatistics*, 2nd ed. (Norwalk, CT: Appleton & Lange, 1994); B. Rosner, *Fundamentals of Biostatistics*, 5th ed. (Duxbury Press, CA: 2000).
18. B. Dawson-Saunders and R. G. Trap, *Basic and Clinical Biostatistics*, 2nd ed. (Norwalk, CT: Appleton & Lange, 1994); B. Rosner, *Fundamentals of Biostatistics*, 5th ed. (Duxbury Press, CA: 2000).

19. B. Dawson-Saunders and R. G. Trap, *Basic and Clinical Biostatistics*, 2nd ed. (Norwalk, CT: Appleton & Lange, 1994); T. D. V. Swinscow and M. J. Campbell, *Statistics at Square One*, 10th ed. (Spain: BMJ Books, 2002); B. Rosner, *Fundamentals of Biostatistics*, 5th ed. (Duxbury Press, CA: 2000).
20. B. Dawson-Saunders and R. G. Trap, *Basic and Clinical Biostatistics*, 2nd ed. (Norwalk, CT: Appleton & Lange, 1994); B. Rosner, *Fundamentals of Biostatistics*, 5th ed. (Duxbury Press, CA: 2000); J. F. Jekel, L. Katz, and J. G. Elmore, *Epidemiology, Biostatistics, and Preventive Medicine* (Philadelphia: Saunders, 2001); H. A. Khan and C. T. Sempos, *Statistical Methods in Epidemiology* (New York: Oxford University Press, 1989).
21. B. Dawson-Saunders and R. G. Trap, *Basic and Clinical Biostatistics*, 2nd ed. (Norwalk, CT: Appleton & Lange, 1994); B. Rosner, *Fundamentals of Biostatistics*, 5th ed. (Duxbury Press, CA: 2000).
22. B. Dawson-Saunders and R. G. Trap, *Basic and Clinical Biostatistics*, 2nd ed. (Norwalk, CT: Appleton & Lange, 1994); B. Rosner, *Fundamentals of Biostatistics*, 5th ed. (Duxbury Press, CA: 2000); H. A. Khan and C. T. Sempos, *Statistical Methods in Epidemiology* (New York: Oxford University Press, 1989).
23. B. Dawson-Saunders and R. G. Trap, *Basic and Clinical Biostatistics*, 2nd ed. (Norwalk, CT: Appleton & Lange, 1994); T. D. V. Swinscow and M. J. Campbell, *Statistics at Square One*, 10th ed. (Spain: BMJ Books, 2002); B. Rosner, *Fundamentals of Biostatistics*, 5th ed. (Duxbury Press, CA: 2000).
24. B. Dawson-Saunders and R. G. Trap, *Basic and Clinical Biostatistics*, 2nd ed. (Norwalk, CT: Appleton & Lange, 1994); T. D. V. Swinscow and M. J. Campbell, *Statistics at Square One*, 10th ed. (Spain: BMJ Books, 2002).
25. B. Dawson-Saunders and R. G. Trap, *Basic and Clinical Biostatistics*, 2nd ed. (Norwalk, CT: Appleton & Lange, 1994); T. D. V. Swinscow and M. J. Campbell, *Statistics at Square One*, 10th ed. (Spain: BMJ Books, 2002); B. Rosner, *Fundamentals of Biostatistics*, 5th ed. (Duxbury Press, CA: 2000).
26. B. Rosner, *Fundamentals of Biostatistics*, 5th ed. (Duxbury Press, CA: 2000).
27. T. Colton, *Statistics in Medicine* (New York: Little, Brown and Company, 1974).
28. B. Dawson-Saunders and R. G. Trap, *Basic and Clinical Biostatistics*, 2nd ed. (Norwalk, CT: Appleton & Lange, 1994).
29. B. Dawson-Saunders and R. G. Trap, *Basic and Clinical Biostatistics*, 2nd ed. (Norwalk, CT: Appleton & Lange, 1994); B. Rosner, *Fundamentals of Biostatistics*, 5th ed. (Duxbury Press, CA: 2000).
30. B. Dawson-Saunders and R. G. Trap, *Basic and Clinical Biostatistics*, 2nd ed. (Norwalk, CT: Appleton & Lange, 1994); T. D. V. Swinscow and M. J. Campbell, *Statistics at Square One*, 10th ed. (Spain: BMJ Books, 2002); B. Rosner, *Fundamentals of Biostatistics*, 5th ed. (Duxbury Press, CA: 2000).
31. B. Dawson-Saunders and R. G. Trap, *Basic and Clinical Biostatistics*, 2nd ed. (Norwalk, CT: Appleton & Lange, 1994); T. D. V. Swinscow and M. J. Campbell, *Statistics at Square One*, 10th ed. (Spain: BMJ Books, 2002); B. Rosner, *Fundamentals of Biostatistics*, 5th ed. (Duxbury Press, CA: 2000).
32. B. C. Cronk, *How to Use SPSS: A Step-by-Step Guide to Analysis and Interpretation*, 3rd ed. (Glendale, CA: Pyrczak Publishing, 2004).
33. B. Rosner, *Fundamentals of Biostatistics*, 5th ed. (Duxbury Press, CA: 2000); T. Colton, *Statistics in Medicine* (New York: Little, Brown and Company, 1974).
34. B. C. Cronk, *How to Use SPSS: A Step-by-Step Guide to Analysis and Interpretation*, 3rd ed. (Glendale, CA: Pyrczak Publishing, 2004); T. Colton, *Statistics in Medicine* (New York: Little, Brown and Company, 1974).
35. J. L. Garb, *Understanding Medical Research: A Practitioner's Guide* (Boston: Little, Brown, and Company, 2000).

36. B. Dawson-Saunders and R. G. Trap, *Basic and Clinical Biostatistics*, 2nd ed. (Norwalk, CT: Appleton & Lange, 1994); L. S. Meyers, G. Gamst, and A. J. Guarino, *Applied Multivariate Research* (Thousand Oaks, CA: Sage Publications, 2006).
37. *STATA, Multivariate Statistics*, Release Version 10 (College Station, Texas: STATA Press, 2007).
38. *STATA, Multivariate Statistics*, Release Version 10 (College Station, Texas: STATA Press, 2007).
39. *STATA, Multivariate Statistics*, Release Version 10 (College Station, Texas: STATA Press, 2007); A. C. Rencher, *Methods of Multivariate Analysis*, 2nd ed. (New York: Wiley, 2002).
40. D. W. Hosmer and S. Lemeshow, *Applied Logistic Regression Analysis*, 2nd ed. (New York: Wiley, 1989).
41. B. Dawson-Saunders and R. G. Trap, *Basic and Clinical Biostatistics*, 2nd ed. (Norwalk, CT: Appleton & Lange, 1994).
42. A. C. Rencher, *Methods of Multivariate Analysis*, 2nd ed. (New York: Wiley, 2002).
43. A. C. Rencher, *Methods of Multivariate Analysis*, 2nd ed. (New York: Wiley, 2002); D. W. Hosmer and S. Lemeshow, *Applied Logistic Regression Analysis*, 2nd ed. (New York: Wiley, 1989); D. G. Kleinbaum and M. Klein, *Logistic Regression*, 2nd ed. (New York: Springer, 2002).
44. D. G. Kleinbaum and M. Klein, *Logistic Regression*, 2nd ed. (New York: Springer, 2002).
45. D. W. Hosmer and S. Lemeshow, *Applied Logistic Regression Analysis*, 2nd ed. (New York: Wiley, 1989); D. G. Kleinbaum and M. Klein, *Logistic Regression*, 2nd ed. (New York: Springer, 2002).
46. D. G. Kleinbaum and M. Klein, *Logistic Regression*, 2nd ed. (New York: Springer, 2002).

5 Study size and statistical power estimations

5.1 Introduction

Clinical or scientific knowledge in medicine and public health is largely based on evidence from samples rather than the entire population. And for statistical inference to be valid and reliable, the sample studies must be representative of the population with the outcome or issues of interest. Samples that are random and are large are more likely to be representative of the entire population, and the inferences from such samples are more likely to be reliable.

The statistical power of a study—or simply, the power—is the ability of the study to detect the minimum between the groups or measurement stages in a study (repeated measures or a paired measure) should such a difference really exist. It is designated by power $= 1 - \beta = P(\text{reject } H_0 | H_1 \text{ true})$. This is the probability of rejecting the null hypothesis if the alternative hypothesis is true. Simply, power reflects the sample size in that the more subjects studied, the higher the power of the test. Therefore, more subjects → higher power.

BOX 5.1 FACTORS ASSOCIATED WITH STUDY SIZE

- Significance level (α)
- Power ($1 - \beta$)
- Size of the difference in response (δ) to be detected

The power of the test will depend on the significance level (α), variance or standard deviation ($\boldsymbol{\sigma}$), effect size ($\boldsymbol{\delta}$), the selected or appropriate statistical test, and the sample size (n). The probability that a clinical trial will have a significant (positive) result—that is, it will have a *p value* of less than the specified significance level (usually 5%)—reflects the power of a study. This probability is computed under the assumption that the treatment difference or strength of association equals the minimum detectable difference. The minimum detectable difference is the smallest difference between the treatments or strength of association that one wishes to be able to detect.

In clinical trials, this is the smallest difference that one believes would be clinically important and biologically plausible. In a study of association, it is the smallest change in the dependent per unit change in the independent that is plausible.

Consider a hypothetical study to examine the difference in the mean hematocrit between two independent groups (those with and without the event of interest); as the variance changes with the fixed sample size ($2n = 32$) and as the significance level changes, the power changes. With $2n = 32$, two-sample test, 81% power, $\delta = 2$, $\sigma = 2$, $\alpha = 0.05$, two-sided test: Variance/Standard deviation: (a) σ: 2 → 1, power: 81% → 99.99%; (b) σ: 2 → 3, power: 81% → 47%, and significance level (α): (a) α: 0.05 → 0.01, power: 81% → 69%; (b) α: 0.05 → 0.10, power: 81% → 94%.

As the difference to be detected (which is termed the effect size) changes, the power of the test changes. As illustrated below, the larger the effect size, the more powerful the study. With $2n = 32$, two-sample test, 81% power, $\boldsymbol{\delta} = 2$, $\boldsymbol{\sigma} = 2$, $\boldsymbol{\alpha} = 0.05$, two-sided test: difference to be detected ($\boldsymbol{\delta}$): (a) $\boldsymbol{\delta}$: 2 → 1, power: 81% → 29%; (b) $\boldsymbol{\delta}$: 2 → 3, power: 81% → 99%. Sample size (n): (a) n: 32 → 64, power: 81% → 98%; (b) n: 32 → 28, power: 81% → 75%. One-tailed versus two-tailed tests, power: 81% → 88%.

BOX 5.2 RANDOM ERROR AND HYPOTHESIS TESTING

- Hypothesis tests are subject to two types of random error.
- Type I—false positive: if there is no treatment effect but investigator wrongly concludes there is.
- Type I error does not depend on the size of the study.
- Type I error can be inflated when multiple tests are performed.
- Examining many outcomes or treatment groups using multiple hypothesis tests can inflate type I errors.
- Multiple subsets, interactions, and exploratory analyses can inflate type I errors.
- Type II—false negative: when investigator fails to detect a treatment effect or difference that is indeed present, small sample size
- Type II errors can easily be corrected by using the appropriate sample size, which is estimated before conducting the study.

The information required for the sample size or power estimation should be prepared in advance and researched diligently. This information includes (a) variables of interest—type of data (continuous, categorical, nominal, binary, etc.), (b) desired power of the study, (c) desired significance level, (d) effect/difference of clinical importance, (e) standard deviations of continuous outcome variables, and (f) direction of the test—one- or two-sided tests.

The design is important in sample size estimation as well, since the test statistic required to indicate the difference in the outcome (mean or proportion) is in part dependent on the type of design to be utilized in conducting the research. The examples of designs to be considered are (a) the randomized controlled trial (RCT), (b) the block/stratified-block randomized trial, (c) the equivalence trial, (d) the nonrandomized intervention study, (e) the observational study, (f) the prevalence study, and (g) the study measuring sensitivity and specificity.

The structure of the data is essential in determining the appropriate sample size. Possible structures include (a) paired data, (b) repeated measures, (c) groups of equal sizes, and (d) hierarchical data. The nonrandomized studies looking for differences or associations require larger samples to allow adjustment for confounding factors. In a survey design or studies involving follow-up, absolute sample size is of interest, implying that investigators must take into consideration the response proportion of the population to be surveyed and the attrition proportion in a follow-up study.

The sample size should be based on the study's primary outcome variable; if secondary outcome variables are considered important, the sample size estimation should accommodate such variables. And as indicated earlier, sample size estimation should be realistic and practical, meaning that the size of the study must be adjusted to reflect loss to follow-up, expected response rate, and lack of compliance.

In this chapter, some of the basic notions of sample size and power estimations are developed and applied to statistical inference. Statistical stability, which is based on probability value and the 95% confidence interval, is stressed in power and sample size estimations. The *p* value is the null hypothesis of obtaining a test statistic as extreme as or more extreme than the observed test statistic. The importance of estimating the sample size before the study actually begins cannot be overstressed, since inappropriate sample sizes will underpower the study, thus limiting the chance of detecting significant differences. The question to be addressed before the commencement of the study is, what sample size is needed to be able to detect a significant difference with probability $1 - \beta$? Power estimation is essential since it informs us how likely it is that a significant difference will be found given that the alternative hypothesis is true; for example, let's say that the true mean μ is different from the mean under the null hypothesis (μ_o). Therefore, if power is too low (<80%), then there will be little chance of finding a significant difference and nonsignificant results are likely to be observed even if real differences exist between the true point estimate, such as the mean of the group being studied and the null mean (μ_o).

5.2 Sample size characterization

Clinical research, including though not limited to clinical trials, is conducted to detect the differences between groups. This implies that such studies must have sufficient statistical power to detect the differences of clinical or public health interest. In clinical trials, sample size is the number of patients or experimental units required for the trial. Sample size estimation, which should be considered early in the planning stage of the study, is necessary in order for the study to detect the effects of treatment with substantial magnitude and clinical relevance. Sample size computation could then be referred to as the process of obtaining an estimate of the needed size of a study.[1]

5.3 Purpose of sample size

The primary function of estimating an appropriate sample size for the study is to be able to detect the difference between treatments or to indicate a difference in terms of predictors associated with outcomes. In equivalence trials or studies, a larger sample size is required to demonstrate equivalence in terms of drug treatment.[2] The importance of estimating the sample size before the study actually begins cannot be overstressed, since inappropriate sample sizes will underpower the study, thus limiting the chance of detecting significant differences. The question to be addressed before the commencement of the study is, what sample size is needed to be able to detect a significant difference with probability $1 - \beta$?

5.4 Sample size computation

Using phase III RCT as an illustration, the following represents a hypothetical study with the objective being to determine if patients with metastatic prostatic adenocarcinoma who undergo proton-beam therapy (PBT) have a different overall survival compared with patients receiving external-beam radiation (EBT). The investigators propose a trial to two-arm randomization in a single institution. If the study is planned for 4 years (48 months), what will be the required sample and information needed for the computation? Assuming the 1:1 ratio between the two arms, the following information will be required for the SS estimation: (a) 80% power to detect a difference between 12-month median survival and 36-month median survival; (b) two-tailed $\alpha = 0.05$; (c) 36 months of follow-up after the last patient has been enrolled; and (d) 48 months of accrual.

Suppose a study is to be conducted to examine the mean systolic blood pressure (normally distributed) among African-American women, and $\mu_o = 120$ mmHg, $\mu_1 = 115$ mmHg, $\sigma^2 = 576$, $\alpha = 0.05$, and $1 - \beta = 0.80$. What is the sample size needed to conduct the study? Using the formula: $\sigma^2(Z_{1-\beta} + Z_{1-\alpha})^2/\mu_o - \mu_1^2$. Substituting, $n = 576\,(Z.8 + Z.95)^2/25 = 23.04\,(0.84 + 1.645)^2 = 23.04\,(6.175) = 142.3$ ($n = 143$).

BOX 5.3 *p* VALUE (SIGNIFICANCE LEVEL): APPROPRIATE OR NOT IN STATISTICAL INFERENCE?

What is *p* value? To address this often-confusing notion in research, a question must be raised: if the null hypothesis is correct, how likely would we be to obtain the observed result or one more extreme?

The significance level, or p value, is the probability of obtaining the observed result (or one further away from the null [1.0]) when the null hypothesis is indeed true. Therefore, if the observed result (or one more extreme) is relatively likely, the null hypothesis would not be rejected.

p Values do not determine clinical or biological significance and are poor measures of the strength of evidence.

When basing inference predominantly on *p* values, an arbitrary level should not be the sole criterion for the declaration of "statistical significance."*

For biological and clinical support, if observed to be strong with large effects estimates, confidence intervals or *p* values indicate significance and the result could be termed "statistically significant."

Studies with no biologic or clinical significance despite a *p* value showing significant difference should be interpreted with caution.

Even when *p* values are smaller than 0.05, the result of the study can be due to type I errors.

If investigators could repeat experiments or studies many times (which is not the case since we usually perform one experiment), the estimates of clinical effects obtained or point estimates would average out close to the true values, given no bias. The probability distribution or uncertainty refers to the estimate obtained and not the treatment effect. Therefore, the *p* value does not directly judge the treatment effect but makes a statement about estimates that might be obtained if the null hypothesis were true.

Given the inadequacy of *p* value in summarizing evidence from data (statistical inference), *p* value should be deemphasized, while the combination of effect size (point estimate) and precision (95% CI) should be highly encouraged in providing evidence on the effect of treatment from the data.

* S. Piantadosi, *Clinical Trials*, 2nd ed. (Hoboken, New Jersey: John Wiley & Sons, 2005).

Using STATA, the sample size is computed as follows:

```
. sampsi 120 115, sd1(24) alpha(0.05) power(0.80) onesample onesided

Estimated sample size for one-sample comparison of mean
  to hypothesized value

Test Ho: m =     120, where m is the mean in the population

Assumptions:

         alpha =   0.0500 (one-sided)
         power =   0.8000
 alternative m =      115
            sd =       24

Estimated required sample size:

             n =   143
```

The above STATA output using a one-sided test for mean of one/a single sample demonstrated the sample size to be 143 subjects.

Sample size estimation can be based on the following study designs:

> **BOX 5.4 INFORMATION NEEDED FOR SAMPLE SIZE ESTIMATION**
>
> - Variables of interest—type of data, e.g., continuous, categorical
> - Desired power
> - Desired significance level
> - Effect/difference of clinical importance
> - Standard deviations of continuous outcome variables
> - One- or two-sided tests

1 Parallel design: This is a design in clinical trials in which the results of a treatment on two separate groups of patients are compared. The sample size calculated for a parallel design can be used for any study where two groups are being compared.

2 Crossover study: This is a design that compares the results of two treatments on the same group of patients. The sample size calculated for a crossover study can also be used for a study that compares the value of a variable after treatment with its value before treatment. The standard deviation of the outcome variable is expressed as either the within-subject

standard deviation or the standard deviation of the difference. The former is the standard deviation of repeated observations in the same individual, and the latter is the standard deviation of the difference between two measurements in the same individual.

3 Association study: This is a design to assess an association and is used to determine if a variable, the outcome, is affected by another, the predictor or independent variable—for instance, a study to determine whether or not developmental motor delay is related to thoraco-lumbar kyphosis progression in children with achondroplasia.

The group assessed could also be used in estimating the sample size of a study, for example, (a) a single- or one-sample proportion study size estimation, (b) a two-sample or two-group comparison study, and (c) a more-than-two-samples comparison study. Using the latter approach to sample size estimation, we present the steps involved in sample-size estimation here. In a properly designed clinical research study, clinical trial, or observation, investigators must ensure that power will be sufficiently high to detect reasonable departures from the null hypothesis; otherwise, it is not worth conducting such a study. It is therefore important for researchers or investigators to consider the factors influencing power ($1 - \beta$—probability of finding significance when indeed there is one) in a statistical test. These factors, which have been stated before but need to be stressed again here, are (a) the statistical test—parametric or nonparametric, parametric tests are more powerful than nonparametric tests, which do not assume the shape of the distribution, distribution-free tests), (b) sample size—the larger the sample size, the larger the power (Figure 5.1). However, increasing the sample size involves tangible costs in time, money, and effort. Therefore, whereas low power occurs because of a small sample, sample size should be large enough but not unnecessarily or wastefully large. What is the sample size required to yield a certain power for a test, given a predetermined type I error rate? This question must be addressed during the conceptualization phase of the study, with the adequate sample expected to be accurately obtained according to the design and/or the groups compared. There are sample size calculators that estimate samples for one or two means and one or two proportions, which are the commonly estimated sample sizes in clinical research.*

Whenever inferences are made from hypothesis tests, two random errors are possible—namely, type I and type II. From Table 5.1, if the null is true but the test rejects it, a type I error has been committed. The *p* value quantifies the type I error, assuming the null hypothesis is true. A type II error has been committed if the alternate hypothesis is true, implying the null hypothesis is false, but the test fails to reject the null hypothesis.

* For example: http://www.rad.jhmi.edu/jeng/javarad/samplesize/, accessed 03/10/09.

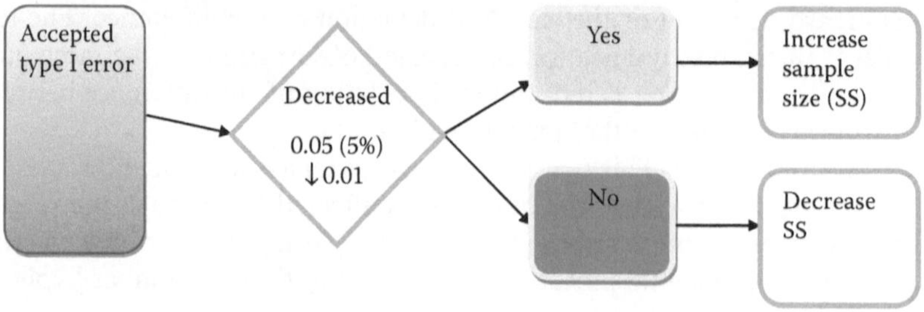

Figure 5.1 Factors affecting the sample size of a study (significance level).

Table 5.1 Hypothesis testing: type I and type II errors

	Significant difference (in universe)—TRUTH	
Test result	*Present (Ho incorrect)*	*Absent (Ho correct)*
Reject H_0	No error $1 - \beta$	Type I error α
Nonrejection of H_0	Type II error β	No error $1 - \alpha$

5.5 Sample size estimation for single- or one-sample proportion hypothesis testing

What is the estimated sample size for comparing a proportion in a single sample with a standard value (Figures 5.2 through 5.4)? The estimate of the study size in this design involves (a) the desired level of significance (α) related to the null hypothesis of no difference in proportion, $\pi_o = \pi_1$; (b) desired level of power ($1 - \beta$); (c) difference between the proportions ($\pi_1 - \pi_0$) that is considered to be clinically significant or be of public health relevance; and (d) a good estimate of population SD, which is $\pi (1 - \pi)$.

With these criteria, we can compute the sample size (n):

$$n = \left[z_\alpha \sqrt{\pi_0(1-\pi_0)} - z_\beta \sqrt{\pi_1(1-\pi_1)} \right]^2 / \pi_0 - \pi_1$$

z_α is the two-tailed z value related to the significance level (α) in the hypothesis, and z_β is the lower one-tailed z value and is related to the alternative hypothesis, the power (β).

For example, a study was planned to examine the prevention of infection in children with neuromuscular scoliosis after spine fusion to correct curve deformities, if the investigators wanted to reduce infection from 30% to 10%, the probability of detecting a 20% difference as 0.8 (80%) and 0.05 significance

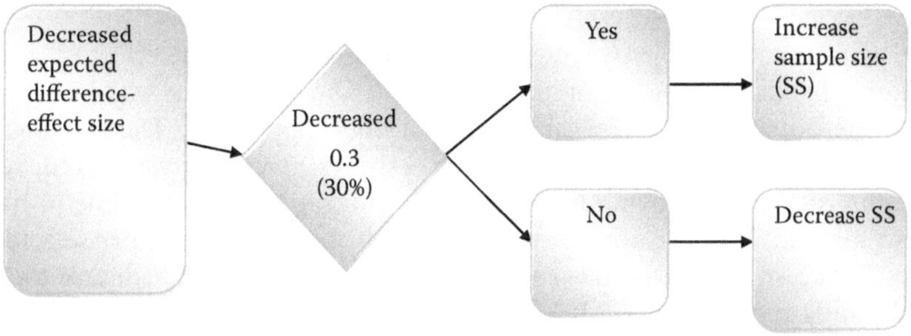

Figure 5.2 Factors affecting the sample size of a study (effect size).

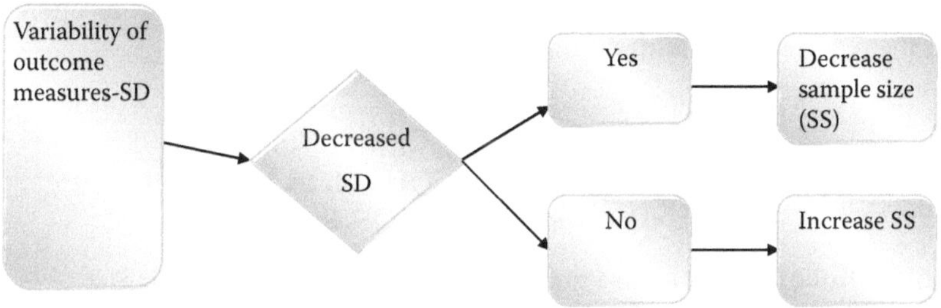

Figure 5.3 Factors affecting the sample size of a study (variability, SD).

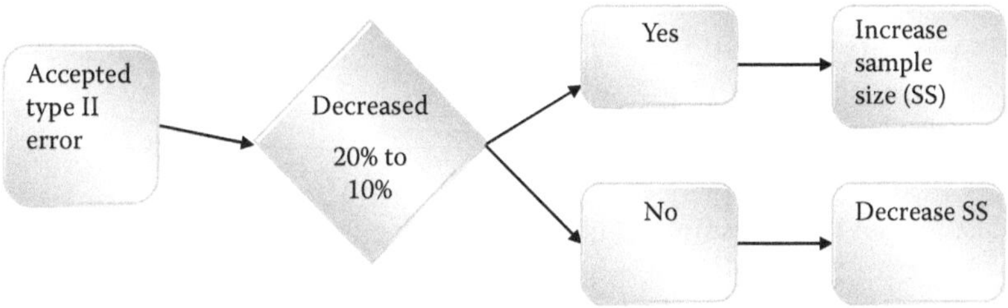

Figure 5.4 Factors affecting the sample size of a study (type II error).

level, what would be an adequate sample size? Using the above formula, the two-tailed z related to $\alpha = 0.05$ is ± 1.96, which is the critical value of the z distribution from the 2.5% in each tail, while the lower one-tailed z value related to β is approximately -0.84, which is the critical value separating the lower 20% of the z distribution from the upper 80%; the sample size $= (1.15/0.20)^2 = 5.75^2 = 34$. Therefore, the investigators will need 34 patients to determine whether infection will decrease by 20% (30% to 10%).

5.6 One-sample estimation of sample size with outcome mean

Let us take an example. A study was planned to look at the effect of a new sedative hypnotic drug on unipolar patients, and the design was one group with the outcome to be measured with a one-sample test. The baseline to sedation time after taking the drug for 21 days (3 weeks) was taken, with the aim of the study being to increase sleep duration from baseline (4 h) to (postintervention measure [21 days after]) 5 h. If the investigators selected a two-sided test, $\alpha = 0.05$, power = 90%, difference = 1 (4 h of sedation to 5 h) and standard deviation = 2 h, what is the required sample size?

$$n = \left(z_{1-\alpha/2} + z_{1-\beta}\right)^2 \sigma^2/\delta^2 = (1.960 + 1.282)^2 2^2/1^2 = 42.04 = 43$$

Using the z value $1 - \alpha/2$ (two-sided test) = 1.96 and the z value for $1 - \beta$ = 1.282, where power = 90%, SD = 2, and the effect size or difference of interest = 1 h, the required sample size is estimated as 43 subjects.

> **BOX 5.5 SAMPLE SIZE EQUATION FORMULA AND RANDOM ERROR RATES**
>
> - Intended error rates are part of the equation of sample size.
> - These error rates are written with normal quantiles for type I and II errors.
> - $z_\beta = (1 - \beta)$ and $z\alpha = (1 - \alpha/2)$.
> - $\alpha = 0.05$, $z_\alpha = 1.96$.
> - $\alpha = 0.01$, $z_\alpha = 2.58$.
> - $\beta = 0.10$, $z_\beta = 1.282$.
> - $\beta = 0.20$, $z_\beta = 0.84$.

Using STATA, the sample number is obtained:

```
Estimated sample size for one-sample comparison of mean to hypothesized value
Test Ho: m = 4, where m is the mean in the population
Assumptions:

          alpha = 0.0500 (two-sided)
          power = 0.9000
          alternative m = 5
          sd = 2
```

```
Estimated required sample size:

      n = 43
```

5.7 Two independent samples: Proportions

Let us consider a study in which the outcome is measured in proportion and is dichotomous—that is, yes or no, success or failure, presence or absence; the sample size estimation will involve a formula for two independent groups with an outcome that is dichotomous, implying proportion.

5.7.1 What are the requirements for the sample size estimation?

To estimate the sample size, the following information is required: (a) setting of the significance level (α), that is, related to the null hypothesis (π_0); (b) power ($1 - \beta$), the desired chance of detecting an actual difference relative to the alternative hypothesis; (c) difference between the two proportions of clinical relevance or significance (proportion in one group vs. the proportion in the other group)—$\pi_1 - \pi_2$; and (d) standard deviation, which is determined by the proportion itself, and is $\pi\ (1 - \pi)$.

5.7.2 How is the sample size computed?

Assuming that the sample size is the same in each group, it is computed as follows:

$$n = \left[z_\alpha \sqrt{2\pi_1(1-\pi)} - z_\beta \sqrt{\pi_1(1-\pi) + \pi_2(1-\pi_2)} / \pi_1 - \pi_2 \right]^2$$

where z_α is the two-tailed z value related to the null hypothesis and z_β is the lower one-tailed z value related to the alternative hypothesis. To illustrate the use of this formula in sample size estimation, we present a hypothetical study to examine the outcome of cervical fusion with instrumentation in pediatric patients with cervical spine instability. Of 32 patients who underwent spine fusion with instrumentation, 27 achieved solid fusion (0.844), while 8 out of 15 who had surgery without instrumentation had solid fusion (0.533). The 95% CI for the difference in proportion was 0.044–0.578, indicative of the difference in proportion with respect to fusion. If the investigator wanted to estimate the sample size needed to detect a significant difference, using $\alpha = 0.05$ and $1 - \beta = 0.90$, what would be the estimated sample size in each group? Substituting in the formula above, we have $(1.997/0.30)^2 = 6.657^2 = 45$ subjects in each group.

The STATA software is used here to estimate the sample based on these specifications:

```
. sampsi 19.15 39.15, sd1(45) sd2(45) alpha(0.05) power(0.80)

Estimated sample size for two-sample comparison of means

Test Ho: m1 = m2, where m1 is the mean in population 1
                   and m2 is the mean in population  2

Assumptions:

       alpha =   0.0500 (two-sided)
       power =   0.8000
          m1 =    19.15
          m2 =    39.15
         sd1 =       45
         sd2 =       45
       n2/n1 =     1.00

Estimated required sample sizes:

          n1 =       80
          n2 =       80
```

Suppose a hypothetical study was conducted to determine the power (ability to detect a minimum difference between two groups, namely, case versus non-case) with respect to the implication of diabetes mellitus (DM) in pediatric dental disorders (Figure 5.5). If the overall sample size is 2355, and case (n = 471) and non-case (1884), what is the expected power if the effect size or difference in proportion is 0.2, type I error tolerance is 0.05, and binomial regression model is used for the hypothesis testing? Using stats syntax:

```
power twoproportions 0.50 0.70, test(chi2) n(2355) nratio(1/4)

Estimated power for a two-sample proportions test
Pearson's chi-squared test
Ho: p2 = p1  versus  Ha: p2 != p1
```

alpha	power	N	N1	N2	nratio	delta	p1	p2
.05	1	2355	1177	1177	1	.2	.5	.7
.05	1	2355	785	1570	2	.2	.5	.7
.05	1	2355	588	1766	3	.2	.5	.7
.05	1	2355	471	1884	4	.2	.5	.7

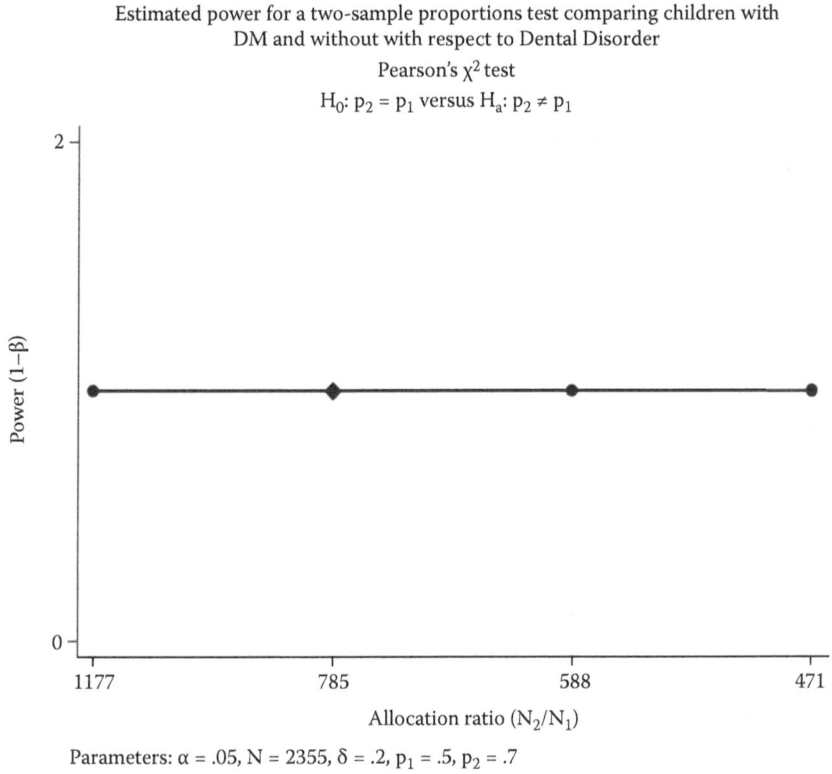

Figure 5.5 Graphical illustration of power estimation

5.8 Two independent group means

Using a similar approach in one sample mean: (a) alpha statement—type I error rate, (b) power—type II error rate, (c) differences between the two means judged to be of clinical relevance or importance, and (d) estimate of standard deviation considered to be good.

$$n = 2\left[(z_{\alpha} - z_{\beta})^{\sigma}/\mu_1 - \mu_2\right]^2$$

where μ1 − μ2 is the magnitude of the difference to be detected between the two groups, σ is the estimate of standard deviation in each group (the assumption is that the standard deviations, σ, in the two groups are equal). For example, let us compare the time taken to develop neurologic complications in patients with skeletal dysplasia who underwent cervical arthrodesis with and without instrumentation. If the investigators wanted to estimate the sample size given the ability to detect the difference of 20 h or more, alpha = 0.05, and 1 − β = 0.80, and the standard deviation is 45 h, what would be the estimated sample size in each group?

```
Using STATA syntax: sampsi 19.15 39.15, sd1(45) sd2(45) alpha(0.05) power(0.80)


Estimated sample size for two-sample comparison of means
Test Ho: m1 = m2, where m1 is the mean in population 1
         and m2 is the mean in population 2
Assumptions:
         alpha = 0.0500 (two-sided)
         power = 0.8000
            m1 = 19.15
            m2 = 39.15
           sd1 = 45
           sd2 = 45
         n2/n1 = 1.00
Estimated required sample sizes:

            n1 = 80
            n2 = 80
```

The estimated sample size using STATA shows that to be able to detect a difference of 20 h between the two groups, if one really existed, there would need to be 80 in each group.

5.9 Prospective cohort or two-group comparison in clinical trials

The sample size and power estimations for prospective or clinical trials involving two groups can be performed using the following equation:

$$n = (p1q1 + p2q2) * K/(p1 - p2)^2$$

where n is the number of subjects in each group, $p1$ is the frequency of outcome in group 1 and $q1 = 1 - p1$, and $p2$ is the frequency of outcome in group 2 and $q2 = 1 - p2$.

$K = (z_\alpha + z_\beta)^2$, where z_α and z_β are normal deviates corresponding to significance level and α and power $(1 - \beta)$. The required sample size would be $2n$.

The power estimation could be performed using the following formula, which, as stated earlier, involves the random error rates, α and β:

$$\text{Power} = z_\beta = (\boldsymbol{p}1 - \boldsymbol{p}2) * \sqrt{\boldsymbol{n}} / \sqrt{(\boldsymbol{p}1\boldsymbol{q}1 + \boldsymbol{p}2\boldsymbol{q}2)} - z_\alpha$$

With the same example, if $n = 160$ and alpha is 0.05, the difference between the groups is 2 h, and the standard deviation is 45 in each group, power should be estimated before conducting the study; thus, if there is really a difference in hours from surgery to onset of infection, will such a difference be detected with the preexisting study size?

Using STATA: sampsi 19.15 39.15, sd1(45) sd2(45) alpha(0.05) n1(80) n2(80)

```
Estimated power for two-sample comparison of means

Test Ho: m1 = m2, where m1 is the mean in population 1
         and m2 is the mean in population 2
Assumptions:
         alpha     = 0.0500 (two-sided)
         m1        = 19.15
         m2        = 39.15
         sd1       = 45
         sd2       = 45

sample size n1 = 80
         n2 = 80
         n2/n1 = 1.00
Estimated power: power = 0.8026
```

5.10 Case–control study

Sample size estimation for case and control studies with equal size can be performed using the following formula. Because proportions are used in this estimation as well as the odds ratio, the random error rates are involved already in the estimation of the relative odds expected.

$$p1 = p2 * \mathrm{OR}/1 + p2(\mathrm{OR} - 1)$$

where $p1$ is the frequency of exposure in cases, $p2$ is the frequency of exposure in controls, and OR is the odds ratio predicted.

BOX 5.6 STATISTICAL POWER AND SIGNIFICANCE

- To assess clinical and statistical inferences, adequate sample size (adequate number of subjects) and power are essential.
- This concern is critical for safety and activities studies (phase II and IIa) as well as comparative studies (phase IIb and phase III) in clinical trials—these phases support therapeutic decisions.
- With a phase I trial, which is dose-finding and dose-ranging, the sample size is often the outcome of the study.
- The necessary size of the study depends on (a) the strength of the association, (b) the frequency of outcome in the control/unexposed group or the frequency of exposure in the control group in case–control studies, (c) the level of statistical significance, and (d) statistical power.
- A type I error is the error that occurs when investigators find a significant difference when there is none in truth (does not exist).
- A type II error or beta occurs when investigators fail to detect a significant difference when indeed there is one in truth (really existed).

5.11 Summary

Sample size and power estimations are used to determine the size of the study and the ability of the study to detect the minimum difference should one exist, respectively. These estimates should be estimated before conducting clinical research. The importance of estimating the sample size before the study actually begins cannot be overstressed, since inappropriate sample sizes will underpower the study, thus limiting the chance of detecting a significant difference. The question to be addressed before the commencement of the study is, what sample size is needed to be able to detect a significant difference with probability $1 - \beta$? The factors influencing sample size are (a) effect size, (b) significance level (alpha or type I error tolerance), (c) power—$1 - \beta$, and (d) variability expressed as the standard deviation or variance. However, in time-to-event outcomes, the number of events must be put into consideration in sample size estimation. Other factors include attrition rate, failure probability, missing variables or incomplete records, interest in subset analysis, prognostic factors adjustment, and highly asymmetric distributions. These factors tend to limit precision even when large samples from large data sets are used in the study.

Power estimation is essential since it informs us how likely it is that a significant difference will be found given that the alternative hypothesis is true—for example, given that the true mean μ is different from the mean under the null hypothesis (μ_o). Therefore, if power is too low (<80%), then there will be little chance of finding a significant difference and nonsignificant results are likely to be observed even if real differences existed between the true point estimate, such as the mean of the group being studied and the null mean, μ_o. Power is influenced by (a) sample size, (b) variability—SD, (c) effect size, and (d) significance level—type I error tolerance.

Questions for discussion

1 Suppose that you are studying the effect of chemotherapy on prostate cancer survival, and chemotherapy is measured on a binary scale, denoted by X, in a time-to-event analysis. The distribution of $X = 0$ and $X = 1$. (a) What sample size is needed to detect the adjusted hazard ratio of $\Delta = 2.5$, power = 0.85, and type I error = 0.05? (b) Suppose the power is changed to 90%, what would be the effect of this change on the sample size? (c) If the attrition rate or the loss to follow-up is 20%, what would be an appropriate size of the study? (d) Suppose the sample size for the study is 256, HR = 1.5, $\alpha = 0.05$. Will there be enough power to detect a significant difference, avoiding type II error (false-negative) results?

2 Suppose 24 children with adolescent idiopathic scoliosis (AIS) are enrolled in a study to determine the effectiveness of titanium instrumentation in correcting spinal deformities, if the mean difference 0.5 unit, two-sided test, significance level = 0.05, mean and SD = 0.61 ± 0.7 and 0.04 ± 0.68 for the treatment and control groups, respectively. (a) Compute the power of the study. (b) What factors may possibly affect this power?

3 Suppose an investigator wishes to estimate the number of subjects needed to study the effect of tumor stage at diagnosis on survival of African-American women diagnosed with breast cancer and treated for the disease, and suppose there is a 90% chance of finding a significant difference using a two-sided test with a significance level of 0.05 and effect size of 0.5 unit is expected. (a) How many subjects are needed in the study? (b) What other information is needed for this computation if any? (c) If the expected effect size increases, what is the impact of that on the sample size?

References

1. B. W. Brown, Jr., Statistical controversies in the design of clinical trials—Some personal views, *Controlled Clinical Trials* 1 (1980):13–27.
2. S. Piantadosi, *Clinical Trials*, 2nd ed. (Hoboken, New Jersey: John Wiley & Sons, 2005).

6 Single sample statistical inference

6.1 Introduction

Clinical research sometimes involves a single group and requires no comparison group. In conducting such a study, which is often encountered in surgical settings, the preoperative, immediate operative, and follow-up measures are used to determine the effectiveness of a surgical procedure. In other clinical settings, a pretest measure is obtained from a single sample before intervention, and the same instrument is used to obtain information from the same sample after intervention. These tests allow one to infer conclusions about the wider population from the data on selected individuals (sample).

Descriptive and inferential statistics are essential in making sense of data collected in clinical research.[1] Clinical research is often conducted on a sample, implying the impossibility of studying the entire population.[2] The inferential statistics allow one to draw inferences on the entire population based on the sample.[3] The application of inferential statistics assumes that the sample has been randomly selected from the larger population in order to provide a valid generalization beyond the targeted population.[4] Simply, statistical inference uses data in hand (collected data) to answer the research question or hypothesis about a clinical setting that goes beyond the data collected or present data and attributes a known degree of confidence to the answer, termed *statistical significance*. We use a test statistic such as the t test to quantify the difference between the actual observation and the one we would expect if the hypothesis of no effect or no difference were true. A statistically significant difference or effect, as we commonly say, refers to an observed effect or difference so large that it could rarely occur by chance. A commonly used test of significance is the p value, which assesses the evidence against the null hypothesis and provides a summary of this evidence in terms of probability. The smaller this value, the stronger the evidence against the null hypothesis of no effect or no difference provided by the data. Strictly, the application of significance level should be restricted to the probability sample, which is the sample selected for the study by chance that results in random variables. To recap, a random variable is a variable whose value is a numerical outcome of randomness (random statistically speaking does not mean haphazard; it is a kind of order or behavior that emerges only in the long run and describes a chance behavior that is unpredictable in the short run but has a regular and predictable pattern in the long run) or random phenomenon, and the probability of any outcome of a random phenomenon is the proportion of times the outcome would occur in a very long series of repetitions.

Hypothesis testing may involve one group of participants in which data are collected or measurement is obtained on one or more occasions—for example, a *single-sample t test* in which information is obtained from a single group and compared with the population mean, and the *repeated-measure analysis of variance* in which measurement is obtained more than two times from the same subject. A *paired t test* is another example in which pre- and post-test measurements are used to determine the effectiveness of an intervention. Because a single group hypothesis testing is about the difference between some norm in the population, a baseline measure, or a pretest, the amount of variation must be addressed by the confidence interval or the significance level.[5]

The test statistics required to assess the variation or quantify error depend on the scale of measurement of the variable and the number of times the data are obtained from the subjects. A t distribution is used to estimate the mean value of a numerical variable, while a standard normal distribution or z (which is a normal distribution with $\mu = 0$ and standard deviation $\sigma = 1$; if each observation x_i in a sample has a normal distribution with μ and standard deviation σ, then $(x_1 - \mu)/\sigma$ will have a standardized normal distribution) is used to estimate the proportion of subjects who have specific characteristics,[6] for example, the presence or absence of solid fusion or union in a group of subjects with skeletal dysplasia who underwent cervical spine fusion for cervical spine instability.

This chapter presents statistical inference when a study is conducted on a single sample. In observational and experimental designs, a single sample could be used to test the null hypothesis of no effect, no difference, or no benefit. Recall that statistics is primarily concerned with the sample (the subset of a population from which data are collected and which is used to draw conclusions about the whole population) and not the population, which is the entire group of individuals or patients about which information is sought. The selection of a sample for a study must follow a probability method (sample chosen by chance) in order for it to be representative of the population. These methods include (a) a simple random sample, (b) a stratified random sample, and (c) a systematic random sample. The test statistic used, the rationale for selecting these tests, and their interpretations are presented as well. In addition, the use of statistical software in the analysis of data on a single sample is presented using the STATA statistical package for illustrative purposes.

6.1.1 Single-sample test techniques

The hypothesis regarding single sample studies could be tested with appropriate test statistics and statistical methods depending on the scale of measurement of the variables and the number of times the measures are taken from the same subject. These tests include (a) a single-sample *t* test, (b) a sign test, (c) a paired *t* test, (d) the Wilcoxon rank-sum test, (e) the repeated-measure analysis of variance, and (f) the Friedman test.

6.1.2 *One-sample tests—Illustrations*

6.1.2.1 *What is a single-sample* t *test?*

This statistic is used to test the null hypothesis of no mean difference between the assumed or postulated mean and the population mean. It assumes normal distribution of a random variable from a random sample. Recall that normal distribution, also termed *normal curve*, involves density curves that are symmetric, single-peaked, and bell-shaped. These curves are described by the mean (μ) and standard deviation (σ). Normal distributions comply with the rule 68–95–99.7, which implies that 68% of the observations fall within one σ and the mean, 95% of the observations fall within 2σ of μ, and 99.7% of the observations fall within 3σ of μ.

6.1.2.2 *What is a sign test?*

The sign test, which is a nonparametric test, estimates the median value of an ordinal variable, as well as a variable that is assumed or assessed to deviate from normal distribution.

6.1.2.3 *What is paired* t *test?*

A paired *t* test (matched group or dependent *t* test) estimates the mean difference between the pretest or the baseline measure and the posttest or the postintervention measure. For example, if a study was conducted to assess the effectiveness of titanium instrumentation in correcting or curing deformities in adolescent idiopathic scoliosis and if investigators wanted to see the differences between preoperative and immediately postoperative main curve angle, a paired *t* test is an adequate test statistic. Why? A nonparametric equivalent of the paired *t* test is the Wilcoxon signed-rank test, which estimates the difference in the median in single-group subjects/participants. For example, if a study was conducted to examine the difference in preintervention and postintervention hematocrit, but the data failed to meet the normality assumption, the Wilcoxon signed-rank test would be appropriate.

6.1.3 *What are the steps in hypothesis testing in studies involving a single sample?*

The steps in the testing of a hypothesis include (a) a statement of the null hypothesis using H_0, which claims that there is no difference between the assumed or postulated mean or proportion and the population mean; (b) an alternative hypothesis, using H_A or H_1, which claims that there is a difference between the assumed mean/proportion and the population mean/proportion; (c) the direction of the test, which could be two-tailed or one-tailed; (d) the decision on the appropriate test statistic—for example, if inference is required about the mean, a single sample *t* test is appropriate, which is the difference between the sample mean and the hypothesized or assumed mean divided by the standard error and presented mathematically as follows:

$$t = X - \mu/\mathrm{SE} \text{ or } t = X - \mu/\mathrm{SD}/\sqrt{n}$$

where X is the sample mean, μ is the hypothesized mean, SE is the standard error of the sample mean, and $\mathrm{SE} = \mathrm{SD}/\sqrt{n}$; and (e) selection of the level of significance for the statistical test—termed alpha (α) or type I error, which is the probability of incorrectly rejecting the null hypothesis when indeed the null hypothesis is *true*. While alpha is conventionally set at 0.05 (5% error), other levels of alpha include 0.01 (1% error) and 0.001 (0.1% error). The above formula for the inference regarding one-sample *t* statistics is contingent on a simple random sample of size *n* that is drawn from an $N(\mu, \sigma)$ population. Please note that the one-sample *t* statistic has the *t* distribution (normal distribution with mean μ and standard deviation $\sigma/\sqrt{n}$, and when σ is not known, standard error, SE, is used and is given by $\mathrm{SD}/\sqrt{n}$) with $n - 1$ degrees of freedom.

6.1.4 How is a single t test computed?

Statistical packages are available for the computation of single-sample *t* test. For example, this is performed by STATA statistical packages using the following syntax or command:

```
ttest varlist = 50
```

where *varlist* is the variable (hypothesized mean) termed μ, H_0: $\mu = 50$.

6.1.5 Drawing and stating the conclusion

The null hypothesis can be rejected as a result of sample evidence, and then the alternative hypothesis is concluded. However, if the evidence is insufficient to reject the null hypothesis, it is retained but not accepted as such—simply the null hypothesis cannot be rejected based on the evidence from the sample. The one-sample *t* test is used to test whether the sample mean differs significantly from the hypothesized value $\mu = 50$. The significance level or *p* value represents the probability of observing a mean of 60 units (granted the calculation showed $n = 60$ units) in a random sample of 100 subjects, if the true mean is 50 units. If the significance level or alpha was set at 0.05 (5%), and the observed $p = 0.10$ (10%), then one is likely to conclude that because the observed *p* value is greater than the alpha chosen for the test, there is no significant difference between the hypothesized mean

(60 units) and the sample mean (50 units), implying that the null hypothesis cannot be rejected—insufficient evidence to reject the null hypothesis.

```
. ttest Mathscore==6

One-sample t test
------------------------------------------------------------------------------
Variable |     Obs        Mean    Std. Err.   Std. Dev.   [95% Conf. Interval]
---------+--------------------------------------------------------------------
Mathsc~e |      60    6.333333    .1026944    .7954674    6.127842    6.538824
------------------------------------------------------------------------------
    mean = mean(Mathscore)                                        t =   3.2459
Ho: mean = 6                                     degrees of freedom =       59

    Ha: mean < 6                 Ha: mean != 6                 Ha: mean > 6
 Pr(T < t) = 0.9990         Pr(|T| > |t|) = 0.0019          Pr(T > t) = 0.0010
```

Notes: The null hypothesis is that the sample mean is not different from the hypothesized mean (6.0), the evidence from the data (mean = 6.3, SD = 2.49, $p = 0.33$) does not support the rejection of the null hypothesis of no difference between the mean. The observed difference between the population mean and the observed mean in the study sample is due to chance, given the 5% significance level.

```
. ttest Mathscore==6, level (90)

One-sample t test
------------------------------------------------------------------------------
Variable |     Obs        Mean    Std. Err.   Std. Dev.   [90% Conf. Interval]
---------+--------------------------------------------------------------------
Mathsc~e |      60    6.333333    .1026944    .7954674    6.161721    6.504945
------------------------------------------------------------------------------
    mean = mean(Mathscore)                                        t =   3.2459
Ho: mean = 6                                     degrees of freedom =       59

    Ha: mean < 6                 Ha: mean != 6                 Ha: mean > 6
 Pr(T < t) = 0.9990         Pr(|T| > |t|) = 0.0019          Pr(T > t) = 0.0010

. ttest Mathscore==6, level (99)
One-sample t test
------------------------------------------------------------------------------
Variable |     Obs        Mean    Std. Err.   Std. Dev.   [95% Conf. Interval]
---------+--------------------------------------------------------------------
Mathsc~e |      60    6.333333    .1026944    .7954674    6.059986    6.606681
------------------------------------------------------------------------------
    mean = mean(Mathscore)                                        t =   3.2459
Ho: mean = 6                                     degrees of freedom =       59

    Ha: mean < 6                 Ha: mean != 6                 Ha: mean > 6
 Pr(T < t) = 0.9990         Pr(|T| > |t|) = 0.0019          Pr(T > t) = 0.0010
```

Note: The *t* test automatically provides the 95% confidence interval (CI) in the output, which can be modified to either 90% or 99% by adding `level (90)` or `level (99)`, respectively, to the syntax, thus: `ttest nummeanScore = 6, level (90)` for 90% CI.

6.2 One-sample group design

We discussed the research question in the first section of this book. The research question refers to a statement that identifies the phenomenon to be investigated. For example, "Does coffee drinking result in pancreatic neoplasm?" As observed earlier in this chapter, research questions could involve *one group of subjects* who are measured on one or two occasions, for example, mean milk consumption and bone density in women 45 years and older. The following are appropriate research questions: (1) Is the mean milk consumption of women 45 years and older different in our sample compared with the National Study on Nutrition sample? In other words, how confident are we that the observed mean milk consumption in our sample is X oz/day? (2) Is the mean bone density (X) in the National Study on Nutrition of women 45 years and older significantly different from our sample?

6.3 Hypothesis statement

The hypothesis tests the mean value of a numerical value (e.g., milk consumption, bone density). This hypothesis testing involves the examination of the mean in one group when the observations are normally distributed (e.g., bone density, milk consumption).

6.4 Test statistic

The test statistic refers to the inferential statistical methods used to assess differences, association, or effect and its application in drawing conclusions from the sample to the targeted population and beyond the targeted population. A one-sample t statistic is given as follows: $t = X - \mu/\text{SD}/\sqrt{n}$ with $n - 1$ degrees of freedom. While robust to normality assumption violation, it assumes that a simple random sample of size n is drawn from $N(\mu, \sigma)$ population. The following are illustrations of single- or one-sample statistical inferences.

6.4.1 One-sample t *test*

As mentioned earlier, a single-sample t test estimates the mean difference comparing the sample to the postulated mean in the population. For example, it answers the research question regarding the mean difference between the systolic blood pressure of Caucasian women, age 35 to 45 years, in the study sample and the known mean systolic blood pressure of women of the same age in the United States.

6.4.1.1 What is the appropriate test statistic in a one-sample hypothesis testing involving the mean?

The t distribution is appropriate for performing the test statistics and obtaining the confidence limits.[7] Simply stated, the single- or one-sample t test compares the mean of a single sample to a known population mean.

6.4.1.2 *When is a one-sample* t *test appropriate?*

The purpose of this test (t) or Student's t test is to answer research questions about means. Therefore, if data are numerical, normality is assumed with respect to their shape and distribution, and only one sample is involved, then a one-sample t test is an appropriate test statistic.

6.4.1.3 *What is the* t*-test formula?*

As stated earlier, the formula for the t test is (statistic − hypothesized value)/estimated standard error of the statistic.[8] Mathematically, it appears as such:

$$t = (X - \mu)/(SD/\sqrt{n}) = (X - \mu)/SE$$

where X is the observed or sample mean, μ is the hypothesized mean value of the population (true mean in the population), and SE is the standard error of the mean (X). Simply, mean (x) − constant (μ)/SD(x), where SD(x) is the sum $\{(x_i - \text{mean}(x)\}^2/(n-1)$.[9]

6.4.2 *Considering statistical significance?*

In the NSN illustration described earlier, to determine whether the observed mean is real (i.e., the observed mean is different from the mean of the National Study of Nutrition [NSN], termed the norm or population mean) and not just a random occurrence, the following factors need to be considered: (1) the difference between the observed mean and the norm (NSN) or population mean, implying much larger or smaller magnitude of the mean difference → greater difference; (2) the amount of variability among subjects, implying less variation—smaller standard deviation in the sample (i.e., homogeneous sample and relatively precise method of measurement); and (3) the number of subjects in the study, implying a larger rather than a smaller sample.

Vignette 6.1: Consider a study conducted to compare the mean vitamin C intake among eighth-grade schoolchildren at New School, Texas, with the population mean (Texas Study of Nutrition, or TSN). If the investigator found a greater standard deviation (SD), what is the probable explanation?

Solution: If the SD is greater in the sample studied (eighth-grade children at New School), it is likely that (1) vitamin C intake varies widely from one child to another or (2) a crude measure device is used to ascertain the vitamin C intake (improper, imprecise, or crude measure).

6.4.2.1 *What is the test assumption—Normality?*

The normal distribution, also referred to as the *Gaussian distribution or bell-shaped curve*, is a continuous probability distribution. This distribution takes any value and is characterized as (1) smooth, (2) bell-shaped curve, (3) symmetric about the mean of the distribution, and (4) symbolized by mean μ, and a standard deviation σ.[10] Simply, normal distributions are a family of distributions that have the same general shape, implying symmetry, where the left side is an exact mirror of the right side, with scores more concentrated in the middle than in the tails (Figure 6.1). If normality is not assumed, observations should be more than 30 subjects, and hence the mean becomes normally distributed above this number regardless of the distribution of the original observations (central limit theorem). Even with the violation of normal distribution, a *t* test could still be performed since it is robust for nonnormal data, implying the drawing of a proper conclusion even when the assumptions are not met, including normality.

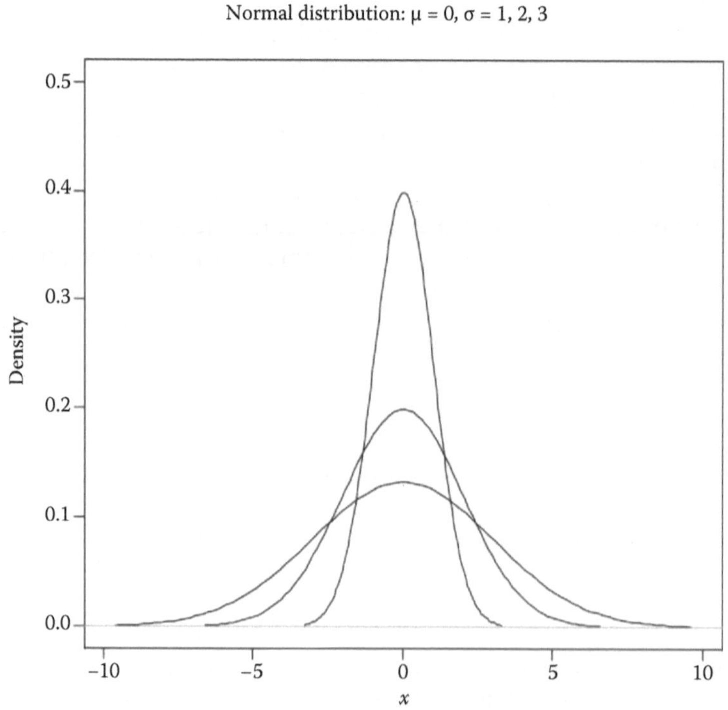

Figure 6.1 Normal distribution curve.

6.4.2.2 *How is one-sample* t*-test result interpreted?*

The null hypothesis assumes the equality of means; a result at significance level (<0.05) is indicative of a significant difference between the sample mean (X) and the population mean (μ). A nonsignificant mean difference implies that the difference may be due to random error or chance, given the significance level ($p > 0.05$); it does not mean that the two means are equal.[10] Simply, it is not possible to be confident about accepting the observed difference because this might be due to random occurrence.

Vignette 6.2: Consider a random sample of systolic blood pressure from 10 African-American women: 145, 136, 151, 140, 139, 148, 138, 136, 147, and 142. Do these data give a good reason for a clinician to believe that the systolic blood pressure of African-American women is greater than 140 mmHg? What is the hypothesis? What is the *t* statistic and its *p* value? What do you conclude from the data?

Solution: To test whether the systolic blood pressure of African-American women differs from the standard systolic blood pressure of 140 mmHg, the null hypothesis H_0: $\mu = 140$ mmHg and H_a: $\mu > 140$ mmHg. Using STATA, the *t* statistic and *p* value are computed as shown below. The syntax: `ttest varlist = = 140`, where `varlist` is the variable, SBP.

```
. ttest sbp ==140

One-sample t test
------------------------------------------------------------------------------
Variable |     Obs        Mean    Std. Err.   Std. Dev.   [90% Conf. Interval]
---------+--------------------------------------------------------------------
     sbp |      10       142.2    1.671991    5.287301    138.4177    145.9823
------------------------------------------------------------------------------
    mean = mean(sbp)                                              t =   1.3158
Ho: mean = 140                                   degrees of freedom =        9

    Ha: mean < 140              Ha: mean != 140              Ha: mean > 140
 Pr(T < t) = 0.8896       Pr(|T| > |t|) = 0.2208         Pr(T > t) = 0.1104
```

The *t* statistic is 1.31 with 9 degrees of freedom. The *p* value of the equality of the SBP mean is 0.22, which is >0.05, the set significance level, implying that we fail to reject the null hypothesis and conclude that the mean SBP of African-American women (142.2 mmHg) is not significantly different from the population mean, $\mu = 140$ mmHg.

6.4.2.3 *How is statistical power estimated in a one-sample* t *test?*

The power of a test, as discussed previously, measures its ability to detect deviations from the null hypothesis. The power of a one-sample *t* test against a specific alternative value of the population μ is the probability that the test will reject the null hypothesis when the alternative hypothesis is true. The power estimation of a one-sample t test utilizes the sample size (n), significance level, $\alpha = 0.05$, μ, and the SD.

BOX 6.1 STATISTICAL POWER AND ELEMENTS INFLUENCING POWER

- Statistical power is the ability of a test to detect deviations from the null hypothesis.
- Statistical power is influenced by
  - (a) Significance level—decrease in α leads to decrease of power.
  - (b) Alternative mean or effect size—as the alternative mean shifts further away from the null (effect size), power increases.
  - (c) Standard deviation—as the SD of the individual observations increases, power decreases.
  - (d) Sample size (n)—as n increases, power increases.

Vignette 6.3: Suppose you wish to determine whether or not the fasting serum cholesterol level (FSCL) in African-American women (AAW) aged 21 to 50 years differs from that of the general US population of women of the same age. If the FSCL is known to be normally distributed with mean 190 mg/dL, and the mean FSCL of 100 AAW of the same age is 181.52 mg/dL with a standard deviation of 40 mg/dL. Using a one-sample t test, calculate the t statistic. On the basis of this evidence, what is your conclusion regarding FSCL among AAW relative to the general US population of women?

Solution: Use the formula: $X - \mu \div SD/\sqrt{n}$. Substituting, $181.52 - 190 \div 40/\sqrt{100} = -8.48/4 = -2.12$. To address whether the obtained value is significantly different, we obtain the confidence interval for the two-sided test with $\alpha = 0.05$. The critical values are $C_1 = t_{99,.025}$, $C_2 = t_{99,.975}$. Using the percentage points of t distribution (*not provided in the appendix*), because $t_{99,.975} < t_{60,.975} = 2.000$, and because $C_2 < 2.000$ ($t = -2.12 < -2.000 < C_1$), the null hypothesis is rejected at a 5% significance level in favor of the alternative hypothesis. On the basis of this evidence, the mean FSCL is significantly lower among AAW compared to the general US population of women.

6.4.2.4 *How do power and study size influence a negative result?*

Because the power of the test is influenced by the sample size, small studies are prone to negative results. Therefore, the smaller the study size, the higher the likelihood of not detecting the effect or difference if one really existed. As pointed out earlier, it is meaningless to report a statistically insignificant finding unless the power of a test was estimated before the study being conducted or post hoc (after the fact).

Vignette 6.4: Using the data in Vignette 6.2, estimate the power of the study. What can you conclude regarding the result?

Solution: The power of a one-sample *t* test for a mean of a normal distribution with known variance ($\mu_1 - \mu_0$) is expressed as follows:

$$\text{Power} = \Phi[z_\alpha + (\mu_1 - \mu_0)/\sigma\sqrt{n}]$$

$\mu_1 = 140$ mmHg, $\mu_0 = 142$ mmHg, $\sigma = 0.05$, assuming that the standard deviation is 5 mmHg and $n = 10$. Power $= \Phi[z_{0.05} + (140 - 142.2)/5\sqrt{10}]$.

BOX 6.2 STUDY SIZE AND ELEMENTS INFLUENCING SIZE

Study size is influenced by (a) standard deviation or variability—sample size decreases as SD increases; (b) significance level—as significance level (type I error tolerance) is set at a lower level, the sample size increases; (c) statistical power—as the sample size increases, the power of a study increases and vice versa; and (d) effect size—as the effect size or the absolute value between the null (μ_0) and the alternative mean (μ_1) increases, sample size decreases.

The power of the study is 40% (*STATA output below*), which is insufficient, given the minimum power requirement of 80.0% ($1 - \beta$). The negative result is indicative of the small size of the study, implying that the test lacked the capacity to detect the minimum difference in SBP comparing the mean SBP of African-American women with that of the general US population of women. Using STATA syntax, `sampsi 140 142.2, sd1(5.0) alpha(0.05) n1(10) onesample onesided`, the power of the study is computed as shown in the following.

```
Estimated power for one-sample comparison of mean
to hypothesized value

Test Ho: m =   140, where m is the mean in the population
```

```
Assumptions:

         alpha = 0.0500 (one-sided)
alternative m =      142.2
            sd =      5
sample size n =      10

Estimated power:

         power = 0.4000
```

6.5 Inference from a nonnormal population—One-sample *t* test

6.5.1 What is the nonparametric alternative to the one-sample t *test?*

The sign test, which is a distribution-free significance test, does not require that the data follow any specific type of distribution, such as Gaussian. This statistic tests the hypothesis of the equality of the median since the data may be skewed. The sign test, called *sign* because it depends only on the sign of the differences of the score and not the relative magnitude, is an example of a nonparametric test.

We recap the three scales of measurement of variables in order to discuss very briefly the application of nonparametric tests in hypothesis testing. The scales of measurement in clinical research can be classified into the following categories:

A Cardinal—pertaining to data that are in a scale where it is meaningful to measure the distance between possible data values. These data are measured on interval (with an arbitrary zero point, such as body temperature) or ratio (with a fixed zero point, such as blood pressure, height, weight, etc.) scale. For example, height is a cardinal variable because a difference of 4 m is twice as large as a difference of 2 m.

B Ordinal variables pertain to data that can be ordered but do not have specific numeric values, for example, the quality-of-life score, the pain score, and the functional score used to measure health outcomes. These variables can be measured on a Likert scale using a five-point score system: much satisfied = 1, slightly satisfied = 2, no difference = 3, slightly unsatisfied = 4, and unsatisfied = 5.

C Nominal variables pertain to data that can be classified into categories without any specific ordering, for example, the types of cerebral palsy: hemiplegic, diplegic, and quadriplegic.

Nonparametric statistical tests are used in any of these scales of measurements and are suited for distribution-free data. For example, if the cardinal dat violates the normality assumption and there is uncertainty on the shape of the distribution, nonparametric tests are appropriate. In addition, ordinal data are suited for nonparametric tests, where comparison, for instance, is required between groups with respect to the health outcomes on the quality of life. Finally, nonparametric methods are useful in making comparisons regarding nominal data.

6.5.2 When is the sign test feasible?

If the investigators intended to determine whether the mean reserved O_2 (which correlates with the walking heart rate) at a baseline with the mean reserved O_2 obtained from a previous cohort are different, a one-sample t test is appropriate, provided the data meet the assumptions, namely, they have the right shape of distribution, are derived from a random sample of reasonable sample size ($n \geq 30$), and are measured on a continuous scale. A violation of these assumptions, especially normality, requires the use of a nonparametric test that is equivalent to the one-sample t test, which is the ***sign test***.

6.5.3 How is the sign test applied?

This test utilizes the binomial distribution, which describes a behavior of a count variable X when (a) the number of observations, n, is fixed; (b) each observation is independent; (c) each observation represents one of two outcomes (success or failure); and (d) the probability of success ($\pi = p$) is the same for each outcome. Once these conditions are met, X has a binomial distribution with parameters n and p, denoted as $B(n,p)$.

6.5.4 When is the sign test appropriate?

The sign test is used to test the hypothesis about medians. Using the example with O_2 reserve, the sign test examines whether the median O_2 reserve is equal to the value of the median O_2 reserve obtained previously from the sample.

6.5.5 How is the sign test computed?

Below is the STATA syntax for the computation of a sign test. We are concerned with whether or not the current median score is equal to that obtained previously from the same sample.

STATA Syntax: signtest med_score=6

```
signtest med_score =6

Sign test

          sign|      observed      expected
      positive| 25               21
      negative| 17               21
          zero| 9                9
           all| 51               51

One-sided tests:
Ho: median of med_score - 6 = 0 vs.
Ha: median of med_score - 6 > 0
        Pr(#positive >= 25) =
        Binomial(n = 42, x >= 25, p = 0.5) = 0.1400

Ho: median of med_score - 6 = 0 vs.
Ha: median of med_score - 6 < 0
        Pr(#negative >= 17) =
        Binomial(n = 42, x >= 17, p = 0.5) = 0.9179

Two-sided test:
Ho: median of med_score - 6 = 0 vs.
Ha: median of med_score - 6 != 0
        Pr(#positive >= 25 or #negative >= 25) =
        min(1, 2*Binomial(n = 42, x >= 25, p = 0.5)) = 0.2800
```

6.5.6 *How is the result of a sign test interpreted?*

The sign test, like the *t* test, shows the right-, left-, and two-tailed probabilities. Unlike the *t* test, which uses the symmetrical *t* distribution, the binomial distributions used here in the sign test have different left- and right-tailed probabilities. However, because we are concerned with whether the median of the current sample O_2 reserve differs from the median of the previous sample's O_2 reserve, we are interested in the interpretation of the two-tailed probability. The interpretation of the sign test is similar to the result obtained with the one-sample *t* test. Since p is >0.05 (5%), we have no reason to reject the null hypothesis of no significant median difference comparing the hypothesized median with the sample median.

6.6 Other types of *t* tests

6.6.1 *A paired sample* t *test (dependent* t *test or* t *test for correlated data)*

6.6.1.1 *What is a paired* t *test?*

A paired, correlated data, or dependent *t* test involves a single group or one-sample hypothesis testing and compares the means of two scores from related samples. This is a very popular test when pre- and posttest measures are involved in a study and the scale of measurement is continuous.

6.6.1.2 *What are the assumptions in a paired* t *test?*

The assumptions for a paired *t* test are (a) both variables (pre- and post-test measures) are at interval or ratio scales, (b) both variables are normally distributed, (c) both are measured with the same scale, (d) data collection utilizes the same instrument, and (e) if different scales are involved, the scores are converted to *z* scores before *t* test analysis.

6.6.1.3 *When is the paired* t *test required in hypothesis testing?*

This test is appropriate when the same subjects are measured on a numerical scale and data are obtained before (baseline measure/pretest) and after (postintervention/posttest data) intervention. For example, if an investigator wanted to determine the effect of treatment with drug A in controlling the plasma glucose level in patients with diabetes mellitus and glycosylated hemoglobin (Hb_{A1c}) is measured in the same subject before and after (30 days after treatment), a paired *t* test is appropriate in determining the mean difference (with a higher level indicative of a poorly controlled plasma glucose level).

6.6.1.4 *How is the paired* t *test computed?*

A paired *t* test, as noted earlier, is adequate for studies using paired samples, in which two sets of measurements are taken from the same subjects. This design, in which each subject becomes its own control, eliminates between-subject variability. A study to examine the effect of dopamine in increasing blood pressure in women with low pulse and low blood pressure may use a paired *t*-test technique if there is no control and BP is measured before the administration of dopamine and 12 h after. In this design, factors that influence BP, such as age, diet, and stress, are not expected to influence the posttreatment BP measure dramatically, implying a significant reduction in confounding factors.

We present the formula for the paired *t* test as $t = d/(\text{SD}/\sqrt{n})$, and d is normally distributed with mean Δ and variance σ_d^2. SD is the sample standard deviation, while $d = (d_1 + d_2 + d_3 + \ldots \ldots + d_n)/n$, and di (difference between the baseline or pretest and posttest measure) $= X_{i2} - X_{i1}$. We are simply testing the hypothesis that H_0 $\Delta = 0$ against H_a: $\Delta \neq 0$, implying that if $\Delta > 0$, then treatment with dopamine is associated with increased pulse and BP; if $\Delta < 0$, then dopamine is associated with decreased pulse and BP; and if $\Delta = 0$, then there is no mean difference between baseline and post or follow-up BP.

Vignette 6.5: Consider a study conducted to determine the effect of dopamine in increasing pulse and systolic blood pressure in postmenopausal women, age 55 to 85 years. The baseline SBPs were 115, 104, 105, 126, 138, 115, 119, 107, 112, and 115, while the follow-up SBPs were 117, 102, 109, 132, 145, 122, 128, 106, 115, and 128. If SD is 4.566, calculate the t statistic and state whether or not dopamine increases SBP.

Solution: Substituting in the paired t-test formula above, $t = 4.80/(4.566/\sqrt{10} = 4.80/1.444 = 3.32$. With df = 9, $t = 2.262$, and because $t = 3.32$, thus greater than $t = 2.262$, the null hypothesis of $\Delta = 0$ is rejected with the two-tailed significance test, $\alpha = 0.05$. We can also use STATA to illustrate this computation, using this syntax: `ttest baselinesbp = = followupsbp`.

```
. ttest sbp_bl== sbp_fu

Paired t test
```

Variable	Obs	Mean	Std. Err.	Std. Dev.	[90% Conf.	Interval]
sbp_bl	10	115.6	3.259857	10.30857	108.2257	122.9743
sbp_fu	10	120.4	4.182503	13.22624	110.9385	129.8615
diff	10	-4.8	1.443761	4.565572	-8.066013	-1.533987

```
     mean(diff) = mean(sbp_bl - sbp_fu)                        t = -3.3247
 Ho: mean(diff) = 0                           degrees of freedom =        9

 Ha: mean(diff) < 0       Ha: mean(diff) != 0         Ha: mean(diff) > 0
 Pr(T < t) = 0.0044     Pr(|T| > |t|) = 0.0089      Pr(T > t) =  0.9956
```

The above output shows $t = -3.32$ and the significance level for the null hypothesis, 0.009, which is <0.05, implying that we reject the null hypothesis of no mean difference in SBP comparing baseline to follow-up SBP after dopamine treatment. We can conclude that dopamine significantly increased systolic blood pressure in postmenopausal women.

Next, we present another example of a paired t test using STATA command. The syntax for the paired t test is `ttest varlist1 = varlist2`, where `varlist1` represents the pretest or baseline measure and `varlist2` represents the posttest or postintervention measure utilized.

```
Paired t test
```

Variable	Obs	Mean	Std. Err.	Std. Dev.	[95% Conf.	Interval]
SBP_1	19	115.3158	2.232211	9.72998	110.6261	120.0055
SBP_3	19	120.4737	2.612798	11.38892	114.9844	125.963
diff	19	-5.157895	.912112	3.975804	-7.074171	-3.241619

```
     mean(diff) = mean(SBP_1 - SBP_3)                          t = -5.6549
 Ho: mean(diff) = 0                           degrees of freedom =       18

 Ha: mean(diff) < 0       Ha: mean(diff) != 0         Ha: mean(diff) > 0
 Pr(T < t) = 0.0000     Pr(|T| > |t|) = 0.0000      Pr(T > t) = 1.0000
```

Note: A study (hypothetical) was conducted to determine the effectiveness of a blood pressure medication in lowering blood pressure in 19 subjects. The systolic blood pressure was measured before and after treatment. A paired *t* test showed a statistically significant difference in the mean SBP comparing pretreatment to posttreatment SBP, $p < 0.001$, which means the rejection of the null hypothesis at the significance level of 0.05.

6.6.1.5 What is the nonparametric alternative to parametric paired t *test?*

Nonparametric tests are also referred to as distribution-free or nonnormal statistical inference tests. These tests do not require the assumption of normality or the assumption of homogeneity of variance as in two-sample or independent-sample *t* tests. They compare medians rather than means and therefore are not sensitive to outliers like parametric tests of means. A gross violation of the normality assumption requires the use of these tests (nonparametric) for that reason. However, parametric tests are preferred since they have more statistical power, and with a small sample size, they are able to detect minimal differences in means, for example, and are therefore more likely to result in the rejection of a false null hypothesis, should the sample data lack evidence in support of the null hypothesis. The low statistical power in nonparametric tests is due to the loss of information from the conversion or ordering data from the lowest to the highest value as is used in these nonparametric alternative tests. Because information was collected in a ratio or interval scale, this conversion or ranking leads to the loss of some data, rendering nonparametric tests less statistically powerful relative to parametric tests.

When data violate the normality assumption and information was obtained from the same individual, before (pretest or baseline) and after intervention (postintervention), the *Wilcoxon signed-rank test* is considered appropriate. Therefore, since the *t* test assumes that variables follow a normal distribution, when data involve outliers or are nonnormal because of the small sample, it is appropriate to utilize a median-based test that does not assume normality, such as the Wilcoxon signed-rank test. While the Wilcoxon signed-rank test is the nonparametric alternative to the paired *t* test, the *Wilcoxon rank-sum test* serves as the nonparametric alternative to the two-independent-sample *t* test.

6.6.1.6 How is the Wilcoxon signed-rank test computed?

This test is based on the sum of ranks, hence rank sum. Consider two ointments used as chemoprophylaxis for urticaria: (a) URTI-A and (b) URTI-B. If the effect of these two ointments is measured on a 10-point scale, with 10 being worst and 1 being best outcome of urticaria, can one test the null hypothesis that these two ointments are equally effective?

This test involves (a) ranking the differences between positive and negatives scores of the two ointments for instance, (b) computation of the rank sum of the positive differences, and (c) test computation using the formula (not presented here because of the ease of computing this with statistical software). Statistical software, including STATA, can be used to compute a nonparametric alternative to the paired *t* test. We present an example of the Wilcoxon signed-rank test using STATA here. The Wilcoxon signed-rank test assumes only that the distributions are (a) continuous and (b) symmetrical. Using this test on the same data used for the paired *t* test provides the same result. Since these two tests provide the same result—the statistically significant effect of the treatment in lowering systolic blood pressure—we can assert the conclusion with more certainty.

```
STATA syntax:  signrank sbp3=sbp1
signrank sbp3=  sbp1

Wilcoxon signed-rank test
             sign | obs      sum ranks        expected
------------------+-----------------------------------
         positive | 0        0                95
         negative | 19       190              95
             zero | 0        0                0
------------------+-----------------------------------
              all | 19       190              190

unadjusted variance          617.50
adjustment for ties          -0.38
adjustment for zeros         0.00
                    ---------
adjusted variance            617.13
Ho: sbp3 = sbp1
       z = -3.824
  Prob > |z|  = 0.0001
```

6.6.2 *One-sample analysis of variance*

This method assumes normal distribution, implying a known shape of the distribution, thus supporting the use of a parametric test, such as analysis of variance (ANOVA). A commonly used example is the repeated-measure ANOVA.

6.6.2.1 *What is repeated-measure ANOVA?*

This test statistic compares how a within-subjects treatment or experimental group performs in three or more experimental settings.[12] It therefore compares whether the mean of any of the individual settings (measurement cycle) differs significantly from the aggregate mean across the treatment setting or conditions.

6.6.2.2 When is repeated-measure ANOVA used as a test statistic?

As noted earlier, in this statistical method, each subject serves as its own control. The subjects are measured to obtain the baseline data as a preintervention measure, and then after an intervention (surgery, medication, education session) or at a later time (during the follow-up period), the subjects are measured again (postintervention measures). This design is appropriate in assessing the effectiveness of an intervention since it controls for extraneous factors that might influence the results if the control group was selected from the source population. Such selection may introduce selection bias into the study, thus compromising the internal validity of the study. Therefore, any differences caused by the treatment may not be influenced by, or masked by, the differences among the study subjects themselves.

6.6.2.3 When is repeated-measure ANOVA appropriate?

The one-way repeated-measure ANOVA is appropriate if (a) the dependent variable is measured on a continuous scale, (b) the dependent variable follows a normal distribution (with a central theorem assumption, $n > 30$ follows a normal distribution), and (c) the independent variable, experimental setting, or condition has three or more categories. For example, a study was conducted to determine the effectiveness of titanium instrumentation in correcting and maintaining correction for curve deformities in adolescent idiopathic scoliosis; if investigators intended to have no control group but to utilize repeat measures of thoracolumbar and thoracic curves during the preoperative (baseline measure establishment) and immediate postoperative periods (6 months, 12 months, and 24 months, measured on a continuous scale—curve angle), with sample size (n) = 41 (assumption of normal distribution), then the repeated-measure ANOVA is an appropriate test statistic.

6.6.2.4 How is the result in repeated-measure ANOVA interpreted?

The effectiveness of instrumentation is demonstrated by the mean curve angles, SD, degrees of freedom, F value (a statistical test for comparing two variances), and the significance level (p value). The model p value is indicative of either acceptance or rejection of the null hypothesis should there occur a large deviation from the mean of any of the three means for instance. It does not, however, illustrate where the large mean difference or statistically significant mean difference occurs. In order to examine in which measurement cycle the significant differences occur, a pairwise multiple comparison is recommended. An example of post hoc or posteriori multiple comparison is that of Bonferroni. This method increases the critical F value (follows F distribution, which is the probability distribution used to test the equality of two estimates needed for the comparison to be accepted as significant). This adjustment depends on (a) the number of comparison, a multiplier that is based on the level of treatment and the degree of freedom, and (b) sample size, an increase implies a higher power, meaning that the null hypothesis is correctly rejected more often than not. Some statisticians prefer to use Tukey's HSD (honestly significant difference) procedure, while others prefer Scheffe's and Dunnett's procedures. Most statistical software today has all these procedures for pairwise comparison, allowing one to select from the menu. We also recommend the use of box plot to examine these mean differences while considering the model p value and a meaningful interpretation of the result.

6.6.2.5 What is the nonparametric equivalent of one-way repeated-measure ANOVA?

The *Friedman test* by ranks is the alternative of the one-way repeated-measure ANOVA.[12] This test does not require the dependent variable to follow a normal distribution and therefore suits the nonparametric method for nonnormal statistical inference. Since this is nonparametric and hence less efficient compared to its parametric counterpart, repeated-measure ANOVA, a larger sample size is required to detect the different or effectiveness in treatment should one really exist. The investigators using this test should ensure that there is an adequate sample (increase power) and hence increase the ability of the study to determine the effectiveness of treatment if it really exists.

The SPSS output of the Friedman nonparametric test for repeated measures given in Table 6.1 is a result of the preoperative and the 3-year and 10-year follow-up of children with cerebral palsy who were diagnosed with stiff knee and treated for the disease with rectus femoris transfer surgery. The toe drag was used to measure the outcome of surgery as an improvement. And since this measure was nonnumeric, measured on a discrete binary scale (nominal scale), a repeated-measure ANOVA was inappropriate in testing the hypothesis of at least one difference in the variance comparing the three variances (baseline, 3 years, and 10 years). The preceding table only presents a subgroup of the patients in this study, $n = 12$, with TD0 and the baseline, preoperative toe drag, TD1 for 3 years postoperative, and

Table 6.1 The effect of rectus femoris transfer in reducing toe drag in children with stiff knee gait

Variable	*Mean rank*	*Chi-square (df)*	*n*	*p*
		19.42	12	<0.0001
Toe drag = 0	2.83			
Toe drag = 1	1.54			
Toe drag = 2	1.63			

Notes: Friedman Test, non-parametric alternative to repeated measure ANOVA.
Abbreviations: TD, toe drag; 0 = preoperative, 1 = 3 years postoperative, and 2 = 10-year follow-up.

TD2 for the 10 years postoperative toe drag. The chi-square value, 19.42; degree of freedom, 2; and the *p* value, <0.0001 are indicative of a significant reduction in toe drag comparing baseline toe drag to the postoperative toe drag.

6.7 Summary

One-sample hypothesis testing is used to examine inference in normal and nonnormal or distribution-free random variables. Such tests are used in study designs in which the same patient is observed repeatedly over time or data are acquired before and after an intervention. In this context, we seek to make inferences about individuals in the target population who are treated in the same way as the sample studied.

The choice of a test statistic depends on (a) distribution and (b) scale of measurement of the variables of interest. In any case, the application of inference assumes that the variables are random. The assumption of distribution, that is, normally distributed data that are symmetric and bell curve–shaped, favors the use of parametric inferential tests, while the distribution-free data are used to demonstrate the comparison between measurements with the less powerful or effective nonparametric tests. The scales of measurement used in clinical research are (a) cardinal—interval and ratio scales, (b) ordinal, and (c) nominal. The parametric inference is applied to cardinal data, and the violation of normality of the cardinal data suggests the use of a nonparametric alternative in this circumstance. Because both ordinal and nominal data are nonnormal, parametric tests are adequate in making inferences about them.

With one-sample hypothesis testing, the mean difference comparing the population to the sample mean can be achieved using a one-sample *t* test (Figures 6.2 and 6.3). And if the normality assumption is violated or the data are ordinal, the sign test remains the nonparametric equivalent. A paired, correlated data, matched, or dependent *t* test is used when data are collected from the same subjects more than once, as illustrated in test and retest, pretest and posttest, preoperative and postoperative measures. The appropriate assumptions for the use of this statistic must be met: (a) random sample implying that a simple random sample from the population was chosen with a known sampling probability, (b) normality assumption, and (c) cardinal scale of measurement. The violation of normality requires the use of the nonparametric alternative, the Wilcoxon signed-rank test, and not the Wilcoxon rank-sum test, as it is commonly erroneously used interchangeably.

A repeated-measure ANOVA is another parametric test used in hypothesis testing involving one sample. This test is necessary when measurements are taken more than twice from the same subject. A paired *t* test is inappropriate when repeated measures are more than two in the study design. The violation of the normality assumption or when data are collected on an ordinal scale suggests the use of the nonparametric equivalent, the Friedman test for repeated-measure ANOVA.

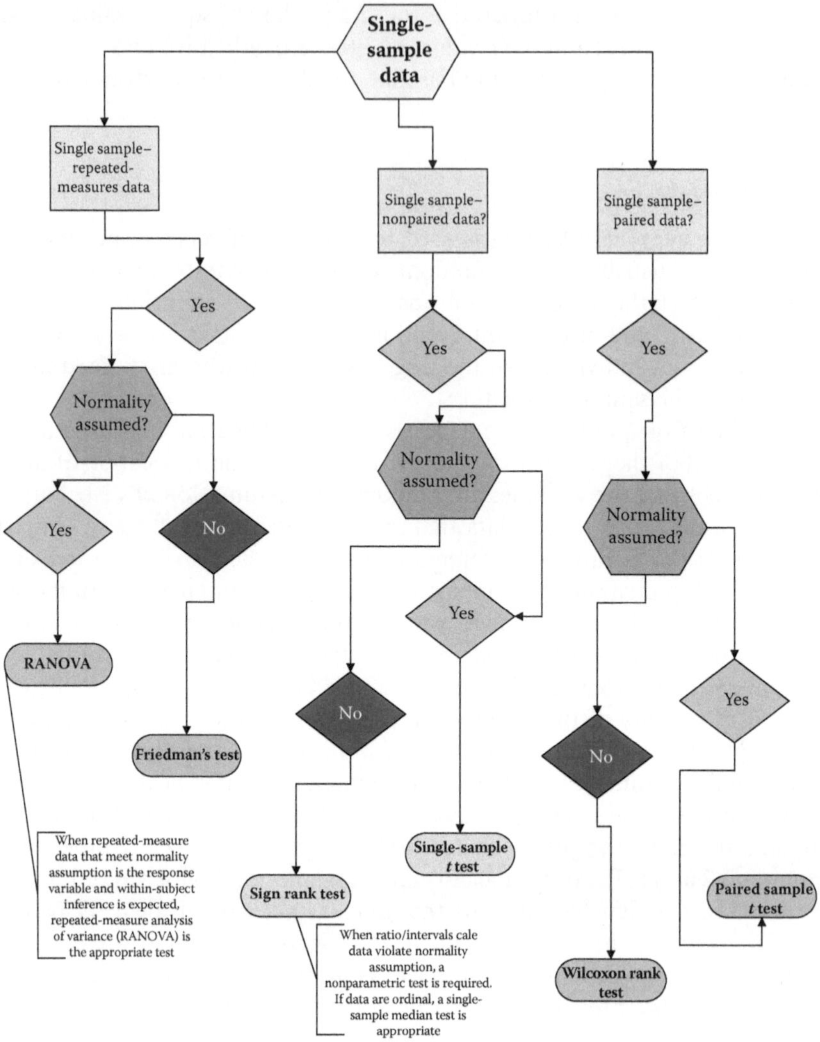

Figure 6.2 Selection of statistical test for one-sample data.

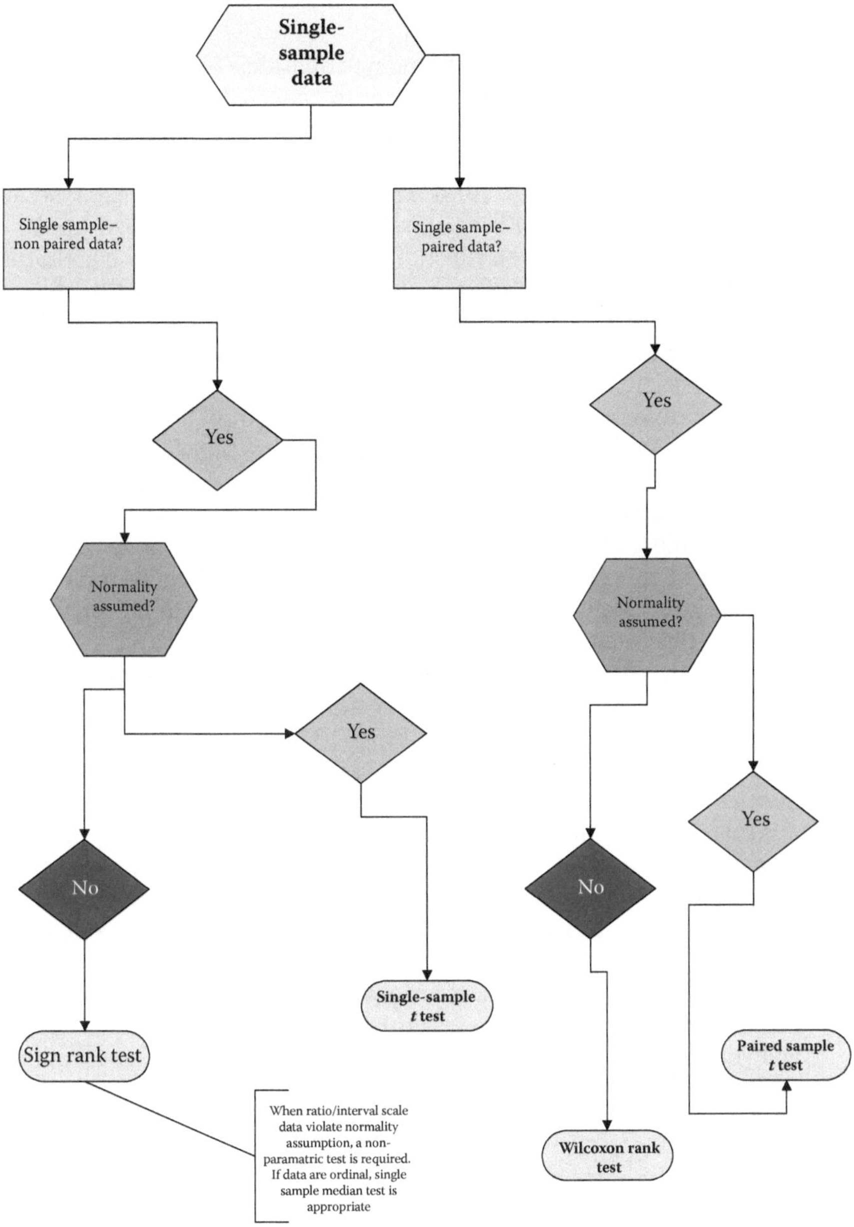

Figure 6.3 One-sample hypothesis testing.

Questions for discussion

1 Sodium restriction favorably affects hypertension. To test the effect of dietary sodium restriction, 12 men were observed for 1 month. The baseline systolic blood pressures were obtained: 117.3, 111.3, 117.4, 122.8, 126.4, 115.8, 133.3, 96.2, 109.9, 123.6, 100.0, and 119.7, while the follow-up SBPs were 108.4, 107.0, 110.4, 126.3, 121.6, 113.2, 128.9, 95.7, 107.7, 123.8, 98.8, and 117.3. Examine the baseline and follow-up data for possible inference on the effect of dietary sodium restriction and SBP lowering. (a) Which test is adequate for the comparison of the SBP difference? (b) Using preferred statistical software, compute the test. (c) What can be concluded based on this evidence regarding the effect of dietary sodium restriction on SBP?

2 The mean duration of hospital stay tends to vary from hospital to hospital given the same diagnosis. Below is the duration of stay of 10 patients in a hospital after diagnosis for chronic bronchitis: 3, 17, 11, 30, 14, 5, 11, 6, 10, and 5 days. If the mean population of hospital stay is 10.0 days and the standard deviation is 2.3 days, determine whether or not the hospital stay of this sample differs from the population mean hospital stay. (a) Which test statistic will be appropriate? (b) What can be concluded based on the evidence from the data?

3 Below are the data on the white blood cells ($\times 10^3$) of 16 patients admitted to the pulmonary and allergy department of a comprehensive treatment center in Nocity: 8, 5, 12, 4, 11, 6, 8, 7, 7, 12, 7, 3, 11, 14, 11, and 9. If white blood cells are known not to be normally distributed in the population, using the appropriate test statistic, determine if the WBC count in this sample differs from that of the population if the population estimate is said to be 7.0×10^3. Second, what can be concluded from these data regarding the WBC counts of this sample relative to the population?

4 Suppose you are to conduct a study on the effectiveness and safety of titanium instrumentation in correcting and maintaining correction of scoliosis in adolescent idiopathic scoliosis, and there are four measurements of main curve during a 2-year follow-up period. (a) Which design will you consider to be appropriate in this study? (b) What assumptions will you consider in the selection of the test statistic for the inference? (c) What distribution will you assume, and how will you interpret the critical value obtained from this test? (d) State the null hypothesis and discuss its rejection and acceptance of the alternate hypothesis.

References

1. D. G. Altman, *Practical Statistics for Medical Research* (London: Chapman & Hall, 1991); P. Armitage and G. Berry, *Statistical Methods in Medical Research*, 3rd ed. (Oxford, UK: Blackwell Scientific Publishing, 1994); B. Rosner,

Fundamentals of Biostatistics, 5th ed. (CA: Duxbury Press: 2000); J. A. Freiman et al., The importance of beta, the type II error and sample size in the design and interpretation of the randomized clinical trial, *N Engl J Med* 299 (1978):690–694.

2. J. A. Freiman et al., The importance of beta, the type II error and sample size in the design and interpretation of the randomized clinical trial, *N Engl J Med* 299 (1978):690–694; W. D. Dupont, *Statistical Modeling for Biomedical Researchers* (Cambridge, UK: Cambridge University Press, 2003).
3. J. A. Freiman et al., The importance of beta, the type II error and sample size in the design and interpretation of the randomized clinical trial, *N Engl J Med* 299 (1978):690–694; W. D. Dupont, *Statistical Modeling for Biomedical Researchers* (Cambridge, UK: Cambridge University Press, 2003); B. Dawson-Saunders and R. G. Trap, *Basic and Clinical Biostatistics*, 2nd ed. (Norwalk, CT: Appleton & Lange, 1994); T. D. V. Swinscow and M. J. Campbell, *Statistics at Square One*, 10th ed. (Spain: BMJ Books, 2002).
4. W. D. Dupont, *Statistical Modeling for Biomedical Researchers* (Cambridge, UK: Cambridge University Press, 2003).
5. W. D. Dupont, *Statistical Modeling for Biomedical Researchers* (Cambridge, UK: Cambridge University Press, 2003); B. Dawson-Saunders and R. G. Trap, *Basic and Clinical Biostatistics*, 2nd ed. (Norwalk, CT: Appleton & Lange, 1994); T. D. V. Swinscow and M. J. Campbell, *Statistics at Square One*, 10th ed. (Spain: BMJ Books, 2002); T. D. V. Swinscow and M. J. Campbell, *Statistics at Square One*, 10th ed. (Spain: BMJ Books, 2002).
6. W. D. Dupont, *Statistical Modeling for Biomedical Researchers* (Cambridge, UK: Cambridge University Press, 2003); B. Dawson-Saunders and R. G. Trap, *Basic and Clinical Biostatistics*, 2nd ed. (Norwalk, CT: Appleton & Lange, 1994); T. D. V. Swinscow and M. J. Campbell, *Statistics at Square One*, 10th ed. (Spain: BMJ Books, 2002); D. A. Freedman et al., *Statistics*, 4th ed. (New York: Norton, 2007).
7. T. Colton, *Statistics in Medicine* (New York: Little, Brown and Company, 1974).
8. B. Dawson-Saunders and R. G. Trap, *Basic and Clinical Biostatistics*, 2nd ed. (Norwalk, CT: Appleton & Lange, 1994); T. D. V. Swinscow and M. J. Campbell, *Statistics at Square One*, 10th ed. (Spain: BMJ Books, 2002); H. A. Khan and C. T. Sempos, *Statistical Methods in Epidemiology* (New York: Oxford University Press, 1989).
9. B. Dawson-Saunders and R. G. Trap, *Basic and Clinical Biostatistics*, 2nd ed. (Norwalk, CT: Appleton & Lange, 1994); H. A. Khan and C. T. Sempos, *Statistical Methods in Epidemiology* (New York: Oxford University Press, 1989).
10. B. Dawson-Saunders and R. G. Trap, *Basic and Clinical Biostatistics*, 2nd ed. (Norwalk, CT: Appleton & Lange, 1994); T. D. V. Swinscow and M. J. Campbell, *Statistics at Square One*, 10th ed. (Spain: BMJ Books, 2002).
11. B. J. Winer, *Statistical Principles in Experimental Designs*, 2nd ed. (New York: McGraw-Hill, 1971).
12. B. Dawson-Saunders and R. G. Trap, *Basic and Clinical Biostatistics*, 2nd ed. (Norwalk, CT: Appleton & Lange, 1994); B. J. Winer, *Statistical Principles in Experimental Designs*, 2nd ed. (New York: McGraw-Hill, 1971).

7 Two independent samples statistical inference

7.1 Introduction

In clinical research, two-sample hypothesis testing is more frequently used relative to one-sample hypothesis testing. In this statistical inference, the underlying parameters of two different populations are compared but the parameters are not assumed to be known, as observed in one-sample *t* test for example. We discussed in previous chapters hypothesis testing when a single or one sample is involved. Specifically, we compared the parameters of the population from which the sample was drawn with that of the larger population, whose parameters were assumed to be known. To recap, single-group hypothesis testing provides an estimation of the proportion (binary or categorical measures), mean (continuous scale variable), or a comparison of the observed continuous or ordered/ranked values to a norm or standard. For example, a one-sample hypothesis testing is appropriate in comparing the mean weight of children (0 to 19 years old) with leukemia with that of same age children in the United States (values of US children 0 to 19 years assumed to be known). Also, when a single group is measured twice (paired sample) or more (repeated measures), which allows us to estimate how much the proportion or mean in the single group changes between measurements, a single-sample hypothesis testing technique is used.

Two independent groups hypothesis testing involves the comparison of means or proportion in two independent groups.[1] Independent groups refer to groups in which information obtained from one is not influenced or dependent on the observation or information from the other.[2] In addition, this hypothesis testing assumes that the groups represent random samples (each study sample with equal chance of being selected from the larger population into the study population or sample) from a larger population in which statistical inference could be drawn.

This chapter presents the rationale and assumptions and study designs suitable for the application of two-sample or independent-sample (when data points in one sample are unrelated to the data points in the second sample) hypothesis testing and examples of hypothesis testing techniques as statistical methods in two-sample statistical inference. A simplified approach is taken in presenting these techniques: when, where, why, and how these tests are used.

Clinical examples and the study design used are presented with the analysis of the inference using the STATA statistical package example.

7.1.1 *What are the examples of two-sample hypothesis tests?*

Two independent groups hypothesis testing involves the use of two-sample or independent sample *t* tests (test the null hypothesis of no mean difference—equality of means) when observations are (a) numerical, meaning that the variables are measured on either an interval or ratio scale—continuous; (b) normality is assumed; and (c) the intent of investigators is to determine whether or not the two means are significantly different. For example, in a retrospective cohort study conducted to examine the risk associated with post-operative pancreatitis, the mean estimated blood loss was compared between cases and noncases using a two-sample *t* test. A nonparametric alternative to the two sample *t* test is the Mann Whitney *U* test despite the fact that the two tests are similar, which is appropriate when (a) the normality assumption of the two-sample *t* test is violated, (b) data are measured on an ordinal scale, and (c) there is a small study sample (small study sizes are more likely to be skewed, thus violating the normality assumption). A *z* distribution can be used to test proportions involving independent groups, as well as a chi-square statistic and Fisher's exact test when the sample sizes are not large, as seen in small, expected, and not observed cell frequency. A disadvantage of the chi-square test is its inability to form a confidence interval, hence dichotomous significance tests (rejection or nonrejection of the null hypothesis of no difference).

7.2 Independent (two-sample) *t* test and nonparametric alternative (Mann–Whitney *u* test)

If a study is conducted using a longitudinal or follow-up design to determine the effect of calcium supplement intake on prostate cancer incidence, will a two-sample *t* test or paired *t* test be adequate in assessing the mean prostate-specific antigen (PSA), assuming the same cohort is measured at baseline and followed for 20 months? The investigators identified a group of older men (65 and older) who were not currently on supplement calcium intake, measured their PSAs, followed them for 24 months and ascertained a subgroup of men who had become calcium supplement users and measured their PSA. Again, is a two-sample test or a paired *t* test an appropriate statistical inference in concluding that calcium is associated or not with prostate cancer risk (PSA as end point)?

Whenever a research question involves the comparison of means in two separate groups, a *t* test for two independent groups is appropriate, and it is widely used in clinical research. In fact, the *t* test or Student's *t* test is the most commonly used statistical technique in clinical research, though it is often erroneously used by researchers. For example, investigators comparing means between three independent samples sometimes use the *t* test by comparing the interventions to the control in a pairwise comparison manner. This approach is inappropriate and should be discouraged. However, if the population standard deviation is known, which is highly unlikely, a z test is equally suitable in testing a hypothesis involving two independent means. Therefore, it is unusual to know the true standard deviation of the target population, but the population standard deviation (σ) termed the *parameter (unknown attributes of the target population)* can be estimated by the sample standard deviation, S, termed *statistic (functions of values in the sample)*, and $(x - \mu)/(S/\sqrt{n})$ has a completely specified distribution, which is a t distribution.[3] This distribution as discussed earlier belongs to the family of bell-shaped distributions, which are symmetric about zero. And t = *difference in sample means/standard error of difference of sample means*. Mathematically, the t statistic ($t_n - 1$) is given as follows:

$$t \text{ statistic} = (x - \mu)/(S/\sqrt{n})$$

and has a t distribution with $n - 1$ degrees of freedom. In comparison to z distribution (discussed earlier as well), the S of a t statistic is greater than that of a standard normal distribution as a result of imprecision in S as an estimate of σ. However, as sample size increases, S becomes a more and more accurate estimate of σ and $t_n - 1$ (t statistic) approaches z statistic (standard normal distribution).[4] We can recall that as sample size increases, we are more confident in the estimates of the population mean, implying that the observed differences between the two samples' means is not due solely to random sampling. In other words, the increase in sample size leads to a reduction in the uncertainty of the estimate of the true population mean as obtained from the sample (standard error): ↑ sample size →↓ standard error of the mean. The SE (standard error) = $\sigma/\sqrt{n}$, where σ is the standard deviation of the population being the source of the sample and n is the size of the study. Likewise, the increase in sample size implies the decrease in the uncertainty in the estimate of the differences of the means between the two independent samples relative to the differences of the means.

The Mann–Whitney U test is a nonparametrize equivalent to independent sample t text. The notion of nonparametric is a misnomer since all statistical test of hypothesis draw inference from the sample data (statistic) to compare with the population parameter. Specifically all hypothesis tests are parametric, implying that a clear and meaningful distinction in statistics should be between parametric as probability distribution-based, and distribution-free (non-shape) based data as parametric and nonparametric, respectively.

7.2.1 Terms explanation

Independent sample refers to the notion that the observations (values/data) from one group do not provide any information about the observations in the second group. For example, if investigators intended to examine the mean differences in age of African-American women and Caucasian women diagnosed with breast cancer in the Surveillance Epidemiology and End Results

(SEER) database of the National Cancer Institute (NCI), the observations on age for African-American women with breast cancer must not provide any information about the observation on the age of Caucasian women diagnosed with breast cancer, in order for the two groups or samples to be termed independent. Graphically, error bars can be used to compare the means of two or more independent groups. This method is fairly accurate when there are relatively large sample sizes, so that $n > 10$ in each sample.[5] However, caution is required in the interpretation of error bars, since the selected standard errors for the graph must consider the sample size. As a rule, when $n > 10$, the 95% CI = mean ± 2SE or 2SD (if data are normally distributed). In terms of the interpretation, whenever there is no overlap between the top of one error bar with the bottom of the other bar, one can be 95% confident or sure that the means in the two groups are significantly different.[6]

7.2.2 *Independent/two-sample* t *test*

7.2.2.1 *What is an independent (two-sample)* t *test?*

A *t* test is a test statistic to examine the null hypothesis of no mean difference in two groups or independent samples when the population standard deviation is unknown, which is the case in clinical research. To examine this hypothesis, the test statistic considers (a) the difference in sample means and (b) the standard error of difference of the sample. Simply, t = difference in sample means/the standard error of the difference of sample means.

7.2.2.2 *When is the independent or two-sample* t *test appropriate?*

An independent *t* test is adequate if a study is conducted to determine the mean differences between two groups and the two groups are said to be independent. For example, consider a retrospective cohort study conducted to examine the factors related to deep wound infection after posterior spine fusion in children with neuromuscular scoliosis in which the age at surgery was a potential predictor variable. Since cases were independent from noncases, a two-sample *t* test was appropriate in determining the mean age at walking between cases and noncases.

7.2.2.3 *What are the assumptions of the independent* t *test?*

An independent samples t *test* compares the means of two samples, with the assumptions that (a) the two groups being compared should be independent of each other, (b) the scores should be normally distributed, (c) dependency must be measured on an interval or ratio scale, (d) the independent samples should have only two discrete levels, and (e) the assumption of equal standard deviations or variance, termed *homogeneous variance*. The assumption of equality of variance could be ignored given the equality of the sample sizes. However, it is essential to test and examine whether or not SDs are similar or equal. If the SDs are not equal, a special *t* test—*t* test with unequal variance—should be used. Using the unequal variance test will adjust the degrees of freedom downward, which renders the null hypothesis more difficult to reject if indeed the null hypothesis of no difference in the two means is true. The independent *t* test is robust to normality, and its violation may not necessarily imply not computing a *t* test. However, this violation may produce a *p* value that is lower than expected, implying a rejection of the null hypothesis of no difference when indeed the null hypothesis is true (no difference between the two means compared).

7.2.2.4 How is the independent t *test computed?*

The intent of the two-sample *t* test computation is to compare the relative magnitude of the differences in the sample means with the amount of variability that would be expected. With the null hypothesis of no difference in mean, the two-sample *t* test is computed by using the formula: $t_{(n1+n2-2)} = (X_1 - X_2)/\text{SD}_\text{p}\sqrt{[(1/n_1)+(1/n_2)]}$, where $(n1 - 1) + (n2 - 1)$ represents the degree of freedom $(_{n1+n2-2})$ and SD_p is the pool standard deviation. Simply, *t* = difference of sample means/standard error of difference of sample means, implying mathematically: $t = X_1 - X_2/\sqrt{S^2x_1 + S^2x_2}$, and in terms of sample standard deviation, $t = X_1 - X_2/\sqrt{S_1^2/n + S_2^2/n}$. Because *t* is a ratio, the smaller the value, the less likely it is that both samples were drawn from a single population (statistically insignificant mean difference). In contrast, the larger the ratio, the more unlikely it is that the samples were drawn from a single population (statistically significant mean difference).

To compute the independent *t* test using STATA, the syntax is `ttest` *y*, by (*x*), or ttest *y*, by (*x*) unequal (where equal variance is not assumed). This syntax performs a two-sample *t* test of the null hypothesis that the population mean of *y* is the same for both categories of variable *x*. Using the sample data from the deep wound infection after posterior spine fusion study, the two-sample *t* test for the age at surgery between cases and noncases was computed as follows:

```
ttest   ageatsurgery,by  (deepwound_infeect)
Two-sample t test with equal variances
```

Group	Obs	Mean	Std. Err.	Std. Dev.	[95% Conf.	Interval]
0	214	**13.86916**	.2348174	**3.435083**	13.4063	14.33202
1	22	**13.94545**	.669358	**3.139567**	12.55345	15.33746
combined	236	13.87627	.2214786	3.402419	13.43993	14.31261
diff		**-.0762957**	**.7633827**		**-1.580277**	**1.427685**

```
    diff = mean(0) - mean(1)                              t =  -0.0999
Ho: diff = 0                             degrees of freedom =      234

    Ha: diff < 0              Ha: diff != 0              Ha: diff > 0
 Pr(T < t) = 0.4602     Pr(|T| > |t|) = 0.9205      Pr(T > t) = 0.5398
```

Note: Data used with permission from the investigative team including the author (LH).

A study on insulin insensitivity on women with hyperthyroidism compared the insulin level among normal and overweight patients (hypothetical). An independent sample *t* test was used to determine the exposure effect of weight in these independent samples (normal versus overweight). The assessment of the effect of weight requires exploratory analysis and visualization of the data.

```
. tabstat  Ins_sen, stat (mean, sd, variance, n)

    variable |      mean          sd    variance         N
-------------+--------------------------------------------
     Ins sen |  .3829286    .2739265    .0750357       112
----------------------------------------------------------

. tabstat Ins_sen, stat (mean, sd, variance, n) by ( Weight)

Summary for variables: Ins_sen
     by categories of: Weight

     Weight |      mean          sd    variance         N
------------+--------------------------------------------
          1 |       .55    .2423169    .0587175        64
          2 |  .1601667    .0990859     .009818        48
------------+--------------------------------------------
      Total |  .3829286    .2739265    .0750357       112
---------------------------------------------------------


. ttest  Ins_sen,  by  ( Weight)

Two-sample t test with equal variances
------------------------------------------------------------------------------
   Group |     Obs        Mean    Std. Err.   Std. Dev.   [95% Conf. Interval]
---------+--------------------------------------------------------------------
       1 |      64         .55    .0302896    .2423169    .4894711     .610529
       2 |      48    .1601667    .0143018    .0990859    .1313951    .1889382
---------+--------------------------------------------------------------------
combined |     112    .3829286    .0258836    .2739265    .3316384    .4342187
---------+--------------------------------------------------------------------
    diff |            .3898333    .0371349                .3162407     .463426
------------------------------------------------------------------------------
    diff = mean(1) - mean(2)                                      t =  10.4978
Ho: diff = 0                                     degrees of freedom =      110

    Ha: diff < 0                 Ha: diff != 0                 Ha: diff > 0
 Pr(T < t) = 1.0000         Pr(|T| > |t|) = 0.0000          Pr(T > t) = 0.0000

. ttest  Ins_sen,  by  ( Weight)  unequal

Two-sample t test with equal variances
------------------------------------------------------------------------------
   Group |     Obs        Mean    Std. Err.   Std. Dev.   [95% Conf. Interval]
---------+--------------------------------------------------------------------
       1 |      64         .55    .0302896    .2423169    .4894711     .610529
       2 |      48    .1601667    .0143018    .0990859    .1313951    .1889382
---------+--------------------------------------------------------------------
combined |     112    .3829286    .0258836    .2739265    .3316384    .4342187
---------+--------------------------------------------------------------------
    diff |            .3898333    .0334963                  .32327    .4563967
------------------------------------------------------------------------------
    diff = mean(1) - mean(2)                                      t =  11.6381
Ho: diff = 0                     Satterthwaite's degrees of freedom =  88.3369

    Ha: diff < 0                 Ha: diff ! = 0                 Ha: diff > 0
 Pr(T < t) = 1.0000         Pr(|T| > |t|) = 0.0000          Pr(T > t) = 0.0000
.
```

```
. tabstat le, stat (mean sd, var sem p50 iqr range min max n)

variable |     mean        sd  variance  se(mean)  p50       iqr  range   min   max    N
---------+-------------------------------------------------------------------------------
      le | 30.67667 3.945451  15.56658   .272262  30.7  5.899998   15.1  23.4  38.5  210
-----------------------------------------------------------------------------------------

. tabstat  le , stat (mean sd, var sem p50 iqr range min max n) by ( race)

Summary for variables: le
     by categories of: race

   race |     mean         sd  variance  se(mean)    p5       iqr  range   min   max    N
--------+--------------------------------------------------------------------------------
      1 | 28.77333  3.416399  11.67178  .3334064  28.7  6.299999     11  23.4  34.4  105
      2 |    32.58  3.506571  12.29604  .3422063  32.2  6.200001   11.6  26.9  38.5  105
--------+--------------------------------------------------------------------------------
  Total | 30.67667  3.945451  15.56658   .272262  30.7  5.899998   15.1  23.4  38.5  210
-----------------------------------------------------------------------------------------
```

The above test assumes unequal variance in the two groups (cases and noncases). Likewise, there is a difference in the sample size of the two samples (22 for cases and 214 for noncases). Assuming unequal standard deviations in the two groups, the STATA syntax is `ttest ageatsurgery,by (deepwound_infeect)unequal`. The inclusion of `unequal` in this syntax causes the Satterthwaite's test for groups with unequal variance to be computed. As indicated in the following, the standard deviations in the cases and noncases are not very similar, and the sample sizes are not equal; it is unlikely that this test provides similar results to the test above that assumes equal variance. Since the degrees of freedom substantially differ when unequal variance is assumed and in our case the absolute value of the t statistic changed from 0.099 to 0.107, in this example, the loss in statistical power due to not assuming equal variance is consequential.[7]

Vignette 7.1: Assuming the life expectancy (le) at 40, 41, 42, 43, 44, 45, 46, 47, 48, 49, 50, 51, 52, 53, and 54 is 38.5, 37.6, 36.7, 35.7, 34.8, 33.9, 33.0, 32.1, 31.2, 30.3, 29.5, 28.6, 27.7, 26.9, and 26.0 for Caucasian females and 34.4, 33.6, 32.7, 31.9, 31.1, 30.3, 29.5, 28.7, 27.9, 27.1, 26.4, 25.6, 24.9, 24.1, and 23.4 for African-American females in the United States, (a) is there any difference in the mean life expectancy between white and black women, age 40 to 54? (b) What evidence can be drawn from these data regarding ethnic/racial disparities in life expectancy among US females?

Solution: Using STATA, the two-sample t test is computed with the output below:

7.2.2.5 Independent sample t *test*

```
. ttest  le, by ( race)

Two-sample t test with equal variances
```

Group	Obs	Mean	Std. Err.	Std. Dev.	[95% Conf.	Interval]
1	105	28.77333	.3334064	3.416399	28.11218	29.43449
2	105	32.58	.3422063	3.506571	31.90139	33.25861
combined	210	30.67667	.272262	3.945451	30.13994	31.2134
diff		-3.806667	.4777708		-4.748561	-2.864773

```
    diff = mean(1) - mean(2)                                      t =  -7.9676
Ho: diff = 0                                     degrees of freedom =      208

    Ha: diff < 0                 Ha: diff != 0                 Ha: diff > 0
 Pr(T < t) = 0.0000         Pr(|T| > |t|) = 0.0000          Pr(T > t) = 1.0000
```

```
. ttest  le, by ( race) unequal

Two-sample t test with equal variances
```

Group	Obs	Mean	Std. Err.	Std. Dev.	[95% Conf.	Interval]
1	105	28.77333	.3334064	3.416399	28.11218	29.43449
2	105	32.58	.3422063	3.506571	31.90139	33.25861
combined	210	30.67667	.272262	3.945451	30.13994	31.2134
diff		-3.806667	.4777708		-4.748564	-2.864769

```
    diff = mean(1) - mean(2)                                      t =  -7.9676
Ho: diff = 0                     Satterthwaite's degrees of freedom =  207.859

    Ha: diff < 0                 Ha: diff != 0                 Ha: diff > 0
 Pr(T < t) = 0.0000         Pr(|T| > |t|) = 0.0000          Pr(T > t) = 1.0000
```

The output above indicates the difference in the mean life expectancy for two independent samples of US women, age 40 to 54. African-American women (2) had a mean life expectancy of 28.8 years for women aged 40 to 54, while Caucasian women had a 32.17-year life expectancy for the same period. The data support the evidence that Caucasian women are more likely to live longer than African-American women (the null hypothesis of no mean life expectancy difference is rejected, $p = 0.019$).

```
ttest LExpect, by(race) unequal

Two-sample t test with unequal variances
```

Group	Obs	Mean	Std. Err.	Std. Dev.	[95% Conf.	Interval]
1	15	32.16667	1.031119	3.993507	29.95514	34.3782
2	15	28.77333	0.9087127	3.519429	26.82434	30.72233
combined	30	30.47	0.7451321	4.081257	28.94603	31.99397

```
diff = mean(1) - mean(2)   t = 2.4690
H0: diff = 0      Satterthwaite's degrees of freedom = 27.5645

Ha: diff < 0               Ha: diff != 0                 Ha: diff > 0
Pr(T < t) = 0.9900         Pr(|T| > |t|) = 0.0200        Pr(T > t) = 0.0100
```

The unequal variance output does not seem to vary from the equal variance test computed above in terms of the statistical stability ($p = 0.02$), which indicates an inclination to accept the equal variance result as inconsequential.

7.2.3 Test of the equality of variance

The Levene test for equal variances is often recommended and is adequate in testing the equality of variances even when more than two groups are involved. However, one must be careful in interpreting this test since the Levene test is strictly a test of the absolute value of the distance each observation is from the mean in that group, thus testing the hypothesis that the average deviations from the mean in each group are similar in the two samples or groups. A statistically significant result of the Levene test of equality of variance implies that, on average, the deviations from the mean in one group are greater than those in the other group or sample.

```
. tabstat  le , stat  (mean sd, var sem p50 iqr range min max n) by ( race)

Summary for variables: le
     by categories of: race
```

race	mean	sd	variance	se(mean)	p50	iqr	range	min	max	N
1	28.77333	3.519429	12.38638	.9087127	28.7	6.299999	11	23.4	34.4	15
2	32.58	3.61232	13.04886	.932697	32.2	6.200001	11.6	26.9	38.5	15
Total	30.67667	4.003333	16.02668	.7309053	30.7	5.899998	15.1	23.4	38.5	30

```
. ttest  le, by ( race)

Two-sample t test with equal variances
```

Group	Obs	Mean	Std. Err.	Std. Dev.	[95% Conf.	Interval]
1	15	28.77333	.9087127	3.519429	26.82434	30.72233
2	15	32.58	.932697	3.61232	30.57956	34.58044
combined	30	30.67667	.7309053	4.003333	29.1818	32.17154
diff		-3.806667	1.302184		-6.474069	-1.139264

```
    diff = mean(1) - mean(2)                                   t =  -2.9233
Ho: diff = 0                               degrees of freedom  =       28

    Ha: diff < 0              Ha: diff != 0               Ha: diff > 0
 Pr(T < t) = 0.0034     Pr(|T| > |t|) = 0.0068        Pr(T > t) = 0.9966
```

Prior to performing unequal variance test, the variance test below must be conducted and interpreted. This test indicates the equality of variance, implying retaining the equal variance test above. However, for illustration purpose, the unequal variance test is conducted below with identical results compared with the equal variance test above.

```
. sdtest le, by ( race)

Variance ratio test

   Group |  Obs       Mean    Std. Err.   Std. Dev.   [95% Conf. Interval]
---------+-----------------------------------------------------------------
       1 |  105   28.77333    .3334064    3.416399    28.11218    29.43449
       2 |  105      32.58    .3422063    3.506571    31.90139    33.25861
---------+-----------------------------------------------------------------
combined |  210   30.67667     .272262    3.945451    30.13994     31.2134
---------------------------------------------------------------------------
    ratio = sd(1) / sd(2)                                   f =    0.9492
Ho: ratio = 1                                degrees of freedom = 104, 104

    Ha: ratio < 1            Ha: ratio != 1              Ha: ratio > 1
  Pr(F < f) = 0.3955     2*Pr(F < f) = 0.7910        Pr(F > f) = 0.6045

. sdtest age, by( Sex)

Variance ratio test

   Group |  Obs       Mean    Std. Err.   Std. Dev.   [95% Conf. Interval]
---------+-----------------------------------------------------------------
       1 |   56   47.92857    1.465592    10.96748    44.99146    50.86568
       2 |   55       37.2    .7065828    5.240158    35.78339    38.61661
---------+-----------------------------------------------------------------
combined |  111   42.61261     .961688    10.13201    40.70677    44.51845
---------------------------------------------------------------------------
    ratio = sd(1) / sd(2)                                   f = 4.3805
Ho: ratio = 1                                 degrees of freedom = 55, 54

    Ha: ratio < 1            Ha: ratio != 1              Ha: ratio > 1
  Pr(F < f) = 1.0000     2*Pr(F > f) = 0.0000        Pr(F > f) = 0.0000
```

The above Stata output illustrates the equality of variance test using "sdtest." The null hypothesis is based on the equality of variance while the alternate states that the variances are not equal, implying the variance is not equal to 1.0. The null hypothesis is rejected implying inequality of the variances comparing male and female with respect to age. The appropriate test in this context is the independent *t* test with unequal variance.

```
. ttest  age, by( Sex) unequal

Two-sample t test with unequal variances

   Group |  Obs       Mean    Std. Err.   Std. Dev.   [95% Conf. Interval]
---------+-----------------------------------------------------------------
       1 |   56   47.92857    1.465592    10.96748    44.99146    50.86568
       2 |   55       37.2    .7065828    5.240158    35.78339    38.61661
---------+-----------------------------------------------------------------
combined |  111   42.61261     .961688    10.13201    40.70677    44.51845
---------+-----------------------------------------------------------------
    diff |        10.72857    1.627027                 7.49017    13.96697
---------------------------------------------------------------------------
    diff = mean(1) - mean(2)                                  t =   6.5940
Ho: diff = 0                      Satterthwaite's degrees of freedom = 79.1821

    Ha: diff < 0                 Ha: diff != 0                Ha: diff > 0
 Pr(T < t) = 1.0000         Pr(|T| > |t|) = 0.0000         Pr(T > t) = 0.0000

.
```

```
. ttest  le, by ( race) unequal

Two-sample t test with unequal variances

------------------------------------------------------------------------------
   Group |  Obs        Mean    Std. Err     Std. Dev.   [95% Conf.  Interval]
---------+--------------------------------------------------------------------
       1 |   15    28.77333    .9087127     3.519429    26.82434    30.72233
       2 |   15       32.58     .932697      3.61232    30.57956    34.58044
---------+--------------------------------------------------------------------
combined |   30    30.67667    .7309053     4.003333     29.1818    32.17154
---------+--------------------------------------------------------------------
    diff |        -3.806667    1.302184                -6.474151   -1.139183
------------------------------------------------------------------------------
    diff = mean(1) - mean(2)                                      t =  -2.9233
Ho: diff = 0                     Satterthwaite's degrees of freedom =   27.981

     Ha: diff < 0                Ha: diff != 0                Ha: diff > 0
  Pr(T < t) = 0.0034       Pr(|T| > |t|) = 0.0068          Pr(T > t) = 0.9966
.

ttest ageatsurgery,by (deepwound_infeect) unequal

Two-sample t test with unequal variances

------------------------------------------------------------------------------
   Group |     Obs       Mean    Std. Err.    Std. Dev.    [95% Conf. Interval]
---------+--------------------------------------------------------------------
       0 |     214   13.86916    0.2348174    3.435083      13.40631    4.33202
       1 |      22   13.94545     0.669358    3.139567      12.55345   15.33746
---------+--------------------------------------------------------------------
combined |     236   13.87627    0.2214786    3.402419      13.43993   14.31261
------------------------------------------------------------------------------
    diff = mean(0) - mean(1)             t = -0.1076
H0: diff = 0        Satterthwaite's degrees of freedom = 26.4474

Ha: diff < 0              Ha: diff != 0              Ha: diff > 0
Pr(T < t) = 0.4576        Pr(|T| > |t|) = 0.9152     Pr(T > t) = 0.5424
```

Note: Data used with permission from the investigative team including the author (LH).

7.2.4 Is there a nonparametric alternative to the independent t *test?*

The Wilcoxon rank-sum test mentioned earlier is the alternative or analog nonparametric test to the two independent samples *t* test. This test is also called the Mann–Whitney *U* Test and the Mann–Whitney–Wilcoxon rank-sum test. The Wilcoxon rank-sum test examines whether or not the two medians are equal—it tests the equality of medians when there are two separate or independent groups. This test is effective and appropriate when the independent *t* test's assumptions are not met and data are ordinal.

Suppose the quality of life (QOL) of children with leukemia who received a full cycle of chemotherapy is compared to that of children who did not complete the cycle because they were too ill to do so, and QOL is measured on a Likert scale: 1 = not satisfied, 2 = slightly unsatisfied, 3 = not sure, 4 = slightly satisfied, and 5 = satisfied. The Wilcoxon rank-sum test is the appropriate statistical inference. The Wilcoxon rank-sum test tests the null hypothesis that H_0: $\text{median}_{CC} = \text{median}_{IC}$, where median_{CC} = median QOL of children who had completed the chemotherapy cycle while median_{IC} is the median QOL of those who did not complete the chemotherapy, and the alternate hypothesis is H_1: $median_{CC} \neq median_{IC}$.

Vignette 7.2: The QOLs of children with leukemia who complete the full cycle of chemotherapy are 5, 5, 4, 3, 5, 4, 4, 5, 4, 4, 3, and 5, and those who did not complete are 4, 3, 3, 2, 2, 1, 4, 3, 3, 1, 2, and 2. (a) Is there a difference in the QOL of those who did and did not complete chemotherapy? (b) What can you conclude from the data?

Solution: Using STATA, the syntax for the Wilcoxon rank-sum test is `ranksum qol, by(chemo) porder`

```
Two-sample Wilcoxon rank-sum (Mann-Whitney) test
   chemo |    obs     rank sum       expected
---------+-----------------------------------
       1 |     12          209            150
       2 |     12           91            150
---------+-----------------------------------
combined |     24          300            300

unadjusted variance 300.00

adjustment for ties -15.91

adjusted variance    284.09

H0: qol(chemo==1)  = qol(chemo==2)
           z       = 3.500
       Prob > |z|  = 0.0005

P{qol(chemo==1)  > qol(chemo==2)}  = 0.910
```

The above output shows a significant difference in the median QOL of the two independent samples. Children diagnosed with leukemia who received the full chemotherapy cycle compared to those who did not complete chemotherapy were more likely to report their QOL as being satisfactory.

7.3 *z* Test for two independent proportions

The difference between two independent proportions could be tested using a *z*-test statistic. For example, if we conducted a study to determine the difference in proportion of diabetic patients with diabetic keto-acidosis (DKA) who developed renal failure and died and those without DKA who developed renal failure and died, with renal failure as our end point, a two-tailed z test is appropriate.

7.3.1 *What is a z test for two independent proportions?*

A z-test statistic is that which allows one to test the difference in proportion when two groups are independent. This distribution, unlike binomial (discrete), is continuous, with a small correction required in order to obtain a more accurate approximation (continuity correction). This continuity correction involves a subtraction of 0.5 (½) from the absolute value of the numerator of the z statistic.

7.3.2 *When is it appropriate to use a z test?*

Comparing two independent proportions involves the use of a z test. However, comparing frequencies of proportion in two groups can be achieved with the chi-square test of independence. And to be precise, the chi-square tests the hypothesis of expected frequencies, which is not the purpose of the z score for the test of two independent proportions. Therefore, the z test is adequate in testing the null hypothesis of equality of two independent proportions.

7.3.3 *How is the z test for two independent proportions computed?*

Remember that the formula for the z test for a single proportion test is $z = \rho - \pi / \sqrt{\pi(1-\pi)/n}$, where the standard error is the square root of $\pi (1 - \pi)$, represented as $\sqrt{\pi(1-\pi)}$.

In using the z test for two independent proportions, the mathematical formula is as follows:

$$z = \rho_1 - \rho_2 / \sqrt{\rho(1-\rho)[(1/n_1)+(1/n_2)]}$$

where ρ_1 is the proportion in one group, ρ_2 is the proportion in the second group, and ρ is the average or pooled proportion denoted by $n_1p_1 + n_2p_2 / n_1 + n_2$.

For example, in the deep wound infection data, if we wanted to test the null hypothesis that the cerebral palsy patients who had deep wound infections (cases) were equal to those who had none (noncases) with respect to the proportion that had skin breakdown after posterior spine fusion, the two independent sample proportion is an appropriate test.

```
. prtest  rodproblem, by (  deepwound)

Two-sample test of proportions                  0: Number of obs =        210
                                                1: Number of obs =         22

------------------------------------------------------------------------------
    Variable |       Mean   Std. Err.      z    P>|z|     [95% Conf. Interval]
-------------+----------------------------------------------------------------
           0 |   .0095238   .0067022                     -.0036123    .0226599
           1 |   .3181818   .0993026                      .1235523    .5128113
-------------+----------------------------------------------------------------
        diff |   -.308658   .0995285                     -.5037303   -.1135857
             |  under Ho:   .0432722    -7.13   0.000
------------------------------------------------------------------------------
        diff = prop(0) - prop(1)                                  z =  -7.1329
    Ho: diff = 0

    Ha: diff < 0                 Ha: diff != 0                 Ha: diff > 0
 Pr(Z < z) = 0.0000         Pr(|Z| < |z|) = 0.0000          Pr(Z > z) = 1.0000
```

With the Z, −7.133, and $p < 0.0001$, one must reject the null hypothesis that there is no difference in the proportion of those who had skin breakdown regardless of whether or not they had deep wound infection. Therefore, one must conclude that those who had skin breakdown were more likely to have deep wound infection.

7.4 Chi-square test of proportions in two groups

The *chi-square* statistic is a distribution-free (nonparametric) statistical technique used to determine if a distribution of observed frequencies differs from the theoretically expected frequencies. This test uses nominal (categorical) or ordinal level data, thus instead of using means and variances, this test uses frequencies, comparing the observed to the expected. Simply, the χ^2 *statistic* summarizes the discrepancies between the expected number of times each outcome occurs (assuming that the model is true) and the observed number of times each outcome occurs, by summing the squares of the discrepancies, normalized by the expected numbers, over all the categories.[8]

7.4.1 Types of chi-square tests

The chi-square test for goodness of fit compares the expected and observed values to determine how well an experimenter's predictions fit the data. *The chi-square test for independence* compares two sets of categories to determine whether the two groups are distributed differently among the categories (Figure 7.1).[9]

7.4.2 What is a chi-square test?

This test is used in comparing frequencies of proportion in two samples or groups and is a test of independence, relationship, or association.[10] It

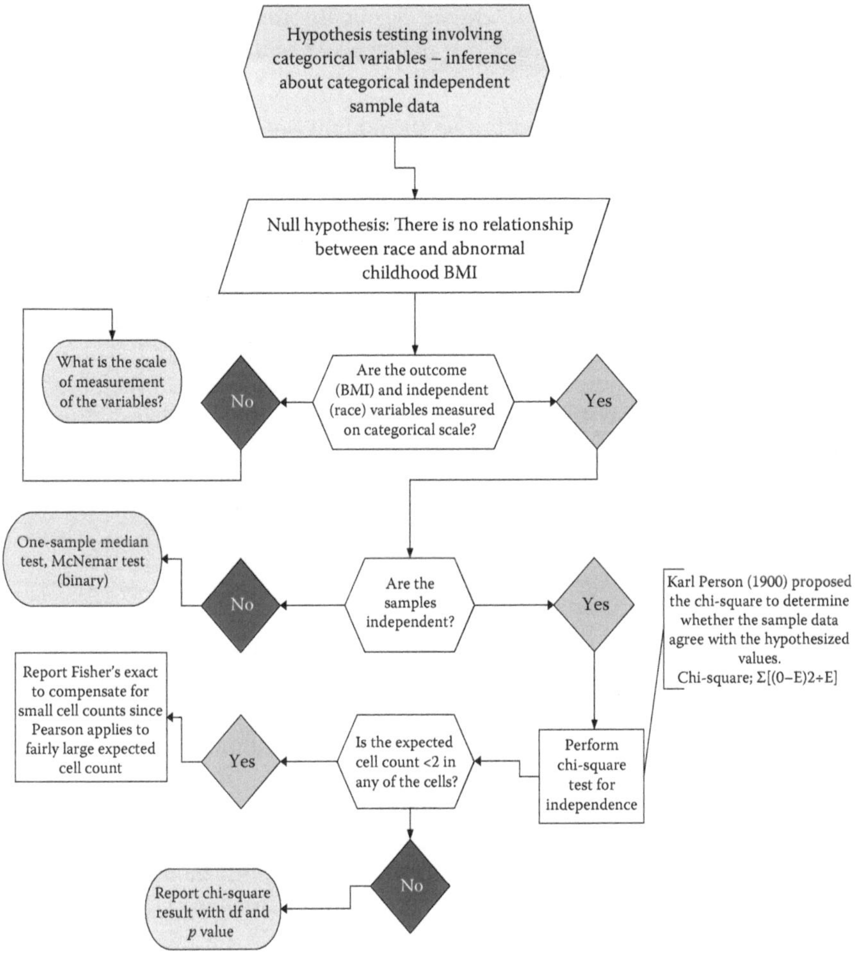

Figure 7.1 Hypothesis testing involving categorical scale—chi-square statistic.

is based on a null hypothesis of no difference/relationship/association or dependency. Unlike the *t* test discussed earlier, the chi-square test is nonparametric, meaning that it is distribution-free. The following are examples of research questions involving two independent proportions and two or more categories that could be tested with a chi-square test: (1) Is there a difference in the proportion of older men treated for prostate problems who received hormonal therapy relative to those who did not receive hormonal therapy? (2) Is there an association or relationship between women with autoimmune disorder and race?

7.4.3 When is it appropriate to use the chi-square statistic to compare proportions in two independent samples or groups?

The chi-square statistic is used to test the equality of these two proportions. For example, the null hypothesis for dependency is that there are no racial differences among women with autoimmune disorders or, simply, women with autoimmune disorders do not differ by race. If investigators conducted a study to examine the association between the types of leukodystrophy and the race/ethnicity of children with this condition, a chi-square statistic would be appropriate. The data from such an investigation can be organized in a row (R) and column (C) contingency table. The intent is to compare the observed with the expected frequency. The greater the difference between the observed and the expected cell counts, the more likely it is that the null hypothesis will be rejected.

7.4.4 What are the assumptions for χ^2 statistic?

The following assumptions and conditions apply to the chi-square statistic:

1 The expected frequency for each category should not be less than 2.
2 No more than 20% of the categories should have expected frequencies of <5.
3 The sample and hence the variable should be randomly drawn from the population.
4 Data should be reported in raw counts of frequency.
5 Measured variables must be independent.
6 Values of independent and dependent variables must be mutually exclusive. Please note that statisticians differ with respect to the smallest cell counts.

7.4.5 How is the chi-square statistic computed?

Chi-square is computed based on the observed and expected frequencies (Table 7.1).

Mathematically, it appears as follows: $\chi^2 = (O - E)^2/E$, where O is the observed frequency, E = the expected frequency → $\chi^2_{(\mathrm{df})} = \Sigma$ (observed frequency − expected frequency)/expected frequency.[11] If no relationship exists, the observed frequencies will be very close to the expected frequency, thus rendering the chi-square value small. If more than 20% of the expected, not the observed, frequency is <5 → Fisher's exact test.[12]

Below is the STATA illustration of how chi-square is computed. In this example, investigators examined the association between the type of cerebral palsy and recurrent surgery for equinus foot deformity.

Table 7.1 Chi-square statistic illustrating the formulae with different degrees of freedom

If x_i ($i = 1, 2, \ldots n$) are independent and normally distributed with mean μ and standard deviation σ, then

$$\sum_{i=1}^{n}\left(\frac{x_i-\mu}{\sigma}\right)^2=\chi^2$$

This is a chi-square distribution with n degrees of freedom (df).
If μ is unknown, chi-square can be estimated using a sample mean:

$$\sum_{i=1}^{n}\left(\frac{x_i-\bar{x}}{\sigma}\right)^2=\chi^2$$

This is a chi-square distribution with $(n-1)$ degrees of freedom.
Using a contingency table, the chi-square test statistic can be computed using the following:

$$\chi^2=\sum_{i=1}^{n}\frac{(O_i-E_i)^2}{E_i}=\chi^2$$

O_i = observed frequency
E_i = expected frequency
This is a chi-square with $n-1$ degrees of freedom.

```
. tab  group cptype, cchi2 chi2 row column exact

                    Cptype
     Group    1          2          3         |     Total

     0        12         78         83        |     173
     |        2.0        4.4        12.8      |     19.2
     |        6.94       45.09      47.98     |     100.00
     |        37.50      44.32      83.00     |     56.17

     1        20         98         17        |     135
     |        2.5        5.6        16.4      |     24.6
     |        14.81      72.59      12.59     |     100.00
     |        62.50      55.68      17.00     |     43.83

     Total    32         176        100       |     308
     |        4.5        10.0       29.2      |     43.8
     |        10.39      57.14      32.47     |     100.00
     |        100.00                100.00          100.00 |
Pearson chi2(2) = 43.8113              Pr = 0.000, implying p <0.0001
since pr is never 0.
        Fisher's exact = 0.000, implying  p <0.0001
```

The expected cell count in the hemiplegic group (1) and nonrecurrence surgery (0) was 2.0, and the Fisher's exact test was reported. However, with or without this adjustment for the small cell count, the significance test indicated a statistically significant difference in the recurrence surgery by the type of cerebral palsy, $p < 0.0001$. With this significance level, $p < 0.0001$, there is an association between the type of cerebral palsy and recurrent surgery for equinus foot deformity.

7.5 Summary

Two-sample statistical inference is used to test the hypothesis when two independent samples are involved (Figure 7.2). The choice of the test statistic

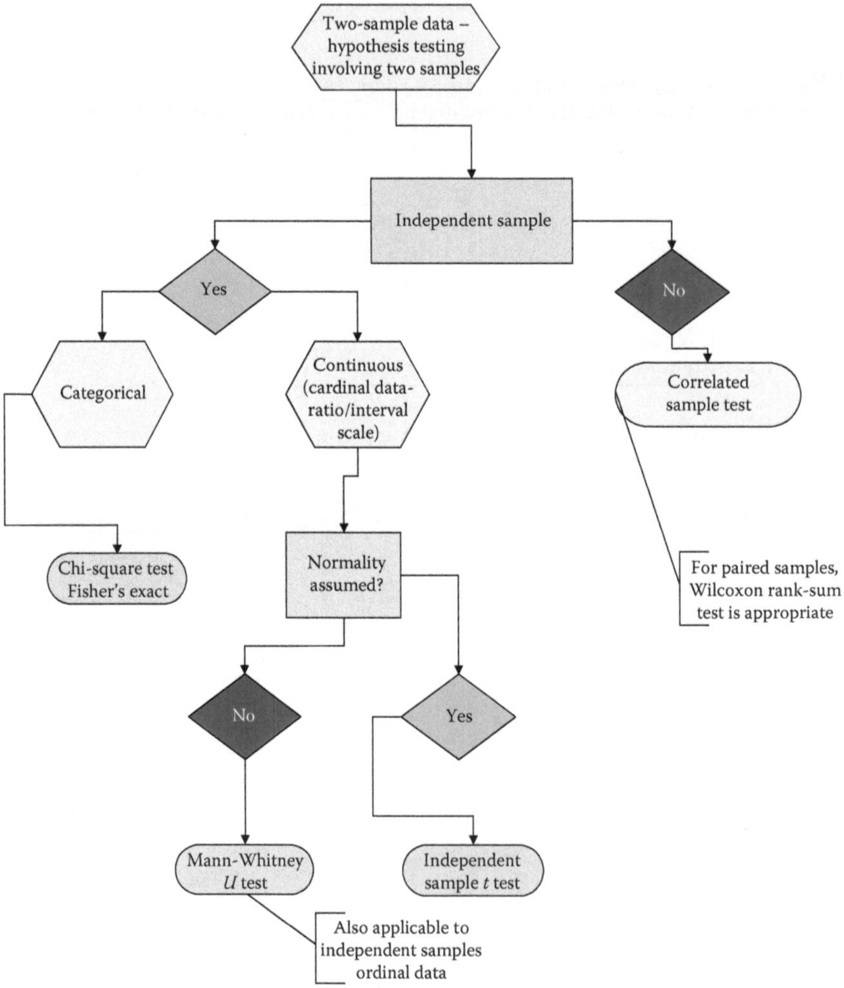

Figure 7.2 Hypothesis testing involving independent or two-sample data.

depends on (a) the scale of measurement of the variable, (b) the shape of the distribution, and (c) the size of the study. The parametric tests are shape-dependent, with normality assumption. An example of a parametric test for a two-sample statistical inference is the independent t test (with and without equal variance). Typically, this test is appropriate when data are measured in a continuous scale, normality is assumed, and the two samples are independent. A nonparametric alternative to the independent t test is the Wilcoxon rank-sum test. This statistical inference tests the equality of the medians of the two independent samples.

A z test for statistical inference involving two samples is used in testing two independent proportions, while a chi-square is used to test the hypothesis regarding frequencies of proportion. Chi-square is a commonly used and abused test in clinical research. This test is appropriate when the two variables are measured on categorical scales, rendering it adequate in testing hypotheses about qualitative variables. There is an assumption regarding expected cell frequency, and where the expected cell count is <2.0, the Fisher's exact test is recommended.

Questions for discussion

1 Suppose you are required to study the effect of a standard drug (A) and a new drug (B) in treating intensive care unit–acquired pneumonia due to mechanical ventilation. If there are 36 patients assigned to drug A and 38 assigned to drug B, the outcome is the number of bacterial counts, and the two groups are administered these two agents for 8 days, (a) what is the appropriate test statistic and why? (b) What are the assumptions of the selected test? (c) How will you interpret the result of this test?

2 A group of investigators decided to study the relationship between the use of recreational steroids and the development of prostate cancer. If they found that of the 116 prostate cancer patients, 16 had used recreational steroids and of 115 men without prostate cancer, 6 had used recreational steroids, (a) what will be an appropriate test statistic to examine this relationship? (b) How will you interpret the result of this test?

3 Consider a hypothetical study conducted to prevent asthmatic attacks among Hispanic children in South Houston. Twenty-two children were selected as participants and 11 were randomized to drug A and 11 to drug B. The number of attacks over 6 months for each participant is given: drug A—4, 0, 3, 4, 4, 3, 3, 4, 5, 3, and 6 and drug B—7, 8, 9, 8, 4, 4, 3, 6, 6, 7, and 3. Test the hypothesis that drug A prevents asthmatic attack. (a) Is a one- or two-sample test appropriate? (b) Is a one-sided test appropriate here? (c) Of these tests, which ones will be appropriate: (i) two-sample t test with equal variance, (ii) two-sample t test with unequal variance, (iii) F test for the equality of two variance, (iv) one-sample t test, or (v) paired t test?

References

1. B. Rosner, *Fundamentals of Biostatistics*, 5th ed. (CA: Duxbury Press, 2000); J. A. Freiman et al., The importance of beta, the type II error and sample size in the design and interpretation of the randomized clinical trial, *N Engl J Med* 299 (1978):690–694; L. D. Fisher and G. van Belle, *Biostatistics: A Methodology for Health Sciences*, 2nd ed. (Hoboken, NJ: Wiley & Sons, 1993).
2. B. Dawson-Saunders and R. G. Trap, *Basic and Clinical Biostatistics*, 2nd ed. (Norwalk, CT: Appleton & Lange, 1994); T. Colton, *Statistics in Medicine* (New York: Little, Brown and Company, 1974).
3. T. Colton, *Statistics in Medicine* (New York: Little, Brown and Company, 1974); W. D. Dupont, *Statistical Modeling for Biomedical Researchers* (Cambridge, UK: Cambridge University Press, 2003).
4. W. D. Dupont, *Statistical Modeling for Biomedical Researchers* (Cambridge, UK: Cambridge University Press, 2003).
5. B. Dawson-Saunders and R. G. Trap, *Basic and Clinical Biostatistics*, 2nd ed. (Norwalk, CT: Appleton & Lange, 1994).
6. B. Dawson-Saunders and R. G. Trap, *Basic and Clinical Biostatistics*, 2nd ed. (Norwalk, CT: Appleton & Lange, 1994).
7. W. D. Dupont, *Statistical Modeling for Biomedical Researchers* (Cambridge, UK: Cambridge University Press, 2003).
8. M. T. Dorak, *Common Concepts in Statistics*, http://dorakmt.tripod.com/mtd/glosstat.html (last accessed February 23, 2006); W. J. Conover, *Practical Nonparametric Statistics* (Hoboken, NJ: Wiley & Sons, 1998); D. L. Katz, *Clinical Epidemiology & Evidence-Based Medicine: Fundamental Principles of Clinical Reasoning & Research* (Thousand Oaks, CA: Sage, 2001); H. A. Khan and C. T. Sempos, *Statistical Methods in Epidemiology* (New York: Oxford University Press, 1989).
9. M. T. Dorak, *Common Concepts in Statistics*, http://dorakmt.tripod.com/mtd/glosstat.html (last accessed February 23, 2006).
10. T. Colton, *Statistics in Medicine* (New York: Little, Brown and Company, 1974); T. D. V. Swinscow and M. J. Campbell, *Statistics at Square One*, 10th ed. (Spain: BMJ Books, 2002); W. J. Conover, *Practical Nonparametric Statistics* (Hoboken, NJ: Wiley & Sons, 1998).; D. L. Katz, *Clinical Epidemiology & Evidence-Based Medicine: Fundamental Principles of Clinical Reasoning & Research* (Thousand Oaks, CA: Sage, 2001); H. A. Khan and C. T. Sempos, *Statistical Methods in Epidemiology* (New York: Oxford University Press, 1989).
11. B. Dawson-Saunders and R. G. Trap, *Basic and Clinical Biostatistics*, 2nd ed. (Norwalk, CT: Appleton & Lange, 1994); T. Colton, *Statistics in Medicine* (New York: Little, Brown and Company, 1974); W. D. Dupont, *Statistical Modeling for Biomedical Researchers* (Cambridge, UK: Cambridge University Press, 2003); H. A. Khan and C. T. Sempos, *Statistical Methods in Epidemiology* (New York: Oxford University Press, 1989).
12. B. Dawson-Saunders and R. G. Trap, Basic and Clinical Biostatistics, 2nd ed. (Norwalk, CT: Appleton & Lange, 1994).

8 Statistical inference in three or more samples

8.1 Introduction

In the previous chapters, we mentioned that when numerical or continuous variables represent the outcome (response or dependent), means are used as appropriate measures of effect. Likewise, when the scale of measurement is continuous, the summary statistics involve the mean and standard deviation. For example, in the study on the prevalence and risk factors in postoperative pancreatitis after spine fusion in patients with cerebral palsy, the mean was used to determine the preoperative Cobb angles, preoperative WBC count, and hematocrit, comparing cases with noncases. In these three measures, the investigators were interested in the differences in these preoperative measures between cases and noncases. The statistical inference used was the two-sample *t* test. Suppose researchers were interested in examining the differences in these three preoperative measures between three groups. The *t* test will not be an adequate test statistic. To examine these differences, the investigators will need a global test in order to determine whether or not any differences exist in the data before testing the combination of the means for individual group differences. Since there are three groups in this situation, simply comparing these three groups will generate three probability values for statistical inference. The test hypothesis will be H_0: $\mu_1 = \mu_2$, H_0: $\mu_1 = \mu_3$, and H_0: $\mu_2 = \mu_3$. Therefore, each comparison will falsely be termed significant at 5%, implying the occurrence of a type I error three times. The probability or chance, which is the product of alpha (0.05 = −5%), and the number of groups (3) declaring one of the comparisons incorrectly significant will be 15%.[1] Consequently, the use of the two-sample *t* test in comparing the differences in the means between three groups inflates the error and results in an invalid statistical inference.

To illustrate how differences between groups could be tested, let us suggest a hypothetical study to examine the effect of diet on abdominal fat as measured by waist circumference. We randomly selected four hundred healthy children, age 12 to 19, and have four groups. Suppose one group (control) continue eating normally; the second group is assigned to spaghetti only; the third group eats vegetables only; and the fourth group eats red meat only. After 3 months, the waist circumference of all participants is measured. The null hypothesis is that diets have no effect on abdominal fat or waist circumference. Since we are not able to examine the entire population, the question is then if we observe differences, how do we decide if these differences are true based on our sample. Secondly, if there are differences, are these differences due to the fact that the different groups of children ate differently or are they simply due to the random variation in waist circumference between individuals. Since the samples are drawn at random from a single population with some variance, we would normally expect the samples to have different means and standard deviations. However, if the hypothesis that diet has no effect on waist circumference is true, then the observed differences would be due to random sampling.

We can start to examine the data by computing the means and standard deviations of the waist circumferences for the total sample and then do the same for each of the four groups. If the samples were all drawn from the same population, the variability within each sample, which is measured by the standard deviation, will be approximately the same. Thus, the variability in the mean values of the sample will be consistent with the variability one will observe within the individual samples. Conversely, if the variability among sample means is much larger than one would expect, from the variability within each sample, then the samples are different. We will then conclude that at least one of the sample means appears to differ from the others. Since the standard deviation or variance, which is the square of standard deviation (a good measure of variability), the analysis of *variance* (ANOVA) measures the variability between samples when two or more groups are observed and assumptions of normality and random samples are met.

Designs that involve multiple observations or more than two group means employ the analysis of variance tool, termed ANOVA. Like we stated above, ANOVA prevents error inflation. Thus, if the model significance level based on the comparison of the variance (F test) indicates a significant mean difference or differences in the means, then comparison between the pairs or combinations of groups becomes feasible.

This chapter presents the statistical inference when two or more groups are compared and explains the rationale and assumptions regarding the selection of appropriate statistical techniques. The parametric test, ANOVA, is presented with its rationale, assumptions, and examples as well as its computation. The different research situations involving the use of ANOVA are discussed with hypothetical data using STATA examples. The nonparametric statistical method analog of ANOVA is presented as the Kruskal–Wallis statistic (based on ranks).

8.2 Analysis of variance (ANOVA)?

The ANOVA is a statistical technique (constructed from variance) used to test the null hypothesis of no difference when two or more than two groups are compared and data are assumed to be normally distributed. This test is based on variability among sample means, which is quantified by the standard deviation and its square, the *variance*. Since these parameters are used to describe normally distributed data, ANOVA is a parametric test. The ANOVA could be termed (a) one-way or single factor, which is one factor (used to compare the mean differences in more than two groups while evaluating the effect of one factor); (b) two-way, which is two factors (used to compare the mean differences in more than two groups while evaluating the effect of two factors); and (c) multiple, which is multiple analysis of variance (MANCOVA). By considering the effect of one or more factors, ANOVA represents a statistical technique for regressing a dependent variable against one or more classification variables.[2] Also, the one-way ANOVA is the generalization of the two-sample t test.

8.2.1 When is one-way ANOVA feasible?

A hypothetical prospective study was conducted to determine the effect of posterior spine fusion in three types of scoliosis. If the investigators measured the thoracic curve as the main curve to assess curve correction at the end of the two-year follow-up and there were no significant mean differences between the three clinical subtypes of scoliosis, a one-way ANOVA is feasible. One-way ANOVA is also feasible in comparing the means of a numerical (continuous) variable when there are two or more than two categories or groups.

8.2.2 What is the hypothesis and possible computation for one-way ANOVA?

ANOVA is based on the null hypothesis of no difference in the means of two or more groups compared. To understand ANOVA, we must consider (a) variation between each subject and the subjects' group means and (b) the variation between each group mean and the grand mean. While the mathematics of ANOVA cannot be presented here because of the focus of this book, applied biostatistics, please note that this complex computation involves (a) the between-group sum of squares, (b) the within-group sum of squares, (c) the between-group degrees of freedom, (d) the within-group degrees of freedom, and (e) the within-group mean square. Considerable variation is expected between the group means and the grand mean if the groups' means are different from each other.[3]

8.2.3 *What are the assumptions of ANOVA?*

The null hypothesis in ANOVA is stated as previously noted: H_0: $\mu_1 = \mu_2 = \mu_3$; the alternative hypothesis is H_1: $\mu_1 \neq \mu_2 \neq \mu_3$. The assumptions of ANOVA are similar to those of a *t* test, as ANOVA is a parametric test. The ANOVA assumptions are (a) *normality*—Gaussian distribution—each sample drawn must be normally distributed; (b) *equal variance*—the population variance is the same in each group, implying that $\sigma_1 = \sigma_2 = \sigma_3$; thus, even if they are different (no effect), the variance must be equal; (c) *random sample/independent observations*, implying that the observation s are independent and that the value of one observation is not related in any manner to the value of another observation. For example, the value of a subject's mean systolic blood pressure must have no influence on that of any other subject; (d) *independent sample* (each sample must be independent of the other samples)—if data consist of repeated measures, one-way ANOVA is inappropriate. This assumption is critical in ANOVA.

The dependent variable or outcome is assumed to be normally distributed within each group or factor (termed *independent categorical variable*). Since ANOVA assumes that data from the study are sampled from populations that follow a Gaussian bell-shaped distribution or are normally distributed, violation of this assumption may benefit from the transformation of such data. The benefit is that such transformation or normalization increases the power of the analyses to detect differences should they really exist. However, ANOVA works well even if the distribution is approximately normally distributed, especially with a large sample. Not all the assumptions above are equally important, since a moderate departure from the normality assumption does not affect the results of the *F* test. In contrast, the *F* test is more influenced by the equality of variances or homogeneity of variances assumption.

8.2.4 *How is ANOVA computed?*

The computation involved in ANOVA is complex, but it is easily achieved today with statistical software such as SPSS, STATA, SAS, R-Plus, and S-Plus. While these packages facilitate this computation, they cannot select the appropriate test or the variables in the appropriate order. Therefore, no matter how sophisticated your package is, knowledge of these assumptions is essential to the understanding of ANOVA and other related statistical tests.

The ANOVA is computed as a ratio termed *F*-test statistic:

$$F = \text{population variance estimated from sample means} \\ /\text{population variance estimated as average of sample variance}$$

BOX 8.1 *F* TEST AND *F* RATIO

- The *F* test is used to test the ratio of the variance among means to the variance among subjects within each group.
- The *F* ratio is obtained by dividing the estimate of the variance of means (mean square among groups) by estimate of the variance within groups (error mean square).
- Based on the null hypothesis that the two variances are equal and that if they are, the variation among means is not much greater than the variation among individual observations within any given group.
- The null hypothesis in one-way ANOVA is rejected when the *F* statistic is large, while a small *F* provides no evidence against the null hypothesis.

Below, we performed the test of normality to test the assumption for the use of ANOVA. We examined the distribution of systolic blood pressure as a dependent variable to be used in testing the mean differences in systolic blood pressure between three groups. This is the first step in examining the assumption of ANOVA.

The STATA output for the test of the shape and distribution of systolic blood pressure shows a normally distributed BP in the overall sample, $p = 0.74$, as well as normally distributed individual samples, group 1, $p = 0.29$, group 2, $p = 0.38$, and group 3, $p = 0.59$.

BOX 8.2 *p* VALUE INTERPRETATION

- The *p* value is the probability or chance of getting a test statistic at least as extreme as the calculated test statistic if the null hypothesis is true.
- This is not the probability that the null hypothesis is true. Since population parameters are fixed numbers, the null hypothesis about the population parameter is either true or false.
- Strictly, as it is commonly incorrectly explained, *p* value is not the probability that the sample results are due to chance or sampling variability.
- For example, Holmes et al.[4] reported a *p* value of 0.81 on the association between female condom use and education level.
- Because their significance level was 0.05, they failed to reject the null hypothesis of no association between female condom use and education level.

- The most appropriate interpretation of this p value is that the probability of getting a test statistic at least as extreme as the calculated test statistic is 0.81, if the null hypothesis is true, implying that 81% of all possible samples produce test statistics at least as extreme as the calculated test statistic if the null hypothesis is true.

Normality test for group differences

```
. sktest SBP

                    Skewness/Kurtosis tests for Normality
                                                                  ------joint------
    Variable |   Obs   Pr(Skewness)   Pr(Kurtosis)   adj chi2(2)      Prob>chi2
-------------+--------------------------------------------------------------------
         SBP |   111      0.6630         0.0000          19.96           0.0000

.  sktest SBP if Race==1

                    Skewness/Kurtosis tests for Normality
                                                                  ------joint------
    Variable |   Obs   Pr(Skewness)   Pr(Kurtosis)   adj chi2(2)      Prob>chi2
-------------+--------------------------------------------------------------------
         SBP |    54      0.0009         0.0644          11.70           0.0029

. sktest SBP if Race==2

                    Skewness/Kurtosis tests for Normality
                                                                  ------joint------
    Variable |   Obs   Pr(Skewness)   Pr(Kurtosis)   adj chi2(2)      Prob>chi2
-------------+--------------------------------------------------------------------
         SBP |    31      0.2631         0.7676           1.44           0.4876

. sktest SBP if Race==3

                    Skewness/Kurtosis tests for Normality
                                                                  ------joint------
    Variable |   Obs   Pr(Skewness)   Pr(Kurtosis)   adj chi2(2)      Prob>chi2
-------------+--------------------------------------------------------------------
         SBP |    26      0.8264         0.1898           1.93           0.3802
```

Notes and abbreviations: Race: 1 = white, 2 = black, and 3 = other. Whereas the sbp was not normally distributed or rather the Gaussian distribution was violated in the overall sample, the test indicated Gaussian distribution for black and other and not white.

The STATA output demonstrates the computation of ANOVA following the test of normality. The assumption of equal variance is examined and indicates the equality of variance, $p = 0.51$. In addition, it is assumed that the data are from random samples and that the samples are independent. The summary or descriptive statistics are presented as mean and standard deviation for the individual groups as well as the overall sample. The ANOVA also presents the between-group ratio, F as 19.44, with df = 2, and $p < 0.001$. We conclude that the samples are not drawn from a single population and reject the null hypothesis that there are no differences in the systolic blood pressure comparing these three groups. Therefore, there is at least a difference in one group mean relative to the others.

```
. oneway SBP Race, tab bon

                    Summary of SBP
   Race   |        Mean    Std. Dev.      Freq.
----------+------------------------------------
        1 |    111.7963    14.195906         54
        2 |   142.45161     9.735977         31
        3 |   134.26923    15.472705         26
----------+------------------------------------
    Total |   125.62162    19.201351        111

                        Analysis of Variance
    Source              SS         df      MS            F     Prob > F
------------------------------------------------------------------------
Between groups     21046.556      2   10523.278     58.25     0.0000
 Within groups    19509.5521    108   180.644001
------------------------------------------------------------------------
    Total         40556.1081    110   368.691892

Bartlett's test for equal variances:  chi2(2) =   6.4197  Prob>chi2 =  0.040

                    Comparison of SBP by Race
                          (Bonferroni)
Row Mean-|
Col Mean |          1            2
---------+----------------------
       2 |    30.6553
         |      0.000
         |
       3 |    22.4729     -8.18238
         |      0.000        0.072
```

The Bonferroni's multiple comparison is comparable to that of Scheffe's performed above. Without these tests, we are unable to determine where the differences are since we are comparing more than two groups, and the ANOVA does not specify this in the model. These posthoc comparisons are clinically meaningful in decision-making since this information is necessary not only for the appraisal of the mean difference (effect size), but for the generalization of the subpopulation mean difference in sbp for the treatment of future patients with comparable characteristics who were not in the sample (target population).

8.2.5 What is post hoc comparison?

Post hoc or a posteriori comparison is a method of comparing the difference between the two means, $\mu 1 = \mu 2$, $\mu 1 = \mu 3$ or $\mu 2 = \mu 3$, after the computed ANOVA is significant (F test and significant probability value, p). It is termed *post hoc* or *a posteriori* since, as its technique implies, it is conducted after the analysis of ANOVA. When the multiple comparison is planned before the analysis, it is termed *a priori* or *planned*, with the most commonly used being the Bonferroni t procedure or Dunn's multiple-comparison procedure.[5]

The post hoc comparisons commonly used and recommended include the following:

a Tukey's HSD (*honestly significant difference*) procedure, a procedure named after the statistician who introduced the stem-and-leaf and box-and-whisker plots. This test is effective for pairwise comparison, but also in comparing all pairs of means.
b Scheffe's procedure is effective for all types of comparison, including pairwise. A higher critical value of this test is used to determine the significance, and compared to Tukey's HSD, it is more conservative and allows the formation of a confidence interval.
c Newman-Keuls
d Dunnett's procedure is used when the intent is to compare several treatment means with a single control mean. Compared to Tukey's HSD or Scheffe's test, it is less conservative, implying a relatively low critical value.

Most statisticians recommend the use of Scheffe's, Tukey's HSD, and Dunnett's procedure as a post hoc multiple comparisons procedure in that order.[6]

```
. oneway SBP Race, tab scheffe

                    Summary of SBP
  Race  |        Mean       Std. Dev.       Freq.
--------+------------------------------------------
      1 |    111.7963      14.195906          54
      2 |   142.45161       9.735977          31
      3 |   134.26923      15.472705          26
--------+------------------------------------------
  Total |   125.62162      19.201351         111

                     Analysis of Variance
    Source             SS         df        MS            F     Prob > F
------------------------------------------------------------------------
Between groups     21046.556      2    10523.278      58.25     0.0000
 Within groups    19509.5521    108   180.644001
------------------------------------------------------------------------
    Total         40556.1081    110   368.691892

Bartlett's test for equal variances:  chi2(2) =   6.4197  Prob>chi2 =  0.040

                    Comparison of SBP by Race
                           (Scheffe)
Row Mean-|
Col Mean |          1            2
---------+--------------------------
       2 |    30.6553
         |      0.000
         |
       3 |    22.4729     -8.18238
         |      0.000        0.077
```

The above ANOVA model indicates statistically significant racial differences in SBP, requiring multiple comparison analysis to determine whether or not there is a statistically significant difference between white (1) and black (2) patients (1 versus 2), white and other (3) patients (1 versus 3), as well as between 1 (white) and 3 (other), and 2 (black) and 3 (other). While whites clinically and statistically significantly differed from black and other, blacks (2), though clinically meaningfully different from other (3) with respect to the mean sbp, was statistically marginally different from other (3), implying marginal but not a strong evidence against the null hypothesis that the mean difference in SPB between 2 and 3 equals zero (*Ho*: μ_2 (black) – μ_3 (other) = 0).

The STATA output above shows Scheffe's multiple comparisons after significant ANOVA. While the model *p* value only indicates that at least the means differ, the post hoc comparison of the means shows a nonsignificant difference between the pairs, group 1 SBP versus group 2 SBP ($p < 0.20$), but a significant difference between group 1 SBP and group 3 SBP ($p < 0.001$) and between group 2 SBP and group 3 SBP ($p < 0.001$).

```
. oneway SBP Race, tab bon
```

Summary of SBP

Race	Mean	Std. Dev.	Freq.
1	111.7963	14.195906	54
2	142.45161	9.735977	31
3	134.26923	15.472705	26
Total	125.62162	19.201351	111

Analysis of Variance

Source	SS	df	MS	F	Prob > F
Between groups	21046.556	2	10523.278	58.25	0.0000
Within groups	19509.5521	108	180.644001		
Total	40556.1081	110	368.691892		

Bartlett's test for equal variances: chi2(2) = 6.4197 Prob>chi2 = 0.040

Comparison of SBP by Race
(Bonferroni)

Row Mean-Col Mean	1	2
2	30.6553 0.000	
3	22.4729 0.000	-8.18238 0.072

The Bonferroni's multiple comparison is comparable to that of Scheffe's performed above. Without these tests, we are unable to determine where the differences are since we are comparing more than two groups, and the ANOVA does not specify this in the model. These posthoc comparisons are clinically meaningful in decision-making since this information is necessary not only for the appraisal of the mean difference (effect size) but also for the generalization of the subpopulation mean difference in sbp for the treatment of future patients with comparable characteristics who were not in the sample (target population).

Graph 8.1 illustrates the median (p50) SBP of the three samples (middle line in the box). The upper line represents the upper quartile (p75) SBP, while the bottom line represents the lower quartile SBP (p25). The boxes are vertical, as is the default in STATA.

The box plot below shows the vertical presentation of the box plot. This is STATA's default and requires no modification in the command. However, where horizontal box plots are required, the modification of the syntax is required: `graph box var, over (group var)`.

Graph 8.2 is termed the dot plot and shows the separate SBP means on separate lines.

Below is the STATA syntax used to construct the graphs: `graph box sbp1, over(group), graph hbox sbp1, over (group), graph dot (mean) sbp1, over (group)`.

Also below are the STATA syntax used to generate Graph 8.3. The graph shows the means as dots and the error lines.

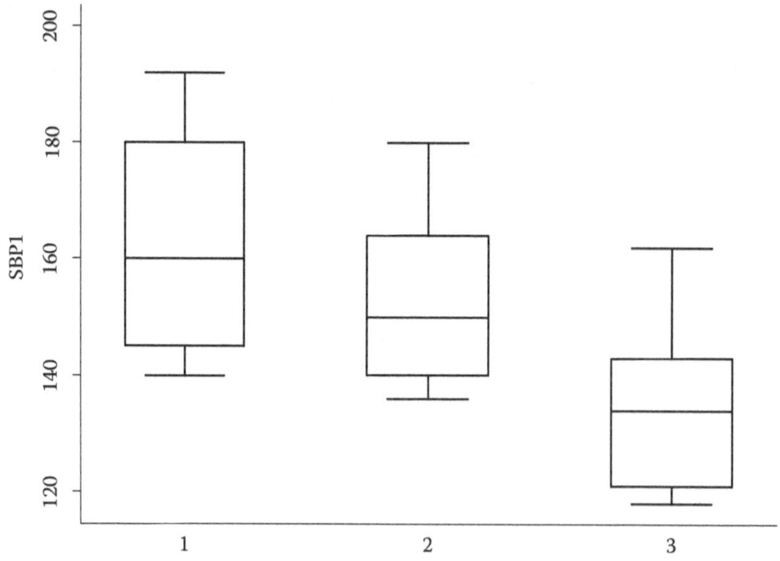

Graph 8.1 Box plot of median systolic blood pressure (SBP) in three independent samples.

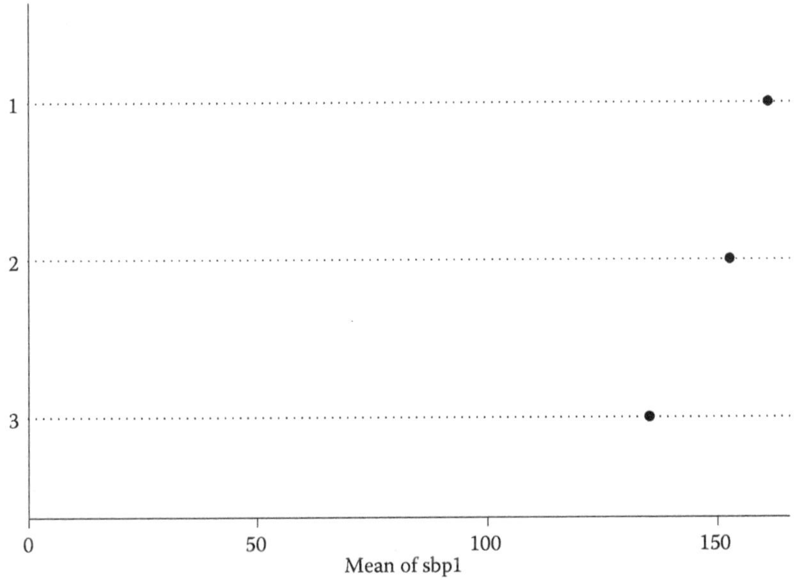

Graph 8.2 Dot lines of systolic blood pressure in three independent samples.

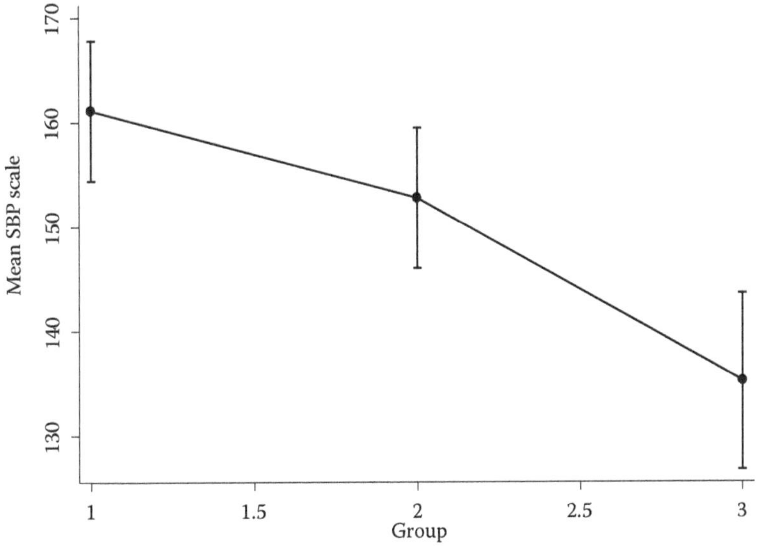

Graph 8.3 The mean values with error line or bars of systolic blood pressure in three independent samples.

```
predict sbp1mean
(option xb assumed; fitted values)
. label variable sbp1mean "Mean SBP Scale"
. predict SEsbp1, stdp
. serrbar sbp1mean SEsbp1 group, scale (2)
. serrbar sbp1mean SEsbp1 group, scale (2) plot
(line sbp1mean group, clpattern(solid)) legend (off)
```

8.3 Other hypothesis tests based on ANOVA

There are other designs where ANOVA is feasible, and examples of these designs include *two-way ANOVA*, which is similar to one-way but involves two factors or two independent variables. For example, if a study was conducted to examine the effect of reactive airway disease (RAD) and gastroesophageal reflux disease (GERD) on the development of postoperative pancreatitis, a two-way ANOVA would be adequate to demonstrate the combined effect of these independent variables in postoperative pancreatitis. The design would address the following questions: (1) Do differences exist between patients with and without postoperative pancreatitis in relation to RAD? (2) Do differences exist between patients with and without postoperative pancreatitis in relation to GERD? (3) Do differences occur that are due to neither RAD nor GERD alone, but the combination of RAD and GERD, termed *interaction*? If after the two-way ANOVA is computed and the graph of interaction is produced and if the lines connecting the RAD and GERD means are parallel, this is interpreted as no interaction, implying an additive effect. However, the intersection of the lines representing the RAD and GERD means is indicative of a multiplicative effect.

```
. gen race_sex = Sex*Race

. anova SBP Race Sex race_sex

                    Number of obs =       111     R-squared     =  0.5777
                    Root MSE      =   12.7718     Adj R-squared =  0.5576
```

Source	Partial SS	df	MS	F	Prob > F
Model	23428.558	5	4685.7116	28.73	0.0000
Race	14057.9512	2	7028.97558	43.09	0.0000
Sex	1583.81077	1	1583.81077	9.71	0.0024
race_sex	6.97902402	2	3.48951201	0.02	0.9788
Residual	17127.5501	105	163.119525		
Total	40556.1081	110	368.691892		

The STATA output above shows a two-way analysis of variance (ANOVA), implying two factors included in the model, namely, race and sex, as well as race and sex interaction. This model indicates significant racial variability in SBP, as well as a statistically significant sex difference that the mean difference in SBP between male and female is not zero (0), and with p = 0.002, the null hypothesis is rejected, implying that there is a very strong evidence against the null hypothesis (($Ho = \mu_1$ (male) – μ_2 (female) = 0)). However, there is no interaction between race and sex as indicated by the low value of the F test (0.02 with 2 degrees of freedom) and the significance (p = 0.98), implying no evidence against the null hypothesis that race and sex interaction influence the observed clinically meaningful and statistically significant differences between racial and sex subgroups in the sample.

The evidence from this model is suggestive of presenting the ANOVA results without interaction. The information below illustrates ANOVA without interaction, indicating the effects of race and sex on the observed SBP in this sample.

```
. anova SBP Race Sex

                    Number of obs =        111     R-squared     =  0.5775
                    Root MSE      =    12.6545     Adj R-squared =  0.5657
```

Source	Partial SS	df	MS	F	Prob > F
Model	23421.579	3	7807.19299	48.75	0.0000
Race	14368.9306	2	7184.46529	44.86	0.0000
Sex	2375.02291	1	2375.02291	14.83	0.0002
Residual	17134.5292	107	160.135786		
Total	40556.1081	110	368.691892		

A randomized factorial design usually involves one or two factors with the possibility of three or more factors. For example, if a study has three factors and two levels, there will be eight treatment groups.

Randomized block designs are effective when variation is attributed to a confounder. Because this design involves controlling for the confounding factor, analysis of covariance (ANCOVA) is adequate. Using the hypothetical SBP data with age groups, sex, and high-density lipoprotein (HDL) as a confounding variable, the ANCOVA was computed to illustrate the confounding effect of HDL on SBP. From this analysis, no significant relationship is shown between HDL and SBP when sex and age are controlled ($p = 0.81$). Because ANCOVA represents a special case of regression, the `regress` option is added to the ANOVA command, which is the extension of the two-way

ANOVA, by encompassing mixed categorical and continuous independent (HDL) variables present in the regression result.

```
. table   Race Sex, contents (mean  SBP ) row col
```

Race	Sex 1	2	Total
1	118	108.6944	111.7963
2	145.4091	135.2222	142.4516
3	138.3125	127.8	134.2692
Total	134.5714	116.5091	125.6216

Note and abbreviation: Race: 1 = white, 2 = black, and 3 = other; Sex: 1 = male and 2 = female. Regardless of the race, the SBP is consistently higher among males and the same observation holds in the total sample.

In this sample, males and females tend to have the same systolic blood pressure (151.72 vs. 151.68). In the old group (1), men seem to have higher SBP, and in the older old group (2), women seem to have higher SBP, with similar observations seen in the oldest old group (3).

```
. anova SBP Race Sex HDL, continuous ( HDL)

                Number of obs =        111     R-squared     =  0.9132
                Root MSE      =    5.76336     Adj R-squared =  0.9099
```

Source	Partial SS	df	MS	F	Prob > F
Model	37035.1834	4	9258.79586	278.74	0.0000
Race	1083.50797	2	541.753983	16.31	0.0000
Sex	44.6444254	1	44.6444254	1.34	0.2489
HDL	13613.6045	1	13613.6045	409.85	0.0000
Residual	3520.92468	106	33.2162706		
Total	40556.1081	110	368.691892		

The above STATA output illustrates ANCOVA model, which is an extension of ANOVA to include a potential confounding variable in the model. Since low level of serum high density lipoprotein (HDL) had been shown to have an adverse effect in the cardiovascular health, this variable was added to the model that initially assesses the association between race and sex. This model indicates a significant association with HDL, $F = 409.9$, $p < 0.0001$.

However, the observed significant association with sbp and sex was removed, F = 1.34, p = 0.25, implying that in this sample of hypertensive patients on a new antihypertensive agent versus standard of care, the association between sex and SBP did not persist after controlling for HDL.

Using the `regress` option: since two-way ANOVA and ANCOVA do not provide descriptive information (provided by the `tabulate` command) about how the SBP, age, sex, and HDL are related, except the explicit model and the parameter estimates, the regression option furnishes such descriptive data as illustrated below.

```
. anova SBP Race Sex HDL, continuous ( HDL) regress

      Source |       SS        df       MS              Number of obs =      111
-------------+------------------------------           F( 4,    106)  =   278.74
       Model |  37035.1834      4   9258.79586           Prob > F      =   0.0000
    Residual |  3520.92468    106   33.2162706           R-squared     =   0.9132
-------------+------------------------------           Adj R-squared =   0.9099
       Total |  40556.1081    110   368.691892           Root MSE      =   5.7634

------------------------------------------------------------------------------
         SBP        Coef.     Std. Err.       t     P>|t|    [95% Conf.  Interval]
------------------------------------------------------------------------------
_cons            267.474     7.007688     38.17    0.000     253.5806    281.3675
Race
           1   -7.395181      1.53937     -4.80    0.000    -10.44713   -4.34323
           2     1.05746     1.566775      0.67    0.501    -2.048825    4.163745
           3   (dropped)
Sex
           1   -1.496824     1.291108     -1.16    0.249     -4.05657    1.062923
           2   (dropped)
HDL            -2.590087     .1279391    -20.24    0.000    -2.843738   -2.336435
------------------------------------------------------------------------------
```

The above STATA output illustrates a similar effect of HDL on SBP and very importantly shows the subgroup results of race and sex effect on SBP.

```
. anova SBP Race Sex  LDL,   continuous ( LDL)

                 Number of obs =      111     R-squared     =  0.8089
                 Root MSE      =  8.55157     Adj R-squared =  0.8017

      Source |  Partial SS    df       MS            F     Prob > F
-------------+----------------------------------------------------
       Model |  32804.3933     4   8201.09831     112.15     0.0000
             |
        Race |  1526.81555     2   763.407774      10.44     0.0001
         Sex |  76.1509439     1   76.1509439       1.04     0.3098
         LDL |  9382.81429     1   9382.81429     128.30     0.0000
             |
    Residual |  7751.71486   106   73.1293854
-------------+----------------------------------------------------
       Total |  40556.1081   110   368.691892
```

In the STATA output above, a similar ANOVA model for SBP was used, controlling for low density lipoprotein (LDL) in this sample. A high level of LDL (>120 milligrams per deciliter) is implicated in cardiovascular disease (CVD) including hypertension. The model indicates a significant effect of LDL on SBP, $F(\mathrm{d}) = 120.3(1)$, $p < 0.0001$. Also, similar to the HDL, there is no significant association with sex, given LDL in the model.

```
. anova SBP Race Sex LDL, continuous ( LDL) regress

   Source |     SS          df       MS                Number of obs  =     111
----------+----------------------------------          F( 4,    106)  =  278.15
    Model | 32804.3933       4   8201.09831            Prob > F       =  0.0000
 Residual | 7751.71486     106   73.12938854           R-squared      =  0.8089
----------+----------------------------------          Adj R-squared  =  0.8017
    Total | 40556.1081     110   368.691892            Root MSE       =  8.5516

-------------------------------------------------------------------------------------
      SBP       Coef.        Std. Err.       t        P>|t|      [95% Conf. Interval]
-------------------------------------------------------------------------------------
_cons       -42.48273       15.20002      -2.79      0.006     -72.61824    -12.34721
Race
        1    -10.1047       2.263029      -4.47      0.000     -14.59138    -5.618026
        2   -1.872056       2.418141      -0.77      0.441     -6.666256     2.922143
        3   (dropped)
Sex
        1   -2.062101       2.020777      -1.02      0.310     -6.068488     1.944285
        2   (dropped)
LDL          1.591331       .1404882      11.33      0.000      1.312799     1.869862
-------------------------------------------------------------------------------------
```

The above STATA output, which is ANOVA extension using egress, indicates a similar but direct association between SBP and LDL in contrast to HDL. However, in these two instances, the association between SBP and sex did not persist.

```
. oneway  SBP  HNT_TX,   tab

          |          Summary of SBP
   HNT_TX |        Mean    Std.  Dev.        Freq.
----------+---------------------------------------
        1 |   113.03077     12.016875           65
        2 |   143.41304     11.971403           46
----------+---------------------------------------
    Total |   125.62162     19.201351          111

                          Analysis of Variance
  Source              SS           df        MS                F        Prob > F
----------------------------------------------------------------------------------
Between groups     24865.0175       1     24865.0175        172.73        0.0000
 Within groups     15691.0906     109      143.95496
----------------------------------------------------------------------------------
   Total           40556.1081     110     368.691892

Bartlett's test for equal variances:   chi2(1) =   0.0008  Prob>chi2 =  0.978
```

Notes: HTN_TX = antihypertensive agent. The test for an equal variance, which is a requirement in ANOVA, indicates that the variance comparing the two treatment groups are equal, justifying the application of ANOVA.

```
. anova SBP HNT_TX Sex LDL,  continuous ( LDL) regress

    Source |     SS          df       MS              Number of obs =     111
-----------+----------------------------------        F( 3,    107) =  127.77
     Model | 31705.7821      3   10568.594            Prob > F      =  0.0000
  Residual | 8850.32605    107  82.7133276            R-squared     =  0.7818
-----------+----------------------------------        Adj R-squared =  0.7757
     Total | 40556.1081    110  368.691892            Root MSE      =  9.0947

------------------------------------------------------------------------------
       SBP      Coef.      Std. Err.       t       P>|t|     [95% Conf. Interval]
------------------------------------------------------------------------------
_cons       -36.17714     23.18042     -1.56     0.122     -82.12961    9.775339
HNT_TX
         1  -7.376525     3.242007     -2.28     0.025     -13.80343    -.949623
         2  (dropped)
Sex
         1  -.6621888      2.26559     -0.29     0.771     -5.153458     3.82908
         2  (dropped)
LDL          1.517217     .2025943      7.49     0.000      1.115598    1.918837
------------------------------------------------------------------------------
```

The above ANOVA model examines the treatment effect of the anti-hypertensive agent (HTN_TX) and sex, controlling for LDL. The HTN significantly reduced SBP and the effect remained after controlling for LDL in this model, with LDL significantly associated with SBP. Since subgroup results are not computed by the two-way ANOVA as in this example, the `regress` command is used to obtain the subgroups effects above.

Nested designs involve the nesting of one or more treatments within levels of another factor.

Repeated measures design involves the relationship among measures that are repeated and is effective in controlling for individual variation, since subjects serve as their own controls (eliminating the variability due to individual differences, and hence increasing the power of the study).[7] The detail of the technique was covered in the chapter on hypothesis testing involving one or a single sample. We would like to mention the interpretation of some of the output of this test from the statistical package that may be used for the computation. Regardless of the software, the test of sphericity means that the investigators wish to examine the assumption of equal variance, and if this is not met, the Greenhouse–Geisser or Huynh–Feldt corrections should be used.

8.3.1 What is the nonparametric alternative to one-way ANOVA?

Whenever the observation for the one-way ANOVA is relatively skewed or when the sample size is relatively small, a nonparametric alternative test is recommended. The alternative to one-way ANOVA is the Kruskal–Wallis nonparametric procedure. This test statistic tests the null hypothesis of equal population medians. Also, if the equal variance is in doubt, and issues with outliers are anticipated, the Kruskal–Wallis test is a safer procedure.[8] However, since Kruskal–Wallis is a *k*-sample generalization of the two-sample rank-sum test and is distribution-free (makes a weaker assumption of similar-shaped distributions within each group), it is a less powerful test compared to one-way ANOVA.[9]

8.3.2 *How is the Kruskal–Wallis test computed?*

The hypothetical systolic blood pressure data used for one-way ANOVA, which met the assumptions for this procedure, are used here to illustrate the computation of Kruskal–Wallis. This test incorporates an exact method of dealing with ties. The result here is the same as that obtained from one-way ANOVA, which is a significant difference in systolic blood pressure by group (old = 1, older old = 2, oldest old = 3). Below is the *STATA syntax:* `kwallis sbp1, by(group)`.

```
kwallis sbp1, by(group)

Kruskal-Wallis equality-of-populations rank test
```

group	Obs	Rank Sum
1	19	626.00
2	19	502.00
3	12	147.00

```
chi-squared =    14.949 with 2 df
probability =    0.0006
chi-squared with ties =   15.115 with 2 df
probability =    0.0005
```

8.4 Summary

Statistical inference involving three or more independent samples can be tested using parametric and nonparametric techniques. The selection of the appropriate test depends on the distribution and scale of measurement of the variable, as well as the size of the study (Figure 8.1). If a mean comparison of two, three, or more groups is expected and data are normally distributed and from independent samples, then the ANOVA is appropriate. This is a variability-based test and computes the ratio (*F*): population variance estimated from sample means divided by the population variance estimated as an average of sample variances—$F = SD^2_{between}/SD^2_{within}$, where $_{between}$ means between the groups' variance, and $_{within}$ means within-group variance. Thus, if $F = \sigma^2/\sigma^2 = 1$, the test concludes that the data are consistent with the null hypothesis, implying that the null hypothesis of no mean difference should not be rejected. The one-way ANOVA involves one factor, while two-way involves two factors and implies interaction, which could be tested for "additivity" or multiplicity. Other designs that ANOVA could be used for include (a) block designs, (b) factorial designs, and (c) repeated measures.

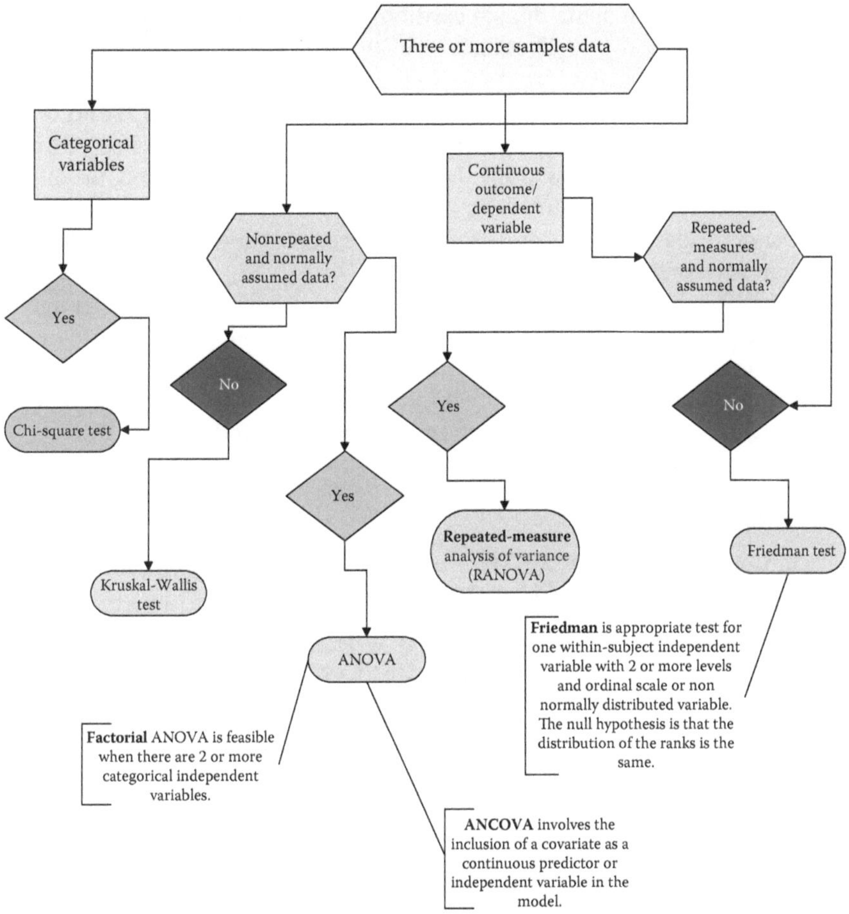

Figure 8.1 Statistical test selection for three or more samples.

If the assumptions for the use of ANOVA are not met and if the study size is relatively small, a nonparametric analog to ANOVA is recommended. The nonparametric alternative to ANOVA is the Kruskal–Wallis test, which examines the median differences in ordered or distribution-free data. A repeated-measure ANOVA discussed earlier (one-sample statistical inference) illustrates the use of ANOVA with a single sample where measurements are taken three times or more from an individual subject. The Friedman test is the nonparametric alternative to repeated-measure ANOVA.

Questions for discussion

1 The following data represent left ventricular ejection fraction (LVEF) from a hypothetical study of the effect of drugs A and B, and no treatment

on patients with acute dilated cardiomyopathy. Group A (drug A): 0.19, 0.24, 0.17, 0.40, 0.40, 0.23, 0.20, 0.20, 0.30, and 0.19; Group B (drug B): 0.24, 0.32, 0.32, 0.28, 0.24, 0.18, 0.22, 0.23, 0.14, and 0.14; and Group C (control): 0.30, 0.07, 0.12, 0.13, 0.17, 0.24, 0.19, 0.07, 0.12, and 0.19. (a) What would be an appropriate statistical test to examine the effect of treatment? (b) Can you show, using the appropriate statistical method, the difference between group A and C? (c) What can be concluded from the data?

2 Using the data in question 1, construct a box plot and error lines. What is your interpretation of these graphs?

3 Suppose you are required to test the effect of a new anti-platelet agent using three independent samples: (a) new agent group, (b) standard drug, and (c) control. If the data are not normally distributed and the sample size is small, what will be the appropriate test statistic to examine this effect? Comment on the limitations of this test including its power.

References

1. B. Dawson-Saunders and R. G. Trap, *Basic and Clinical Biostatistics*, 2nd ed. (Norwalk, CT: Appleton & Lange, 1994).
2. B. Dawson-Saunders and R. G. Trap, *Basic and Clinical Biostatistics*, 2nd ed. (Norwalk, CT: Appleton & Lange, 1994); W. D. Dupont, Statistical Modeling for Biomedical Researchers (Cambridge, UK: Cambridge University Press, 2003); B. C. Cronk, *How to Use SPSS. A Step-by-Step Guide to Analysis and Interpretation*, 3rd ed. (Glendale, CA: Pyrczak Publishing, 2004); T. D. V. Swinscow and M. J. Campbell, *Statistics at Square One*, 10th ed. (Spain: BMJ Books, 2002); D. A. Freedman et al., *Statistics*, 4th ed. (New York: Norton, 2007).
3. B. Dawson-Saunders and R. G. Trap, *Basic and Clinical Biostatistics*, 2nd ed. (Norwalk, CT: Appleton & Lange, 1994); W. D. Dupont, Statistical Modeling for Biomedical Researchers (Cambridge, UK: Cambridge University Press, 2003); B. C. Cronk, *How to Use SPSS. A Step-by-Step Guide to Analysis and Interpretation*, 3rd ed. (Glendale, CA: Pyrczak Publishing, 2004); T. D. V. Swinscow and M. J. Campbell, *Statistics at Square One*, 10th ed. (Spain: BMJ Books, 2002).
4. L. Holmes, Jr., G. O. Ogungbade, D. D. Ward, O. Garrison, R. J. Peters, S. C. Kalichman, J. Lahai-Momohe, E. J. Essien, Potential markers of female condom use among inner city African-American women, *AIDS Care* 20(4) (2008):470–477. doi: 10.1080/09540120701867016.
5. B. Dawson-Saunders and R. G. Trap, *Basic and Clinical Biostatistics*, 2nd ed. (Norwalk, CT: Appleton & Lange, 1994); T. D. V. Swinscow and M. J. Campbell, *Statistics at Square One*, 10th ed. (Spain: BMJ Books, 2002).
6. T. D. V. Swinscow and M. J. Campbell, *Statistics at Square One*, 10th ed. (Spain: BMJ Books, 2002).
7. B. Dawson-Saunders and R. G. Trap, *Basic and Clinical Biostatistics*, 2nd ed. (Norwalk, CT: Appleton & Lange, 1994); T. D. V. Swinscow and M. J. Campbell, *Statistics at Square One*, 10th ed. (Spain: BMJ Books, 2002).
8. L. C. Hamilton, *Statistics with Stata* (Belmont, CA: Thomson, 2004).
9. P. Armitage and G. Berry, *Statistical Methods in Medical Research*, 3rd ed. (Oxford, UK: Blackwell Scientific Publishing, 1994); B. Rosner, *Fundamentals of Biostatistics*, 5th ed. (CA: Duxbury Press, 2000); J. A. Freiman et al., The importance of beta, the type II error and sample size in the design and interpretation of the randomized clinical trial, *N Engl J Med* 299 (1978):690–694.

9 Statistical inference involving relationships or associations

9.1 Introduction

Bivariate or *univariable* analysis refers to the analysis of the relationship between *one* independent (X) and *one* dependent variable (Y). For example, if an investigator decides to examine the relationship between the height and weight of 100 high school children, she or he may wish to determine if weight (Y) depends on height (X).[1] *Multivariable analysis* refers to the analysis between a single dependent variable and more than one independent variable (e.g., a study to determine the impact of race/ethnicity and gender in the development of colorectal cancer).[2] The independent variables are age (X_1) and race (X_2), while the dependent variable is colorectal cancer (Y). *Multivariate analysis* is the technique that involves more than one dependent and more than a single independent variable.[3] This term is *not* interchangeable with multivariable analysis, and it is often used incorrectly.

The relationship between variables can be tested linearly when variables meet certain assumptions involving shape; thus, normally distributed data can be assessed for a linear relationship using the linear regression model as well as the correlation coefficient. These models, which are based on t test and chi-square distributions, examine the variables of interest for a significant relationship. The linear regression model goes beyond mere association to assess whether or not the independent/predictor/explanatory variable can be used to predict the outcome/response/dependent variable that is continuous.

When variables do not meet the assumption of normality (violate Gaussian distribution or the bell-shaped curve), the relationship between variables can be tested using the nonparametric alternative to the Pearson correlation coefficient, which is the Spearman correlation coefficient, also termed Spearman Rho.[4] A correlation coefficient is really a measure of a linear relationship between two variables if the variables are measured on a numerical scale. However, unlike the simple linear relationship, there is no specific dependent or independent variable in correlations coefficient analysis. For example, investigators conducted a study to examine the correlation between radiographic measures of the surgically treated clubfoot (talo-calcaneal angle) and pedobarographic measure (heel impulse) obtained from the gait analysis of foot pressure. Since the data on the two variables were numerical, normality tests were performed on the sets of the two variables of interest. The data were observed not to violate normality, and Pearson correlation was used to examine the significant linear relationship between these radiographic and pedographic measures. In this context, the intent of the investigators was not to determine whether or not the radiographic measure (independent/explanatory) predicts the pedographic measure as an outcome or response variable in the relationship but simply to determine if a correlation, which is a form of relationship, exists. Consider another example. If investigators wanted to examine the linear relationship between systolic blood pressure (SBP) and age measured in years, the two variables are measured on a continuous scale and are normally distributed; the Pearson correlation coefficient is adequate once these assumptions are met. And if the investigators also intended to assess whether or not SBP can be predicted based on the subject's age, then the simple linear regression is appropriate.

A correlation could also be performed using an ordinal or binary and a numerical (continuous) variable. Let us consider a situation in which investigators wanted to determine if there was a significant difference in age at surgery (numerical variable) by postoperative deep wound infection (binary variable). A correlation coefficient could be used. This analysis provides the same results that could be obtained from an independent or two-sample *t* test, where the later test will be most appropriate to provide data on different mean ages at surgery for those with and those without deep wound infection. To illustrate this, we use the data in this study (data used with permission).

STATA syntax: pwcorr ageofsurgery deep_wound, obs sig

```
pwcorr ageofsurgery deep_wound, obs sig

             |          age of surgery                  deep wound
ageofsurgery    |        1.0000
             |          66
             |
deep_wound      |        -0.0803                        1.0000
             |0.5216
             |          66                              66
```

The significance level in the above correlation is greater than 0.05, implying that the null hypothesis of no significant difference in age by deep wound infection should not be rejected. The following STATA output shows a similar relationship, using a two-sample or independent-sample *t* test. The probability level is used to test the null hypothesis of no mean age difference by deep wound infection.

```
. ttest  LDL, by ( Sex)

Two-sample t test with equal variances
------------------------------------------------------------------------------
   Group |     Obs        Mean    Std. Err.   Std. Dev.   [95% Conf. Interval]
---------+--------------------------------------------------------------------
       1 |      56    115.0607    1.234629    9.239121    112.5865     117.535
       2 |      55      104.26    .7081993    5.252146    102.8401    105.6799
---------+--------------------------------------------------------------------
combined |     111     109.709    .8784149    9.254675    107.9682    111.4498
---------+--------------------------------------------------------------------
    diff |            10.80071     1.42996                7.966578    13.63485
------------------------------------------------------------------------------
    diff = mean(1) - mean(2)                                      t =   7.5532
Ho: diff = 0                                     degrees of freedom =      109

    Ha: diff < 0                 Ha: diff != 0                 Ha: diff > 0
 Pr(T < t) = 1.0000         Pr(|T| > |T|) = 0.0000          Pr(T > t) = 0.0000
```

The above STATA output examines the mean difference in LDL comparing female to male patients with hypertension ($n = 111$) on a new antihypertensive drug relative to the standard of care. While the research question is whether or not males and females differ in LDL serum level, the null hypothesis indicates no difference in mean serum LDL comparing male to female patients ($\mu 1$ (male) $- \mu 2$ (female) $= 0$). The mean difference in this output is 10.8 mg/dl, which is clinically meaningful (effect size), while the significant or precision estimate (p value) is < 0.0001, implying a strong evidence against the null hypothesis at a significance level of 0.05 (type I error tolerance).

One of the rationale and assumption of an independent sample t test is equal variance. This must be tested prior to accepting this result; otherwise, an independent sample t test with unequal variance is required. The STATA output below on summary statistics demonstrates the variances between men and women with respect to LDL.

```
. tabstat  LDL, stat (mean, sd sem var n) by ( Sex)

Summary for variables:  LDL
     by categories of:  Sex

     Sex |       mean         sd   se(mean)   variance         N
---------+--------------------------------------------------------
       1 |   115.0607   9.239121   1.234629   85.36136        56
       2 |     104.26   5.252146   .7081993   27.58504        55
---------+--------------------------------------------------------
   Total |    109.709   9.254675   .8784149   85.64902       111
------------------------------------------------------------------
```

The above STATA output clearly indicates unequal variance, which violates one of the independent t test assumptions, requiring a test with unequal variance.

```
. ttest  LDL, by ( Sex) unequal

Two-sample t test with unequal variances

------------------------------------------------------------------------------
   Group |     Obs        Mean    Std. Err.   Std. Dev.   [95% Conf. Interval]
---------+--------------------------------------------------------------------
       1 |      56    115.0607    1.234629    9.239121    112.5865     117.535
       2 |      55      104.26    .7081993    5.252146    102.8401    105.6799
---------+--------------------------------------------------------------------
combined |     111     109.709    .8784149    9.254675    107.9682    111.4498
---------+--------------------------------------------------------------------
    diff |            10.80071    1.423326                7.971927     13.6295
------------------------------------------------------------------------------
    diff = mean(1) - mean(2)                                      t =   7.5884
Ho: diff = 0                     Satterthwaite's degrees of freedom =  87.4996

    Ha: diff < 0                 Ha: diff != 0                 Ha: diff > 0
 Pr(T < t) = 1.0000         Pr(|T| > |t|) = 0.0000          Pr(T > t) = 0.0000
```

The above STATA output corrects for an equal variance assumption, with the null hypothesis of no mean difference between male and female in serum LDL. Similar to equal variance output above, there remains a clinically meaningful mean difference, 10 mg/dl, which is different from 0 mg/dl, as well as a statistically significant difference, $p < 0.0001$, implying that the chance of obtaining a mean difference in serum LDL of 10.8 mg/dl or a value as extreme as this magnitude is less than 1%, if indeed the population parameter is different from the sample statistic (10.8 mg/dl).

The same p value is obtained with the two-sample t test performed with equal variance assumption. The same statistical inference could be drawn here, that with 0.05 as the set significance level, the p value in this test (0.52) implies that we fail to reject the null hypothesis of no significant difference with age at surgery, comparing those with and without deep wound infection by the age at surgery. Assuming inequality of variance, we performed a two-sample t test and obtained the same statistical inference but with a slight difference in the significance level compared to that obtained with the correlation analysis. Therefore, the closest approximation of the Spearman correlation coefficient in this example is the t test with equal variance.

```
STATA syntax: ttest ageofsurgery, by(deep_wound) unequal

Two-sample t test with unequal variances

Group    | Obs      Mean       Std. Err.    Std. Dev.    [95% Conf. Interval]
       0 | 44     14.51818    0.5313857     3.524814     13.44654    15.58982
       1 | 22     13.94545     0.669358     3.139567     12.55345    15.33746
combined | 66     14.32727    0.4170188     3.387876     13.49443    15.16012

       diff = mean(0) - mean(1) t = 0.6701
Ho: diff = 0 Satterthwaite's degrees of freedom = 46.7437

      Ha: diff < 0 Ha: diff != 0 Ha: diff > 0
Pr(T < t) = 0.7470              Pr(|T| > |t|) = 0.5061      Pr(T > t) = 0.2530
```

While correlation and regression assess linear relationships and are similar in some respects (the slope of the regression line has the same negative or positive sign as the correlation), the two differ in that correlation is scale-independent, but regression is scale-dependent, which affects the values of *a* and *b* in the regression equation.[5] For example, the correlation between the pedobarograph and the x-ray are the same regardless of what measure is used to assess the pedobarograph. However, the equation, because of regressing pedograph on the x-ray (predicting x-ray measured in angles or measured in *x* unit vs. *y* unit) gives different values for the constant (a) and the slope (b) in the equation:

$$\text{Simple linear regression} \rightarrow \grave{Y} = a + bX$$

where $\grave{Y}$ is the predicted pedobarograph (response or regressand), *a* is the constant, *b* is the coefficient of regression, and *X* is the x-ray (independent or regressor). Please note that unlike this complete model ($\Upsilon = \beta_0 + \beta_1 X_1 + \varepsilon$), in this regression equation, because it describes the relationship, the error term (ε) is not used (simplification of the relationship). Consider a study to assess the proliferative and prognostic marker in hepatocellular carcinoma. The investigators first wanted to assess the linear relationship between these two markers, assuming an inverse relationship before testing their relationship with clinicopathologic covariates.

```
STATA syntax: regress  p27tum agnor

  Source |       SS       df       MS              Number of obs =      40
---------+------------------------------           F(  1,     38) =    7.78
   Model |  6819.37465     1  6819.37465           Prob > F      =  0.0082
Residual |  33293.5414    38  876.145825           R-squared     =  0.1700
---------+------------------------------           Adj R-squared =  0.1482
   Total |   40112.916    39  1028.53631           Root MSE      =    29.6

------------------------------------------------------------------------------
  p27tum |      Coef.   Std. Err.       t     P>|t|      [95% Conf. Interval]
---------+--------------------------------------------------------------------
   agnor |  -9.633796    3.453133    -2.79    0.008     -16.6243    -2.643293
   _cons |   97.93353    23.95502     4.09    0.000     49.43912     146.4279
------------------------------------------------------------------------------
```

The above STATA output indicates an inverse linear relationship between the proliferative marker (p27tum) and prognostic marker (agnor). This method (simple regression) of analysis is appropriate because the two variables are assumed to be normally distributed and are both measured on a continuous scale. However, since the proliferative marker was not normally distributed, sktest, $p = 0.005$, a robust regression is suggested. The use of robust regression with the STATA syntax `rreg` is described below in other examples involving the stiff knee gait and the kinematics.

```
. regress  LDL HDL

      Source |       SS       df       MS              Number of obs =     111
-------------+------------------------------           F(  1,   109) =  588.32
       Model |  7948.71635     1  7948.71635           Prob > F      =  0.0000
    Residual |  1472.67537   109  13.5107832           R-squared     =  0.8437
-------------+------------------------------           Adj R-squared =  0.8423
       Total |  9421.39172   110  85.6490156           Root MSE      =  3.6757

------------------------------------------------------------------------------
         LDL |      Coef.   Std. Err.      t    P>|t|     [95% Conf. Interval]
-------------+----------------------------------------------------------------
         HDL |  -1.379894   .0568902   -24.26   0.000    -1.492649   -1.267139
       _cons |   183.1206   3.046652    60.11   0.000     177.0822     189.159
------------------------------------------------------------------------------
```

The above STATA output illustrates a simple linear relationship between HDL and LDL. The significant regression line is obtained in this output indicative of the feasibility of using patients' serum HDL to predict their serum LDL level: Serum LDL = 183.1 – 1.38 (HDL). The coefficient of determination provided by R-squared of 0.84 is indicative of 85% changes in LDL as a function of HDL, implying that increasing HDL on average results in 84% reduction in LDL in this sample.

```
. rreg LDL HDL

   Huber iteration 1:  maximum difference in weights = .62796098
   Huber iteration 2:  maximum difference in weights = .1484032
   Huber iteration 3:  maximum difference in weights = .04888443
Biweight iteration 4:  maximum difference in weights = .27234337
Biweight iteration 5:  maximum difference in weights = .03553642
Biweight iteration 6:  maximum difference in weights = .04432487
Biweight iteration 7:  maximum difference in weights = .00988001

Robust regression                                      Number of obs =     111
                                                       F( 1,   109)  =  994.28
                                                       Prob > F      =  0.0000

------------------------------------------------------------------------------
         LDL |      Coef.   Std. Err.      t    P>|t|     [95% Conf. Interval]
-------------+----------------------------------------------------------------
         HDL |  -1.321647   .0419143   -31.53   0.000     -1.40472   -1.238575
       _cons |   178.7614   2.244643    79.64   0.000     174.3126    183.2103
------------------------------------------------------------------------------
```

With the normality assumption requirements for simple linear regression, a robust SE/variance analysis is required to adjust for the assumption violation. Above and below are examples of how to apply this method in linear regression model.

```
. regress LDL HDL, robust

Linear regression                               Number of obs =      111
                                                F(  1,   109)  =   785.46
                                                Prob > F       =   0.0000
                                                R-squared      =   0.8437
                                                Root MSE       =   3.6757
```

LDL	Coef.	Robust Std. Err.	t	p>|t|	[95% Conf.	Interval]
HDL	-1.379894	.049236	-28.03	0.000	-1.477478	-1.28231
_cons	183.1206	2.723784	67.23	0.000	177.7222	188.5191

The following STATA output with the robust regression demonstrates a statistically significant indirect or inverse relationship between the tumor proliferative marker (p27) and tumor prognostic marker (agnor) – $\beta = -10.46$, $t = -2.87$, and $p = 0.007$. Also note the value of F ratio, 8.21, confirming the relationship between the two statistics (t and F): $F = t^2$.

```
STATA syntax: rreg p27tum agnor
Huber iteration 1:   maximum difference in weights = .41297509
Huber iteration 2:   maximum difference in weights = .02492165
Biweight iteration 3:   maximum difference in weights = .12620827
Biweight iteration 4:   maximum difference in weights = .00112964

Robust regression                             Number of obs   =        40
                                              F(  1,     38)  =      8.21
                                              Prob > F        =    0.0067
```

p27tum	Coef.	Std. Err.	t	P>|t|	[95% Conf.	Interval]
agnor	**-10.45858**	3.649444	**-2.87**	**0.007**	**-17.8465**	**-3.070667**
_cons	102.6055	25.31687	4.05	0.000	51.3542	153.8568

Besides simple linear regression, which involves just one independent variable (x), linear regression can be performed with more than one independent variable. *This method is termed multivariable (not multivariate) linear regression.* The intent of this analysis is to assess simultaneously how each variable in the model influences or could be used to predict the outcome while maintaining others at constant, implying controlling for the effect (assuming that x_2, x_3, and x_4 are important confounders) of x_2, x_3, and x_4 in order to determine how x_1 predicts the outcome Y. Therefore, multiple or multivariable linear regression is an extension or generalization of simple linear regression in which there are two or more repressors or independent or predictor variables. However, since simple linear regression only assesses a linear association, how linear is multiple linear regression? For example, if investigators in a study to assess the outcome of posterior spine fusion in correcting curve deformities in pediatric patients with neuromuscular scoliosis intended to determine how estimated blood loss could be used to predict parked blood cells given intraoperatively, as well as control for cell saver given during surgery, a multivariable linear regression would be an adequate statistical analysis method. Thus, predicted parked red blood cells (Y) = a (constant) + (β_1) regression coefficient1 (estimated blood loss $-x_1$) + (β_2) regression coeficient2 (cell saver $- x_2$). This equation could be simply written as $Y = a + m_1X_1 + m_2X_2$ (mathematical model) or by using a probabilistic model:

$$Y = \beta_0 + \beta_1 X_1 + \beta_2 X_2 \quad \text{or} \quad Y = a + b_1 X_1 + b_2 X_2$$

where Y is the predicted parked red blood cells, b_1 is the coefficient of regression for estimated blood loss, and X_1 is the estimated blood loss. Likewise, b_2 is the coefficient of regression for cell saver while X_2 is the cell saver. The linear risk model of this function is

$$\boldsymbol{R}(\boldsymbol{x}_1) = \alpha + \beta_1 \boldsymbol{x}_1$$

$$\boldsymbol{R}(\boldsymbol{x}_1 + 1) = \alpha + \beta_1(\boldsymbol{x}_1 + 1), \text{ and } \boldsymbol{R}(\boldsymbol{x}_1) = \alpha + \beta_1 \boldsymbol{x}_1, \text{ then } \beta_1 = \boldsymbol{R}(\boldsymbol{x}_1 + 1) - \boldsymbol{R}(\boldsymbol{x}_1)$$

where β_1 is the difference in risk between subpopulations defined by having $X_1 = x_1 + 1$ and the subpopulation defined by having $X_1 = x_1$ and the difference does not depend on the reference level x_1 for X_1 where comparison is made.

While regression function (commonly referred to as regression) and model (estimates the true regression function) specification are introduced in this chapter, detailed discussion of model specification is presented in intermediate and advanced epidemiologic and biostatistics texts.[6] We saw earlier the importance of a scale of measurement in selecting linear regression function and correlation (numeric or continuous response variables). Recollect that when considering a regression function $E(Y \mid X = x)$, Y is the response variable (regressand) and x is the regressor or covariate. For example, in the previous illustration on age at surgery and postoperative deep wound infection, if Y is deep wound infection and x is age at surgery, $E(Y \mid X = x)$ represents the average age of subjects (regressor), given deep wound infection, x (regressand). Regression analysis can be performed with binary outcome or regressand, such as binomial and logistic regression functions and models.

With a binary outcome, let us consider a hypothetical prospective cohort study conducted to assess the risk of developing endometrial carcinoma among women aged 18 to 30 years diagnosed with polycystic ovarian syndrome (POS). If we consider the regressand to be endometrial carcinoma and it is indicated by Y, and $Y = 1$ (presence of the disease or outcome) and $Y = 0$ (absence of disease or outcome), then the $E(Y \mid X = 1)$ is the average of the endometrial cancer among women aged 18 to 35 years with POS and $E(Y \mid X = 0)$ is the average of endometrial cancer among women aged 18 to 35 years without POS and $E(Y \mid X = x)$ is a binary regression.

In epidemiologic studies, logistic regression is suitable for obtaining the odds ratio in case–control studies while binomial regression is appropriate for risk ratios from prospective or retrospective cohort designs.[7] However, where the prevalence of disease or outcome of interest is low, the odds ratio approximates the risk ratio, and logistic regression is an adequate method for estimating the effect of an explanatory or regressor on a regressand or outcome with a binary scale of measurement.

In a logistic regression technique, the probability of the outcome is predicted given the value of an explanatory variable, which may be measured on a continuous, binary, or categorical scale called a *mixed scale*. Consider $\pi\,[x]$ to be the probability that a child with neuromuscular scoliosis who has skin breakdown (x) after posterior spine fusion develops a deep wound infection, the probability function will be presented as follows:

$$\pi[\boldsymbol{x}] = \exp[\alpha + \beta\boldsymbol{x}] / (1 + \exp[\alpha + \beta\boldsymbol{x}])$$

And the probability of not developing deep wound infection is presented as follows:

$$1 - \pi[x] = 1 + \exp[\alpha + \beta x] - \exp[\alpha + \beta x]/1 \\ + \exp[\alpha + \beta x] = 1/1 + \exp[\alpha + \beta x]$$

where α and β are unknown parameters associated with the target population. The odds of developing deep wound infection are represented by $P/1 - P = \pi\,[x]/1 - \pi\,[x]$, and the log odds of developing deep wound infection are as follows:

$$\text{Log}\left[\pi[\boldsymbol{x}]/1 - \pi[\boldsymbol{x}]\right] = \alpha + \beta\boldsymbol{x}, \text{ thus logit } [\pi] = \log[\pi/(1 - \pi)]$$

Finally, exp $[\beta]$ = odds ratio, which is the measure of the effect or point estimate in a logistic regression technique utilizing case–control design.

Regression is also used in analyzing time-to-event data. A Cox regression (the proportional hazard model or Cox proportional hazard model) is used in the failure-time model, where the event may be death from a specific cause, overall death, or even system failure.[8] This technique involves *censored data*, implying data where the event beyond a particular temporal point was not observed.

In practice, understanding survival data involves examining censoring (those who survived their follow-up interval, but for whom, it is not known how much longer they lived thereafter or who were lost to follow-up), truncation, survival probability, survival function and Kaplan–Meier survival curve, probability density function, cumulative probability of failure as

Kaplan–Meier failure estimates, Nelson–Aalen hazard estimates, and equality of survival using several test statistics including the most commonly used log-rank test and hazard rate. The distribution of the data is essential, and most survival data are nonnormal in distribution; they are right skewed, with varying degrees of censoring, thus requiring the use of nonparametric or semiparametric tests to determine whether the survival curves are statistically different from one another. Briefly, let us consider a cohort of cerebral palsy pediatric patients with equinus foot deformity who underwent surgery for correction and recurrence as the end point (outcome)—not a very good measure of end point. If investigators followed these patients forward in time to determine recurrence surgery and follow-up continues for each subject until recurrence, the study ends, or further observation becomes impossible, then these individuals are said to be censored. In this demonstration, recurrence surgery may not occur for all subjects during the follow-up, and for such subjects, we assume that the recurrence surgery did not occur while the subjects were being followed and the investigators did not know whether or not recurrence surgery would occur at some later time. However, we can still determine the survival function as well as the median survival but not the mean survival since all the events did not occur at the end of the study.

Survival and cumulative mortality function can be determined using this equation:

$$S[t] = \Pr[t_i > t]$$

which is the probability of surviving until at least time t, where t_i is the time that recurrence occurred and t is the number of subjects who are known to have had recurrence by this time.

The Kaplan–Meier (KM) survival function is a method of generating tables and plots of survival or hazard functions for time-to-event data. The KM is *events dependent only on time*. Because KM models survival based only on time dependence, without covariate effects, it is assumed that event probabilities depend only on time. All subjects are assumed to behave similarly, and computed survival functions are assumed to describe all subjects. This further implies that censored and uncensored cases behave the same. If the censored cases (those for whom the event has not yet happened) are different from the uncensored cases, results may be biased. This is a strong assumption that may be violated in the real world, which is why event history and Cox regression models, which do take covariates into account, are now the more common approach for time-to-event data. The *median survival time* is the time at which half the subjects have reached the event of interest. If the survival curve does not fall to 0.5 (50%), the median time cannot be computed. Rather than classifying the observed survival times into a life table, we can estimate the survival function directly from the continuous survival or failure times. Intuitively, imagine that we create a life table so that each time interval contains exactly one case. Multiplying out the survival probabilities across the "intervals" (i.e., for each single observation), we would get for the survival function:

$$S(t) = \prod_{j=1}^{t} \left[(n-j)/(n-j+1)\right]^{\delta(j)}$$

In this equation, $S(t)$ is the estimated survival function, n is the total number of cases, and $\prod$ denotes the multiplication (geometric sum) across all cases less than or equal to t; $^{\delta(j)}$ is a constant that is either 1 if the jth case is uncensored (complete) or 0 if it is censored. This estimate of the survival function is also called the *product-limit estimator* and was first proposed by Kaplan and Meier. Also, survival function can be simply expressed as follows:

$$S(t) = \Pr\{T > t\} = 1 - F(t)$$

where $F(t) = \Pr\{T\ t\}$, giving the probability that the event has occurred by duration t. This function gives the probability of being alive at duration t, or more generally, the probability that the event of interest has not occurred by duration t.

To determine the effect of covariates and the combined effects of risk factors on the recurrence surgery, the Cox proportional hazard model is adequate. This model allows the independent as well as joint effects of several variables to be assessed. Cox regression, which implements the proportional hazards model or duration model, is designed for analysis of time until an event or time between events. One or more predictor variables, called covariates, are used to predict a status (event) variable. The proportional hazard model is the most general of the regression models because it is not based on any assumptions concerning the nature or shape of the underlying survival distribution. The model assumes that the underlying hazard *rate* (rather than survival time) is a function of the independent variables (covariates); no assumptions are made about the nature or shape of the hazard function (distribution-free). Thus, in a sense, Cox's regression model may be considered to be a semiparametric method. The model may be written as follows:

$$h\{(t), (z_1, z_2 \ldots z_m)\} = h_0(t) * \exp(b_1^* z_1 + \ldots + b_m^* z_m)$$

where $h(t, \ldots)$ denotes the resultant hazard, given the values of the m covariates for the respective case ($z_1, z_2, \ldots, z_m$) and the respective survival time (t). The term $h_0(t)$ is called the *baseline hazard*; it is the hazard for the respective individual when all independent variable values are equal to zero. We can linearize this model by dividing both sides of the equation by $h_0(t)$ and then taking the natural logarithm of both sides:

$$\log\left[h\{(t),\ (z \ldots)\}/h_0(t)\right] = b_1^* z_1 + \ldots + b_m^* z_m$$

Simply, this model represents the instantaneous risk or probability of reaching the end point (recurrence surgery or death) at a particular time. We assume proportional hazards, implying that the hazard ratio for a given explanatory variable or covariate is constant at all times.[9]

This chapter presents the simplified approach to understanding hypothesis testing involving these relationships: (a) correlation analysis, (b) simple linear regression, (c) multiple linear regression, (d) binomial regression, (e) logistic regression (univariable and multivariable), (f) Cox regression (univariable and multivariable), and (g) Poisson regression. Examples of hypothetical studies and their analyses are presented along with their interpretations in order to encourage the understanding of outputs from statistical packages.

9.2 Correlation and correlation coefficients

A sample correlation coefficient is a method used to quantify a linear relationship, implying the use of one variable, (x) to predict another (y), and is measured by sample covariance. However, because unadjusted measures without sample covariance are influenced by observations variability (correlation), requiring such measures as correlations coefficient which adjusts for x and y. For example, if s_x and sy denote the SD of x_i and y_i, mathematically: $r = s_{xy}/s_x s_y$.

9.2.1 What is a correlation coefficient?

This is a statistical technique involving the assessment of the relationship between two variables, but neither is considered dependent. This technique is applicable to normally distributed as well as distribution-free data. The Pearson correlation coefficient, also termed Pearson product-moment correlation coefficient, is used for normally distributed variables. If either of the two variables is not normally distributed, a Pearson correlation is considered inappropriate.[10] Therefore, an alternate approach to analysis involves (1) transformation of either one or both variables in order to achieve near-normal distribution and (2) utilization of the Spearman rank correlation coefficient, which is a nonparametric test. This test allows for the strength of the trends between two variables measured on an ordinal scale to be quantified. Here, we present the nonparametric analog of the Pearson correlation coefficient using STATA illustration.

```
STATA syntax: spearman pkf0 rom0 vkf0, stats(rho obs p)pw
```

The STATA syntax above is used to obtain a nonparametric correlation coefficient given that the peak knee flexion (`pkf`), velocity of knee flexion (`vkf`), and the range of motion (`rom`) are not normally distributed in this sample of children with stiff knee gait.

```
|       pkf0          rom0          vkf0
pkf0    |1.0000
|       100
|       |
rom0|   0.3537        1.0000
|       100           100
|       0.0003
|
vkf0|0.0221           0.0984        1.0000
|       90            90            90
|        0.8365       0.3560
```

Because of multiple comparisons, the correct p value is required, hence the use of Bonferroni, which simply multiplies the uncorrected p value from the uncorrected output by 3 (3 p values) above to derive the corrected p value. This approach is termed *adjustment* or correction for multiple comparison.

STATA syntax: spearman pkf0 rom0 vkf0, stats(rho obs p) pw bon

```
      |     pkf0         rom0          vkf0

pkf0  |  1.0000
|           100
|           |
rom0  |  0.3537       1.0000
|           100          100
|        0.0009
|
vkf0  |  0.0221       0.0984        1.0000
|           90           90            90
|        1.0000      1.0000
```

The STATA syntax bon, obs, p, or pw indicates the Bonferroni correction for multiple comparison—obs for number of observations, p for probability value or significance, and pw for pairwise correlation. In both uncorrected and corrected p values, there remains a significant correlation between the range of motion and the peak knee velocity, $p < 0.05$.

9.2.2 When is the correlation coefficient appropriate?

This technique is adequate in assessing a relationship between two numerical measurements made on the same subjects. The correlation coefficient, also termed Pearson product moment, is the measure of the linear relationship and is designated by r. Because the relationship between the two variables is assumed to be measured in a numeric scale, the violation of this assumption requires an alternative method called the Spearman *rank* correlation coefficient, which is the nonparametric alternative to the Pearson correlation coefficient.

9.2.3 How is the correlation coefficient computed?

Consider a study conducted to examine the correlation between oxygen reserve and walking heart rate. If the investigators wanted to determine the linear relationship between these two variables, assuming the variables are measured in a numeric scale and meet the Gaussian distribution assumption, the Pearson correlation technique would be adequate in determining such a relationship. How could this be computed? Using STATA, we first test the data for normality. Here, we present STATA output for the test of normality of the sample data.

STATA syntax: sktest vo2reserve walkhr

Skewness/Kurtosis tests for Normality

Variable	Pr(Skewness)	Pr(Kurtosis)	joint adj chi2(2)	joint Prob>chi2
vo2reserve	0.907	0.020	5.25	**0.0726**
walkhr	0.310	0.674	1.30	**0.5227**

Since the significance level is >0.05, the two variables are normally distributed, which meets the assumptions for the Pearson correlation coefficient analysis. Below is the STATA output for the Pearson correlation coefficient.

STATA syntax: pwcorr walkhr vo2reserve, sig

	walkhr	vo2res~e
walkhr	1.0000	
voreserve	**-0.8579**	1.0000
	0.0000	

```
. sktest SBP HDL LDL age
```

Skewness/Kurtosis tests for Normality

Variable	Obs	Pr(Skewness)	Pr(Kurtosis)	joint adj chi2(2)	joint Prob>chi2
SBP	111	0.6630	0.0000	19.96	0.0000
HDL	111	0.0001	0.7025	12.98	0.0015
LDL	111	0.0313	0.0000	37.51	0.0000
age	111	0.0002	0.6744	11.64	0.0030

The above STATA output illustrates the normality test for SBP, HDL, LDL, and age of 111 patients. The purpose is to ensure that the distribution of the data meet the normal probability distribution for the intended estimation test and/or hypothesis testing. The result, which is based on the null hypothesis of the data or the random variable, is normal (Ho = data are normal; alternative hypothesis H1 = data are not normal). When the significance test at 5% type one error tolerance is >0.05 (5%), there is evidence against the null hypothesis, implying that the data are normal (reject the null hypothesis and accept the alternative that the distribution of the data follows normal or fit Gaussian probability function).

```
. pwcorr SBP age HDL LDL, obs sig star(5) bonferroni
```

	SBP	age	HDL	LDL
SBP	1.0000			
	111			
age	0.7153*	1.0000		
	0.0000			
	111	111		
HDL	-0.9410*	-0.7453*	1.0000	
	0.0000	0.0000		
	111	111	111	
LDL	0.8767*	0.7613*	-0.9185*	1.0000
	0.0000	0.0000	0.0000	
	111	111	111	111

The correlation coefficient assuming a linear relationship fits the data. The above STATA output illustrates the correlation between these variables, namely, age, SBP, LDL, and HDL. There is a significant direct/positive strong correlation between LDL and SBP, and age, while a very strong, indirect, and statistically significant correlation is observed with HDL.

```
. spearman SBP age HDL LDL, bonferroni
(obs=111)
```

	SBP	age	HDL	LDL
SBP	1.0000			
age	0.5951	1.0000		
HDL	-0.9994	-0.5946	1.0000	
LDL	0.9051	0.7376	-0.9057	1.0000

The above STATA data on the model that fits these data (Spearman correlation coefficient) illustrate a similar correlation coefficient and the direction of the relationship. This model assumes no normal probability distribution, and is hence suitable for distribution-free analysis for linear relationship without any assumption of the predictor in the model.

The $r = -0.86$ shows a strong negative linear relationship between oxygen reserve and heart rate at walking (Graph 9.1). The significance level, <0.001 is indicative of the rejection of the null hypothesis that r is not significantly different from zero. In general, the r is interpreted as follows: (1) correlation coefficient, r, is between -1.0 and $+1.0$, with r close to 0.0 considered to be a weak relationship; (2) 1.0 or -1.0 = strong relationship; (3) >0.7 = strong correlation; (4) 0.3 to 0.7 = moderate correlation, and (5) <0.3 = weak correlation.[11]

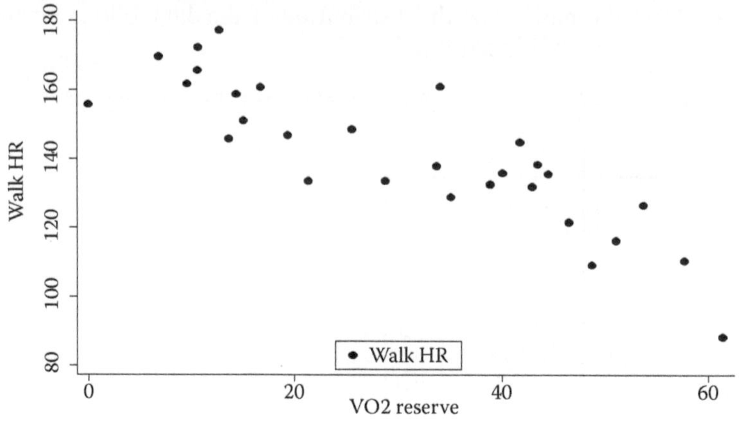

Graph 9.1 Scatter plot of the correlation between volume of reserved 0_2 and walking heart rate. **Note:** The graph of the sample data illustrates a strong negative linear relationship between walking heart rate and volume of reserved oxygen—as reserved oxygen increases, the walking heart rate decreases.

Consider another example of data on stiff knee gait for the correlation between peak knee flexion (pkf0), range of knee motion (ROM0), time to peak knee flexion (tipkf0), maximum velocity of knee flexion (mvkf0), and velocity of knee flexion (vkf0). The correlation coefficients are presented with the significance level and observations (sample size). The output indicates a statistically significant (r is different from 0) moderate positive relationship or correlation between peak knee flexion and the range of motion, $r = 0.37$ (0.4), $p = 0.0001$. Because the null hypothesis for the correlation coefficient is that the correlation coefficient is zero, we reject the null hypothesis that the observed $r = 0.4$ from the data is zero, and conclude that 0.4 is significantly different from 0.0.

STATA syntax: pwcorr pkf0 rom0 tipkf0 mvkf0 vkf0, sig obs

	pkf0	rom0	tipkf0	mvkf0	vkf0
pkf0	1.0000				
	100				
rom0	**0.3713**	1.0000			
	0.0001				
	100	100			
tipkf0	0.0913	0.1559	1.0000		
	0.3688	0.1234			
	99	99	99		
mvkf0	-0.0270	-0.0572	0.0105	1.0000	
	0.8002	0.5925	0.9219		
	90	90	90	90	
vkf0	0.0350	0.0637	-0.0680	0.3819	1.0000
	0.7434	0.5510	0.5240	0.0002	
	90	90	90	90	90

Since the correlation coefficient is based on the assumption that the variables are normally distributed, this normality could be tested graphically by using quantile normal plot or normal probability plot. The above result indicates the uncorrected correlation coefficient, and since we had five correlations of interest, the corrected significance level is required. To obtain this adjustment, we used the Bonferroni correction (bon). Thus, the individual significance level is multiplied by five to obtain the corrected p value. For example, the uncorrected p value for the correlation between peak knee flexion and range of motion was 0.0001, the corrected p value from Bonferroni = (0.001 * 5 = 0.0014). Therefore, in either uncorrected and corrected tests or adjustment for multiple comparisons, the coefficient is significantly different from zero, $p < 0.05$.

```
.STATA syntax: pwcorr pkf0 rom0 tipkf0 mvkf0 vkf0, sig obs bon
      |        pkf0     rom0       tipkf0     mvkf0       vkf0

      pkf0|1.0000
      |       100

      rom0|0.3713       1.0000
      |       0.0014
      |       100       100

    tipkf0|0.0913       0.1559     1.0000
      |       1.0000    1.0000
      |       99        99         99

     mvkf0|-0.0270      -0.0572    0.0105      1.0000
      |       1.0000    1.0000     1.0000
      |       90        90         90          90

      vkf0|0.0350       0.0637     -0.0680     0.3819      1.0000
      |       1.0000    1.0000     1.0000      0.0020
      |       90        90         90          90          90
```

We can test the normality of the range of motion of the knee (ROM0) and the peak knee flexion (pkf0) by using these two tests:

```
STATA Syntax: swilk pkf0 rom0 *(for Shapiro-Wilk) sfrancia pkf0
rom0 *(for Shapiro-Francia) sktest pkf0 rom0 *(for skewness and
kurtosis)
```

Below is the output of the normality test for the three variables, based on the STATA commands above.

```
Shapiro-Wilk W test for normal data
Variable| Obs  W         V      z      Prob>z
pkf0    |  100  0.95593  3.639  2.865  0.00208
rom0    |  100  0.97380  2.163  1.712  0.04346
```

```
Shapiro-Francia W' test for normal data
Variable| Obs   W'        V'      z       Prob>z
pkf0    |   100  0.95177  4.358   2.897   0.00189
rom0    |   100  0.97805  1.984   1.377   0.08427

Skewness/Kurtosis tests for Normality

Variable| Pr(Skewness)  Pr(Kurtosis)  adj chi2(2)  Prob>chi2
pkf0    |   0.001          0.003         15.61       0.0004
rom0    |   0.128          0.057          5.70       0.0578
```

The above three tests for normality, skewness-kurtosis (sktest), Shapiro-Wilk (swilk) and Shapiro-Francia (sfrancia) are used to test the normal distribution of ROM and PKF and indicate that these variables are not normally distributed in this sample (Graph 9.2). *Since the null hypothesis for normality tests states that the distribution is normal, $p < 0.05$ indicates that the distribution is not normal, rejecting the null hypothesis of normally distributed data.*

9.2.4 r *Interpretation*

r takes values from −1 to +1, with $r = 0$ implying no relationship between x and y, and −1 meaning a negative or inverse relationship (negative slope), while 1 reflects a positive slope. Specifically, the closer r is to + 1, the more accurate the application of one variable, x to predict the other variable, y.

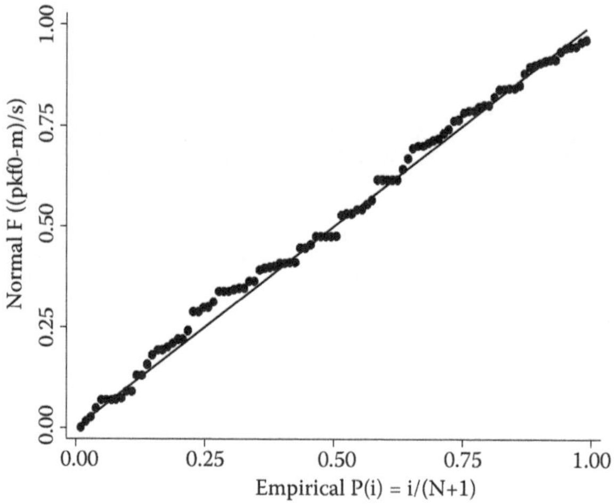

STATA syntax: pnorm pkf0

(a)

Graph 9.2 (a) Normal probability (pnorm) as diagnostic text for the variable of interest, PKFO. Quantile–normal emphasize the tails of the distribution while the normal probability plots places focus on the center of the distribution. (*Continued*)

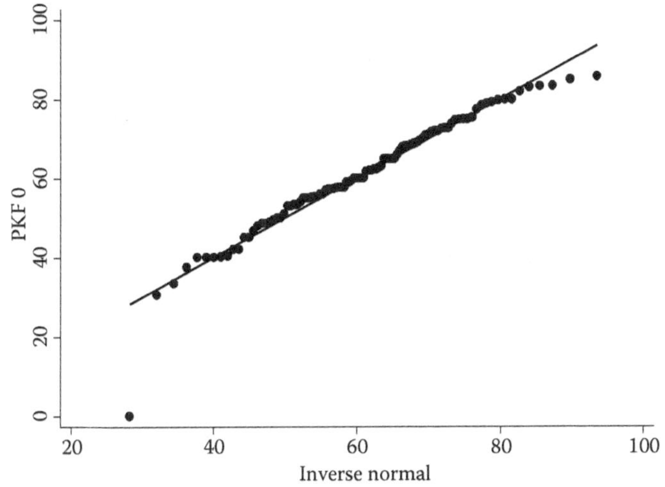

STATA syntax: qnorm pkf0

(b)

Graph 9.2 (Continued) (b) Quantile normal (qnorm) as diagnostic text for the variable of interest, PKFO. Quantile–normal emphasize the tails of the distribution while the normal probability plots places focus on the center of the distribution.

9.3 Simple linear regression

9.3.1 What is a simple linear regression?

A simple linear regression is a method for examining a relationship between a single response or dependent variable and one predictor, explanatory, or independent variable, with the response variable measured as continuous while the independent could be continuous or binary but not categorical (Figure 9.1).[12] Therefore, in a simple linear regression, the relationship between a normally distributed response or dependent variable and a continuous one is examined.

9.3.2 When is simple linear regression feasible?

If the intent of an investigator is to examine the linear relationship between a continuous dependent variable and usually one independent variable, then this method is adequate. Also, if the intent of the investigators is to determine whether or not the independent variable (continuous) could be used to predict the response or outcome variable, given that the outcome or dependent variable is measured on a continuous scale and is normally distributed, then simple linear regression is an adequate method. Recall the following:

Simple linear regression → $\hat{Y} = a + bX$

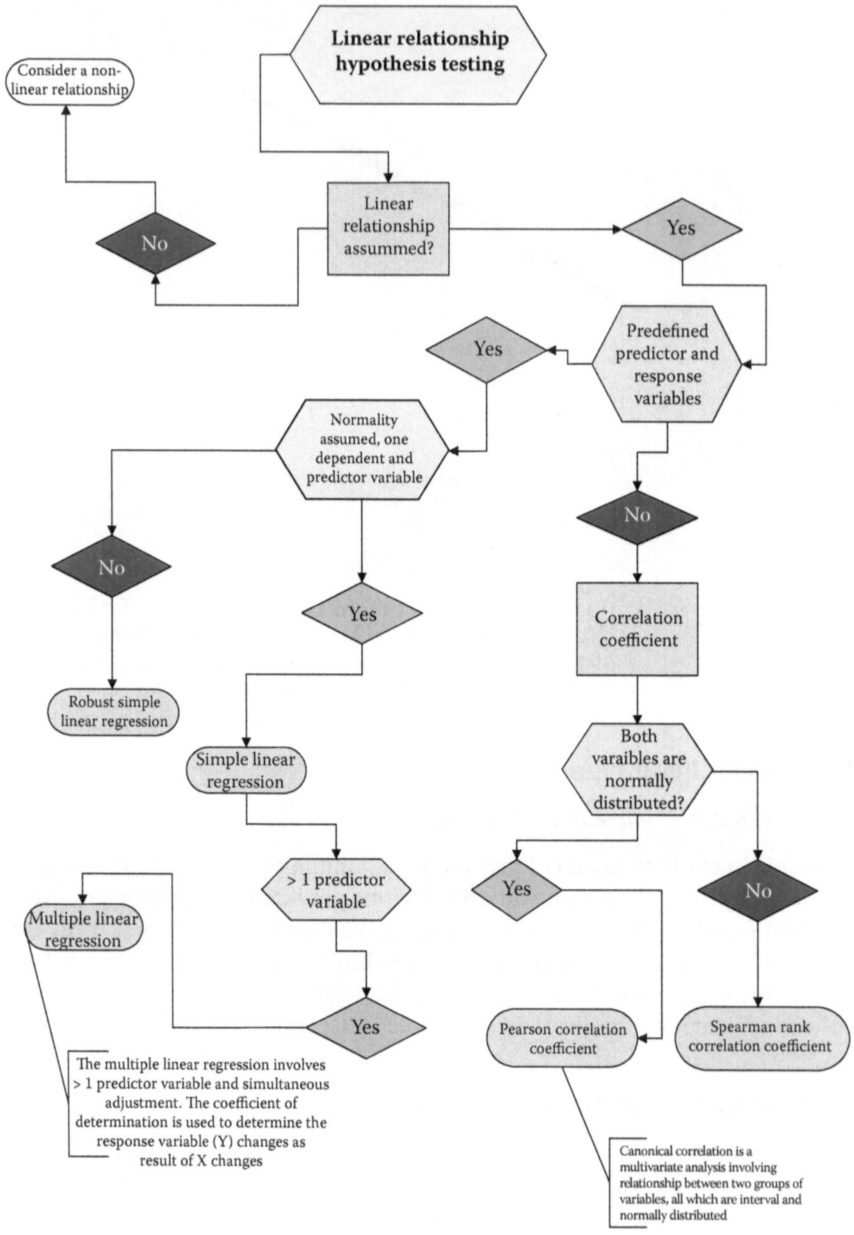

Figure 9.1 Hypotheses testing involving linear relationship.

9.3.3 How is simple linear regression computed?

Consider a study conducted to examine the relationship between range of motion and the peak knee flexion in children with stiff knee gait. Since the investigators wanted to see if peak knee flexion could be used to predict the range of motion of the knee, a simple linear regression is an adequate statistical inference. A linear graph, termed a two-way scatterplot, could be used to graphically illustrate this relationship (Figures 9.2 through 9.4).

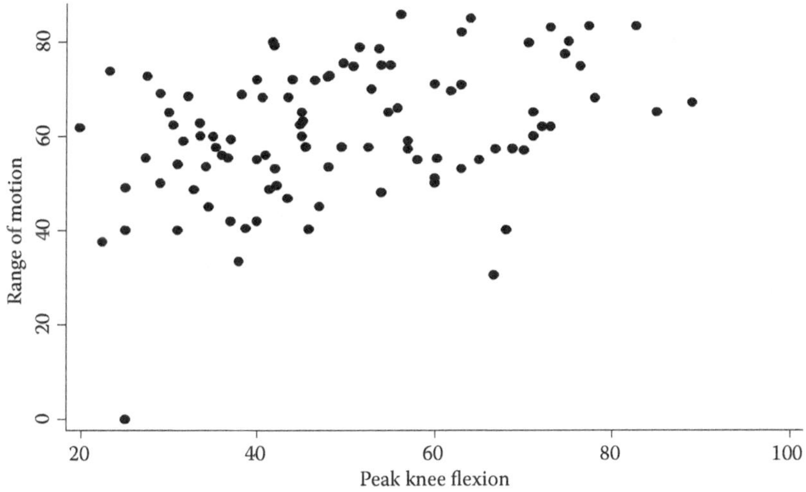

Figure 9.2 Range of motion of the knee by peak knee flexion.

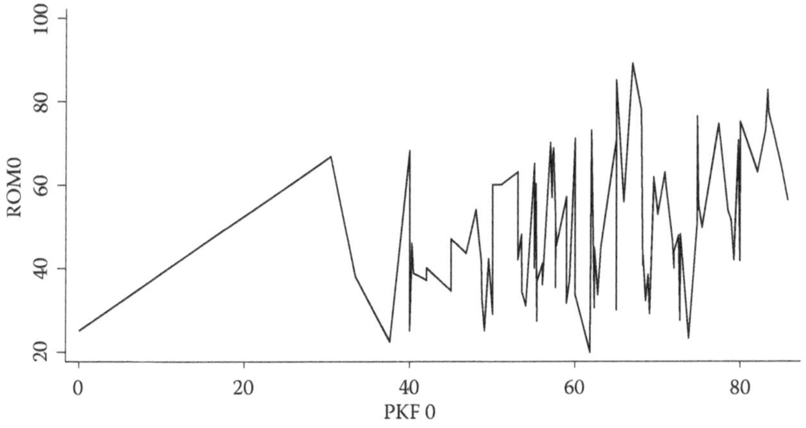

Figure 9.3 Line plot of range of motion by peak knee flexion.

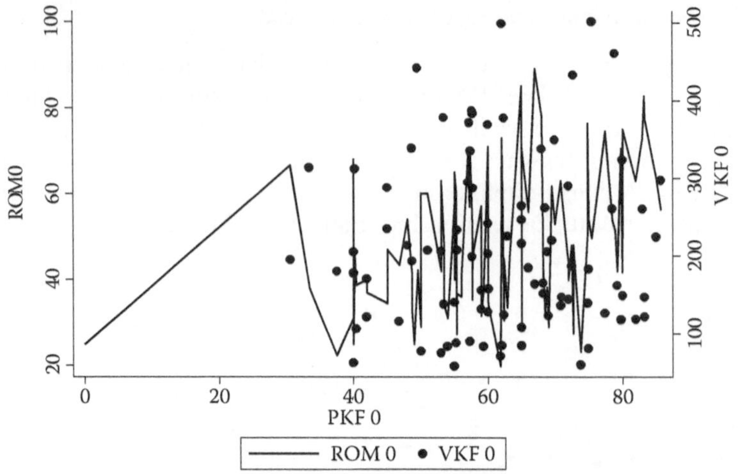

Figure 9.4 ROM and velocity of knee flexion by peak knee flexion.

```
STATA syntax: twoway (scatter pkf0 rom0), ytitle(range of motion,
size(medium)) xtitle(peak knee flexion,size(medium))
```

```
STATA syntax: twoway (line rom0 pkf0, sort)
```

```
STATA syntax: twoway (line rom0 pkf0, sort) (scatter vkf0 pkf0,
sort yaxis(2))
```

We can compute the simple linear regression using peak knee flexion to predict the range of motion of the knee in children with the STATA statistical package. Below is the STATA output of the relationship between knee range of motion and the peak knee flexion in this sample.

STATA syntax: pwcorr pkf0 rom0 tipkf0 mvkf0 vkf0, sig obs

	pkf0	rom0	tipkf0	mvkf0	vkf0
pkf0	1.0000 100				
rom0	**0.3713** **0.0001** 100	1.0000 100			
tipkf0	0.0913 0.3688 99	0.1559 0.1234 99	1.0000 99		
mvkf0	-0.0270 0.8002 90	-0.0572 0.5925 90	0.0105 0.9219 90	1.0000 90	
vkf0	0.0350 0.7434 90	0.0637 0.5510 90	-0.0680 0.5240 90	0.3819 0.0002 90	1.0000 90

```
STATA syntax: regress rom0 pkf0

  Source |       SS       df       MS              Number of obs =     100
---------+------------------------------           F(  1,   109) =   15.67
   Model |  3562.16533     1  3562.16533           Prob > F      =  0.0001
Residual |  22274.1805    98  227.287556           R-squared     =  0.1379
---------+------------------------------           Adj R-squared =  0.1291
   Total |  25836.3458    99   260.97319           Root MSE      =  15.076

------------------------------------------------------------------------------
    rom0 |      Coef.   Std. Err.      t     P>|t|     [95% Conf. Interval]
---------+--------------------------------------------------------------------
    pkf0 |   .4275568   .1080002     3.96    0.000     .2132339    .6418796
   _cons |   23.22742   6.747237     3.44    0.001     9.837744    36.61709
```

Because the outcome variable is not normally distributed, the *robust regression* was used, which is a weighted least square analysis. Simply, the robust regression eliminated gross outliers.

```
STATA syntax: rreg rom0 pkf0    * rreg means robust regression

   Huber iteration 1: maximum difference in weights = .39621995
   Huber iteration 2: maximum difference in weights = .03014185
Biweight iteration 3: maximum difference in weights = .15081295
Biweight iteration 4: maximum difference in weights = .00769687

Robust regression                                      Number of obs =     100
                                                       F(  1,    98) =   14.88
                                                       Prob > F      =  0.0002

------------------------------------------------------------------------------
    rom0 |      Coef.   Std. Err.      t     P>|t|     [95% Conf. Interval]
---------+--------------------------------------------------------------------
    pkf0 |   .4401077   .1141079     3.86    0.000     .2136642    .6665512
   _cons |   22.05167   7.128814     3.09    0.003     7.904769    36.19857
------------------------------------------------------------------------------
```

```
. sfrancia BMI AHI OAI 02SN METC02

                   Shapiro-Francia W' test for normal data

Variable |   Obs       W'          V'        z       Prob>z
---------+---------------------------------------------------
     BMI |   495    0.77305     81.201     9.639    0.00001
     AHI |   505    0.74352     93.398     9.959    0.00001
     OAI |   505    0.68428    114.973    10.415    0.00001
    02SN |   505    0.89320     38.891     8.036    0.00001
  METC02 |   505    0.94374     20.487     6.629    0.00001

.  swilk  BMI  AHI  OAI 02SN  METC02
                    Shapiro-Wilk W test for normal data

Variable |   Obs       W          V          z       Prob>z
---------+---------------------------------------------------
     BMI |   495    0.77384     75.392    10.386    0.00000
     AHI |   505    0.74566     86.328    10.721    0.00000
     OAI |   505    0.68279    107.669    11.253    0.00000
    02SN |   505    0.88913     37.632     8.725    0.00000
  METC02 |   505    0.94647     18.170     6.974    0.00000
```

The STATA output above demonstrates the normality test for the baseline (preoperative polysomnographic parameters) variables for powered intracapsular tonsillectomy and adenoidectomy (PITA). Of the preoperative parameters, namely, apnea hypopnea index (AHI), obstructive apnea index (OAI), oxygen saturation nadir (O2SN), mean EtCO2 level (METCO2), and BMI, none followed normal frequency distribution.

```
. spearman AHI OAI 02SN METC02 BMI, stats(rho obs p) star(0.05) bonferroni

+-------------------+
| Key               |
|-------------------|
|   rho             |
|   Number of obs   |
|   Sig. Level      |
+-------------------+

             |      AHI         OAI          02SN      METCO2          BMI
-------------+--------------------------------------------------------------
         AHI |   1.0000
             |      495
             |
             |   0.8693*     1.0000
             |      495         495
             |   0.0000
             |
        O2SN |  -0.2611*    -0.3244*      1.0000
             |      495         495          495
             |   0.0000      0.0000
             |
      METCO2 |  -0.1151     -0.0472      -0.3138*      1.0000
             |      495         495          495          495
             |   0.1039      1.0000       0.0000
             |
         BMI |   0.0357     -0.0550      -0.1058       0.1181       1.0000
             |      495         495          495          495          495
             |   1.0000      1.0000       0.1849       0.0856
```

The above STATA output illustrates the use of a nonparametric method to examine the data for correlation prior to the choice of model in examining how BMI could be used to predict METCO2, and METCO2 to predict O2SN.

```
. pwcorr AHI OAI 02SN METC02 BMI, star(5) bonferroni

             |      AHI         OAI        02SN      METC02         BMI
-------------+------------------------------------------------------------
         AHI |   1.0000
         OAI |   0.9130*     1.0000
        02SN |  -0.3024*    -0.3265*     1.0000
      METC02 |  -0.0211      0.0135     -0.2871*     1.0000
         BMI |   0.0614     -0.0209     -0.1037      0.0739      1.0000
```

Parametric method illustrating the correlation between the polysomnographic measures and BMI.

```
. regress O2SN METCO2

      Source |       SS       df       MS              Number of obs =     505
-------------+------------------------------           F(1,    109)  =   45.19
       Model |  6379.07591     1  6397.07591           Prob > F      =  0.0000
    Residual |  71201.0746   503  141.552832           R-squared     =  0.0824
-------------+------------------------------           Adj R-squared =  0.0806
       Total |  77598.1505   504  153.964584           Root MSE      =  11.898

------------------------------------------------------------------------------
        O2SN |      Coef.   Std. Err.      t    P>|t|     [95% Conf. Interval]
-------------+----------------------------------------------------------------
      METCO2 |   -.501418   .0745879    -6.72   0.000    -.6479602   -.3548758
       _cons |   109.1745   4.314397    25.30   0.000      100.698    117.6509
------------------------------------------------------------------------------
```

Nonrobustic simple linear regression between O2SN and METCO2, implying the use of METCO2 to predict O2SN.

```
. rreg O2SN METCO2

   Huber iteration 1:  maximum difference in weights = .76940631
   Huber iteration 2:  maximum difference in weights = .07458172
   Huber iteration 3:  maximum difference in weights = .01808082
Biweight iteration 4:  maximum difference in weights = .29375833
Biweight iteration 5:  maximum difference in weights = .02655531
Biweight iteration 6:  maximum difference in weights = .00584214

Robust regression                                      Number of obs =     505
                                                       F( 1,   503)  =   51.60
                                                       Prob > F      = 0.0000

------------------------------------------------------------------------------
        O2SN |      Coef.   Std. Err.      t    P>|t|     [95% Conf. Interval]
-------------+----------------------------------------------------------------
      METCO2 |  -.4612734   .0642118    -7.18   0.000    -.5874298    -.335117
       _cons |   108.3024   3.714212    29.16   0.000     101.0051    115.5997
------------------------------------------------------------------------------
```

With the violation of the normality assumption required in simple linear regression, the robust regression is used, which forces normality on the sample distribution by addressing the outliers. There is a negative or inverse relationship/correlation between O2SN and METCO2, as well as regression equation, implying that METCO2 could be used to predict O2SN: O2SN = 108.3 – 0.46(METCO2).

```
. regress O2SN METCO2, robust

Linear regression                                      Number of obs =     505
                                                       F(1,   503)   =   29.86
                                                       Prob > F      =  0.0000
                                                       R-squared     =  0.0824
                                                       Root MSE      =  11.898

------------------------------------------------------------------------------
             |               Robust
        O2SN |      Coef.   Std. Err.      t    p>|t|     [95% Conf. Interval]
-------------+----------------------------------------------------------------
      METCO2 |   -.501418   .0917611    -5.46   0.000    -.6817002   -.3211358
       _cons |   109.1745   5.157451    21.17   0.000     99.04167    119.3073
------------------------------------------------------------------------------
```

The above STATA output illustrates a robust method, and the result is comparable to the previous (`rreg` syntax) method, except for the distinctive attribute of robust standard error and variance.

```
. regress METCO2 BMI

      Source |       SS           df       MS      Number of obs   =       495
-------------+----------------------------------   F(1, 493)       =      2.71
       Model |  137.164442         1  137.164442   Prob > F        =    0.1004
    Residual |  24961.7446       493  50.6323421   R-squared       =    0.0055
-------------+----------------------------------   Adj R-squared   =    0.0034
       Total |  25098.9091       494  50.8075083   Root MSE        =    7.1156

------------------------------------------------------------------------------
      METCO2 |      Coef.   Std. Err.      t    P>|t|     [95% Conf. Interval]
-------------+----------------------------------------------------------------
         BMI |   .0811913    .049329     1.65   0.100    -.0157298    .1781123
       _cons |   55.84081   1.013806    55.08   0.000      53.8489    57.83273
------------------------------------------------------------------------------
```

The above STATA output demonstrates a nonrobust method of using BMI to predict METCO2. In this sample, while BMI correlates directly with METCO2, it could not be used to predict METCO2.

```
. rreg METCO2 BMI

   Huber iteration 1:  maximum difference in weights = .79039779
   Huber iteration 2:  maximum difference in weights = .0416558
Biweight iteration 3:  maximum difference in weights = .2882931
Biweight iteration 4:  maximum difference in weights = .00471249

Robust regression                                      Number of obs =     495
                                                       F( 1,   493)  =    4.55
                                                       Prob > F      =  0.0333

------------------------------------------------------------------------------
      METCO2 |      Coef.   Std. Err.      t    P>|t|     [95% Conf. Interval]
-------------+----------------------------------------------------------------
         BMI |   .0950825    .044554     2.13   0.033     .0075433    .1826217
       _cons |   55.10698   .9156704    60.18   0.000     53.30788    56.90607
------------------------------------------------------------------------------
```

The above robust method is indicative of the use of BMI to predict METCO2, implying the feasibility of regression equation: METCO2 = 55.11 + 0.10 (BMI). The robust linear regression (not shown) with the same data which generates a robust standard error indicates a statistically marginally prediction of METCO2 by BMI: METCO2 = 55.84 + 0.08 (BMI).

9.3.4 How is the result of simple linear regression interpreted?

The above outputs (nonrobust) show a significant positive linear relationship between the range of motion and peak knee flexion, β (slope) = 0.43, $p < 0.001$, and 95% confidence interval (CI) = 0.21–0.64. In other words, the slope, 0.43, is statistically significantly different from zero ($t = 3.96$, df = 98, $p = 0.0001$). Simply, a significant regression equation is obtained, showing that peak knee flexion could be used to predict the range of motion of the knee: *range of motion (Y) = 23.23 + 0.43 (peak knee flexion)*, with R^2 (*coefficient of determination* called a pseudo square) = 0.137, meaning that a 13.8% change in the range of motion (response variable) is the result of a change in the peak knee flexion (independent variable).

9.4 Multiple/multivariable linear regression

9.4.1 What is multiple linear regression?

In this method, more than one independent variable is used to predict one outcome (dependent or response) variable. This model may include discrete independent variables provided there is a continuous independent variable in the model.

9.4.2 When is it feasible to use multiple linear regression?

A multiple linear regression is appropriate in predicting the response or outcome variable when there is more than one independent variable, and the response variable is measured on a continuous scale and assumed to be normally distributed. However, because regression analysis is robust, violation of normality of the dependent variable does not necessarily negate the utilization of this method.[13]

9.4.3 How is multiple regression analysis computed?

Consider a study performed to predict the maximum velocity of knee flexion where independent variables were measured in continuous scales. The investigators wanted to assess whether or not the range of motion, peak knee flexion, and time to peak knee flexion could simultaneously be used to predict the maximum velocity of knee flexion. First, the response variable has to be tested for normal distribution using the normality test. The skewness and kurtosis normality test is as follows:

```
STATA syntax: sktest mvkf0
```

The output below indicates that the maximum velocity of knee flexion is normally distributed, $p = 0.11$, which means that we should not reject the null hypothesis of normal distribution; that is, the data, variable distribution, or the shape is normal.

Skewness/Kurtosis tests for Normality				
			—— joint ——	
Variable	Pr(Skewness)	Pr(Kurtosis)	adj chi2(2)	Prob>chi2
mvkf0	0.038	0.847	4.45	**0.1080**

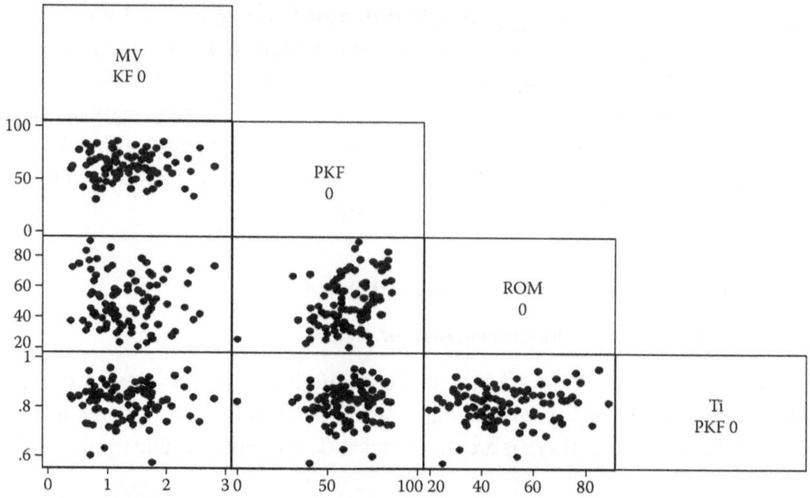

Graph 9.3 Correlation matrix.

Graph 9.3 shows the variables to be used in the regression model.

STATA Syntax: graph matrix mvkf0 pkf0 rom0 tipkf0

The relationship between the maximum velocity of peak knee flexion is shown with peak knee flexion in the second row, range of motion in the third row (column 1), and time to peak knee flexion in the fourth row (column 1).

Below is the STATA output for the multiple linear regression with the maximum velocity of the peak knee flexion (mvkf0) as the response or dependent variable.

STATA syntax: regress mvkf0 pkf0 rom0 tipkf0

```
  Source |       SS        df       MS              Number of obs  =       90
---------+------------------------------            F(  3,    86)  =     0.11
   Model |  .094268202      1   .031422734          Prob > F       =   0.9545
Residual |   24.740844     86   .287684233          R-squared      =   0.0038
---------+------------------------------            Adj R-squared  =  -0.0310
   Total |  24.8351122     89   .279046205          Root MSE       =   .53636

-------------------------------------------------------------------------------
   mvfk0 |      Coef.   Std. Err.       t     P>|t|      [95% Conf. Interval]
---------+---------------------------------------------------------------------
    pkf0 |  -.0003613   .0046934    -0.08     0.939     -.0096914    .0089688
    rom0 |  -.0018705   .0037476    -0.50     0.619     -.0093204    .0055794
  tipkf0 |   .1604612   .7943862     0.20     0.840     -1.418726    1.739649
   _cons |   1.303317   .6717327     1.94     0.056     -.0320429    2.638678
```

The data show no significant linear relationship between maximum velocity of knee flexion and peak knee flexion, while range of motion and time to peak knee flexion are constant and similar for other predictors when other covariates are maintained at constant, $F(3, 86) = 0.11$, $p = 0.95$. For example, the slope for the peak knee flexion showed a very small positive slope ($t = -0.08$, $p = 0.94$). While the outcome or response variable (maximum velocity of peak knee flexion) was normally distributed but the independent variables were not, robust regression, which, as explained earlier, eliminates the gross outliers before using the ordinary least square regression residual to calculate case weight, was used. This method results in weighted least square regression, thus eliminating gross outliers. With this, the researcher's intent was to assess whether or not the utilization of robust regression would result in the slope or beta coefficient that is significantly different from zero.

```
STATA syntax: rreg mvkf0 pkf0 rom0 tipkf0
```

In the robust regression, the result is similar to the regression performed above, that ROM, time to peak knee flexion, and peak knee flexion cannot be used to predict maximum velocity of knee flexion in these samples—$F(3, 86) = 0.21$, $p = 0.89$. The peak knee flexion showed a very small positive insignificant slope ($t = 0.06$, $p = 0.95$).

```
   Huber iteration 1:  maximum difference in weights = .45787602
   Huber iteration 2:  maximum difference in weights = .05462326
   Huber iteration 3:  maximum difference in weights = .00884795
Biweight iteration 4:  maximum difference in weights = .1585585
Biweight iteration 5:  maximum difference in weights = .00538792

Robust regression                                     Number of obs =       90
                                                      F( 3,    86)  =     0.21
                                                      Prob > F      =   0.8908

------------------------------------------------------------------------------
       mvkf0 |      Coef.   Std. Err.      t    P>|t|     [95% Conf. Interval]
-------------+----------------------------------------------------------------
         BMI |   .0003027   .0048453     0.06   0.950    -.0093295    .0099348
        rom0 |  -.0029322   .0038689    -0.76   0.451    -.0106233    .0047588
      tipkf0 |   .1746899   .8200996     0.21   0.832    -1.455614    1.804994
       _cons |   1.280384   .6934759     1.85   0.068    -.0982006    2.658968
------------------------------------------------------------------------------
```

9.5 Logistic regression technique

Logistic regression is a commonly used statistical method in biomedical sciences and public health. This technique allows one to assess a relationship or association and not necessarily a causation, which is judgment beyond mere statistical inference.

9.5.1 What is logistic regression?

This is a statistical technique or method used to assess the relationship or association between one or more independent variables with a binary outcome variable (absence or presence of a disease or event of interest). The independent variable might be binary, categorical, or continuous, hence the mixed scale of measurement with regard to the independent variable. For example, investigators conducted a study to examine the role of intraoperative and other factors, including postoperative skin breakdown and residual postoperative Cobb angle in children with neuromuscular scoliosis, and the development of deep wound infection after posterior spine fusion with rod instrumentation. The cases were ascertained before the ascertainment of their controls, and the controls were comparable to the cases except for the deep wound infection. This design is a retrospective case–control study, which is appropriate for the use of the unconditional logistic regression method of statistical inference. Unconditional logistic regression implies that there were no matched controls, meaning that the controls were not matched to the cases by any factor, such as age or gender. When the point estimate is the odds ratio and the scale of measurement of the dependent variable is binary, the logistic regression technique is a recommended statistical technique.

9.5.2 When is it feasible to use the logistic regression technique?

In the example with the deep wound infection, because the outcome variable (deep wound infection) was measured on a binary scale (absence or presence), the logistic regression would be an adequate statistical technique. Thus, logistic regression is a feasible analytic technique if the intent of the investigators is to assess the relationship or association and/or to determine whether or not the independent variable, such as disease risk factors, could be used to determine the outcome (disease or an event of interest). Therefore, in order for logistic regression to be performed, the outcome variable, also termed *dependent* or *response*, must be measured on a binary scale (0 = absence and 1 = presence) (Figure 9.5). The independent variables, also termed *predictor* or *explanatory variable*, could be numerical (continuous) or discrete (categorical or binary). For example, if a study was conducted to examine the association between alcohol consumption and peptic ulceration, with alcohol consumption as the independent variable measured in a categorical scale while peptic ulcer is measured in a binary scale, logistic regression is an adequate method for a valid statistical inference.

9.5.3 How is logistic regression computed?

This analytic method is distribution-free, meaning there is no assumption of normality. However it is essential to be aware of the coding of each variable, outcome and independent, for the interpretation of the results or output. For this calculation, we will address the univariable and multivariable logistic regression methods through model building using the STATA statistical package. The analysis from the logistic regression yields an odds ratio (AD/BC) as shown earlier in the two-by-two table for a case–control estimate of

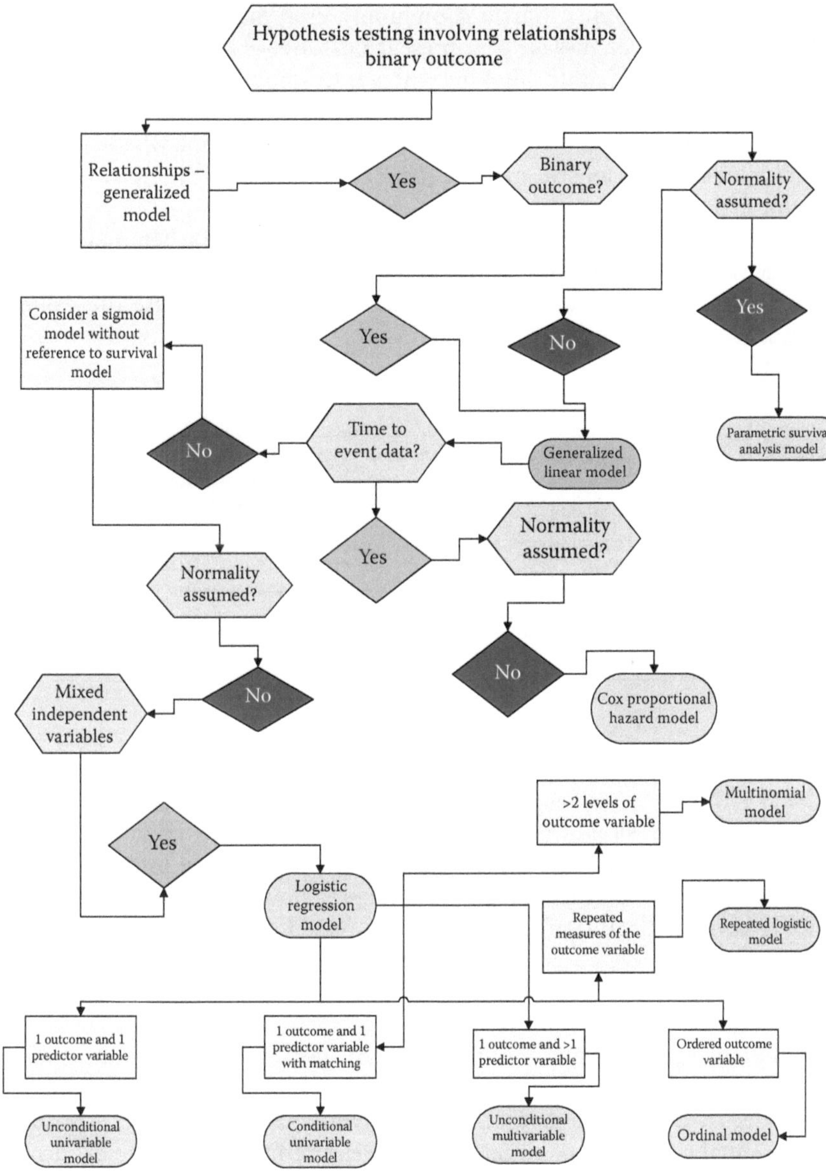

Figure 9.5 Hypothesis testing involving binary outcomes—logistic, binomial, and cox proportional hazard model.

effect measure or point estimate. Commonly used and interpretable codes include (a) absence of disease = 1, presence of disease = 0; low level of x = 0, high level of x = 1; no to smoking = 0, yes to smoking = 1; normal blood pressure level = 0, and abnormal blood pressure level = 1. For example, systolic and diastolic blood pressure could be used to determine whether or not an individual is hypertensive, and the same holds true with the LDL-to-HDL ratio for hyperlipidemia.

The univariable logistic regression analysis is performed when there is one response variable measured on a binary scale and one predictor variable measured on a binary, categorical, or continuous scale. We will use the wound infection data to illustrate the application of the univariable logistic regression model.

STATA syntax: logistic deep_wound skin_abrasion

```
Logistic regression                           Number of obs   =        66
                                              LR chi2(1)      =     11.68
                                              Prob > chi2     =    0.0006
Log Likelihood = -36.167498                   Pseudo R2       =    0.1391
```

deep_wound	Odds Ratio	Std. Err.	z	P>|z|	[95% Conf.	Interval]
skin_abrra~n	**20.06667**	22.27958	2.70	0.007	**2.277218**	**176.8259**

The output above showed that compared to neuromuscular scoliosis patients without skin abrasion/breakdown after posterior spine fusion, those who had skin abrasion/breakdown were 20 times as likely to develop deep wound infection, odds ratio (OR) = 20.07, 95% confidence interval (CI) = 2.28–176.82. This point estimate is significant, though with widened confidence interval, indicative of imprecise measurements.

9.6 Model building and interpretation

To simultaneously examine the predictors of deep wound infection, a multivariable model is required and involves model building. Model building commences with variable specification, implying that the outcome, exposure, and potential confounding variable effect measure modifier variables should be specified. Next, the investigator should identify variables that are biologically or clinically relevant to the outcome of interest. Further interaction should be considered between the exposure variable, such as skin abrasion/breakdown in our example, and other potential predictors. The rationale is to assess for variables or the interacting variables (interaction) that may change or influence the relationship of the exposure (skin abrasion/breakdown) and outcome (deep wound infection). There are two known traditions in model building: (1) *backward technique*—involves the introduction of the specified variables, including interaction into the model, and (2) *forward technique*—which involves stepwise adding of variables (terms and interactions) one at a time and retaining in the model only those terms and interactions that are significant at a predetermined significance level.

Consider model building on the association between deep wound infection (outcome) and skin abrasion/breakdown (exposure) and other potential predictors. Model building will involve (1) variable specification—deep wound infection as outcome, skins abrasion/breakdown as the exposure, age, sex, packed red blood cells, cell saver, and the product term for age and skin abrasion/breakdown, and (2) introduction of the outcome and exposure into the model.

STATA syntax: logistic deep_wound skin_abrasion

```
Logistic regression                          Number of obs   =        66
                                             LR chi2(1)      =     11.68
                                             Prob > chi2     =    0.0006
Log Likelihood = -36.167498                  Pseudo R2       =    0.1391
```

deep_wound	Odds Ratio	Std. Err.	z	P>|z|	[95% Conf.	Interval]
skin_abrra~n	20.06667	22.27958	2.70	**0.007**	2.277218	176.8259

```
. xi:logit  DM  FMH

Iteration 0:   log likelihood = -74.940827
Iteration 1:   log likelihood = -65.148552
Iteration 2:   log likelihood = -65.042811
Iteration 3:   log likelihood = -65.042636
Iteration 4:   log likelihood = -65.042636

Logistic regression                             Number of obs =     111
                                                LR chi(1)     =   19.80
                                                Prob > chi2   = 0.0000
Log Likelihood = -65.042636                     Pseudo R2     = 0.1321
```

DM	Coef.	Std. Err.	z	P>|z|	[95% Conf.	Interval]
FMH	1.821612	.4341689	4.20	0.000	.9706569	2.672568
_cons	-1.386294	.3370999	-4.11	0.000	-2.046998	-7.7255906

The above STATA output illustrates the relationship between family history of diabetes (FMI) and diabetes (DM). The logit is transformed to odds ratio in the STATA output below.

```
. xi:logit  DM  FMH, or

Iteration 0:  log likelihood = -74.940827
Iteration 1:  log likelihood = -65.148552
Iteration 2:  log likelihood = -65.042811
Iteration 3:  log likelihood = -65.042636
Iteration 4:  log likelihood = -65.042636

Logistic regression                               Number of obs =     111
                                                  LR chi(1)     =   19.80
                                                  Prob > chi2   =  0.0000
Log Likelihood = -65.042636                       Pseudo R2     =  0.1321
```

DM	Odds Ratio	Std. Err.	z	P>|z|	[95% Conf.	Interval]
FMH	6.181818	2.683953	4.20	0.000	2.639678	14.4771
_cons	.25	.084275	-4.11	0.000	.1291219	.4840386

The above STATA output indicates clinically meaningful (effect size) and a statistically significant association between the family history of diabetes (DM) and the prevalence of diabetes. Compared to patients without family history, those with family history are six times as likely to have diabetes. The null hypothesis claims that there is no difference in the proportion of family history comparing those with and without diabetes ((Ho = P1 (FMH) – P2(no-FMH) = 0)). With $p < 0.0001$, there is strong evidence against the null hypothesis with a significance level of 0.05, implying the rejection of the null, that chance alone cannot explain the observed magnitude of effect of FMH on DM.

```
. proportion  DM  if  FMH==1

Proportion estimation              Number of obs     =     56
```

	Proportion	Std. Err.	[95% Conf.	Interval]
DM				
0	.3928571	.0658539	.260883	.5248313
1	.6071429	.0658539	.4751687	.739117

Above is the STATA output for exploratory analysis prior to confirmatory analysis for the hypothesis testing. The proportion of those with family history of diabetes is higher in this sample among those with DM compared to those without.

```
. tabodds  DM FMH
```

FMH	cases	controls	odds	[95% Conf.	Interval]
0	11	44	0.25000	0.12912	0.48404
1	34	22	1.54545	0.90397	2.64216

```
Test of homogeneity (equal odds): chi(1)   =  18.91
                                  Pr>chi2 = 0.0000

Score test for trend of odds:     chi2(1) =  18.91
                                  Pr>chi2 = 0.0000
```

```
. tabodds  DM FMH, or
```

FMH	Odds Ratio	chi2	P>chi2	[95% Conf.	Interval]
0	1.000000	.	.	.	.
1	6.181818	18.91	0.0000	2.416337	15.815207

```
Test of homogeneity (equal odds): chi2(1) =  18.91
                                  Pr>chi2 = 0.0000

Score test for trend of odds:     chi2(1) =  18.91
                                  Pr>chi2 = 0.0000
```

The tabulation analysis (nonpredictive model) indicates the number of cases (DM) and non-DM (controls) with FMH (34 versus 22) in this sample. The odd of the exposure given DM is higher among cases compared to controls (1.55 versus 0.25) and the odds ratio is 6.18, $p < 0.0001$. The null hypothesis for the equality of the odds implies that no difference in the exposure odds is rejected at 5% (0.05) significance level.

Model Building Using Backward Technique:

$$\text{logit } P(\text{DWI} = 1 | X) = \beta_0 + \beta_1\text{SA} + \beta_2\text{AGE} + \beta_3\text{SEX} + \beta_4\text{RBC} + \beta_5\text{CS} + \beta_6\text{SAA}$$

STATA Syntax: logit DWI SA AGE SEX RBC CS SAA

```
Logistic regression                             Number of obs   =         35
                                                LR chi2(6)      =      23.27
                                                Prob > chi2     =     0.0007
Log likelihood = -11.456742                     Pseudo R2       =     0.5038
```

DWI	Coef.	Std. Err.	z	P>|z|	[95% Conf.	Interval]
SA	-10.75584	10.56436	-1.02	0.309	-31.4616	9.949918
AGE	-.6216451	.4161613	-1.49	0.135	-1.437306	.1940161
SEX	.8091246	1.223385	0.66	0.508	-1.588665	3.206914
RBC	-.0088093	.0050038	-1.76	0.078	-.0186167	.000998
CS	.0057924	.0036763	1.58	0.115	-.0014131	.0129979
SAA	1.021696	.7848095	1.30	0.193	-.5165024	2.559894
_cons	11.04203	8.030465	1.38	0.169	-4.697391	26.78145

```
. xi:logistics  DM  FMH  Sex  i.Race  age,  level (99)
i.Race            _IRace_1-3          (naturally coded; _IRace_1 omitted)

Logistic regression                               Number of obs   =        111
                                                  LR chi2(5)      =      90.59
                                                  Prob > chi2     =     0.0000
 Log likelihood = -29.643331                      Pseudo R2       =     0.6044
```

DM	Odds Ratio	Std. Err.	z	P>|z|	[99% Conf.	Interval]
FMH	2.598801	2.025135	1.23	0.220	.3491743	19.34211
Sex	.7075883	.53008	-0.46	0.644	.1027415	4.873216
_IRace_2	159.7769	168.9623	4.80	0.000	10.48418	2434.968
_IRace_3	11.79798	9.489862	3.07	0.002	1.485909	93.67492
age	1.132434	.0598034	2.36	0.019	.9884085	1.297446
_cons	.0003498	.0010093	2.76	0.006	2.07e-07	.5913014

The above STATA output illustrates the adjusted logistic regression model, implying the confounding effects of sex, race, and age in the association between the FMH of DM and DM. While the unadjusted model indicates a clinically meaningful effect of FMH on DM, as well as a statistically significant difference in the odds of exposure (FMH) comparing DM with non-DM, the model with adjusted indicated age, race, and sex as positive confounding as seen in the point estimates (adjusted OR, 2.60, 99% CI, 0.35–19.34, $p = 0.22$).

The syntax `logit` is used by STATA to run logistic regression (unconditional). The outcome variable is the deep wound infection (DWI), and the exposure variable is skin abrasion (SA), while the covariates are age (AGE), sex (SEX), packed red blood cells (RBC), and cell saver (CS), and SAA is the product of SA and AGE. The SAA represents the interaction term and is introduced in the model. The output produced includes the iteration (not shown). The logit is based on the dependent variable coded as zero (0) for absence of deep wound infection and one (1) for the presence of deep wound infection.

The above STATA output indicates the log likelihood of −11.46 based on the iteration history (not shown). The regression coefficient estimates, standard error, the test statistic (z), the p value for the Wald test, and the 95% confidence interval are generated. (STATA default could be set to 90% or 99% CI). The interval label `cons` for constant is shown as well as the likelihood ratio test statistic (23.27), and the corresponding p value (0.0007) for the likelihood ratio test comparing the full model with six regression parameters to a reduced model containing only the intercept. The test statistic follows a chi-square distribution with six degrees of freedom under the null hypothesis. The following is the STATA output with the odds ratio. OR = e(exponent)$^{\beta}$.

STATA Syntax: logit DWI SA AGE SEX RBC CS SAA, or

```
Logistic regression                              Number of obs   =         35
                                                 LR chi2(6)      =      23.27
                                                 Prob > chi2     =     0.0007
Log likelihood = -11.456742                      Pseudo R2       =     0.5038
```

DWI	Odds Ratio	Std. Err.	z	P>|z|	[95% Conf.	Interval]
SA	.0000213	.0002252	-1.02	0.309	2.17e-14	20950.5
AGE	.5370602	.2235037	-1.49	0.135	.2375668	1.214116
SEX	2.245941	2.747649	0.66	0.508	.204198	24.70274
RBC	.9912293	.0049599	-1.76	0.078	.9815555	1.000998
CS	1.005809	.0036977	1.58	0.115	.9985879	1.013083
SAA	2.777902	2.180124	1.30	0.193	.5966036	12.93445

The `or` option added to the syntax above is used to obtain exponentiated coefficients as the odds ratio (or). Also in STATA, the `logistic` syntax without the `or` syntax produces similar output. The standard errors and the 95% CI are those for the odds ratio estimates. The odds ratio produced by the logit or logistic syntax must be interpreted with caution especially when continuous variables and interaction terms are included in the model specification and building.

STATA Syntax: vce

Covariance matrix of coefficients of logit model

e(V)	SA	AGE	SEX	RBC	CS	SAA
SA	111.60563					
AGE	3.3130275	.17319023				
SEX	-2.883925	-.00970793	1.4966697			
RBC	-.03799043	.0015325	-.00173444	.00002504		
CS	-.02426434	-.00088261	.00171574	-.000017	.00001352	
SAA	-8.1941146	-.25802177	.24369701	-.00306118	.00198176	.61592593
_cons	-60.65636	-3.2068317	-1.7596699	-.03048614	.01661754	4.6916588

e(V)	_cons
_cons	64.488371

The `vce` syntax above is used to generate a variance–covariance matrix of the parameter estimates, which is used after running the regression. The likelihood ratio test below is performed using STATA syntax `lrtest`. This test is used here to perform a likelihood ratio on the SAA interaction term. STATA saves the full model in memory by the syntax, `lrtest, saving (1)`.

STATA Syntax: logit DWI SA AGE SEX RBC CS

```
Logistic regression                               Number of obs   =         35
                                                  LR chi2(5)      =      21.66
                                                  Prob > chi2     =     0.0006
Log likelihood = -12.258271                       Pseudo R2       =     0.4691
```

DWI	Coef.	Std. Err.	z	P>|z|	[95% Conf.	Interval]
SA	4.67941	2.014123	2.32	0.020	.7318017	8.627017
AGE	-.4358683	.2970971	-1.47	0.142	-1.018168	.1464312
SEX	.5629871	1.131493	0.50	0.619	-1.654698	2.780672
RBC	-.0069186	.0033196	-2.08	0.037	-.0134248	-.0004123
CS	.0045958	.0025135	1.83	0.067	-.0003305	.0095221
_cons	7.906475	5.93409	1.33	0.183	-3.724126	19.53708

The `or` option in the syntax below is used to obtain exponentiated coefficients as the odds ratio (or). Thus, odds ratio = e^{β}. Using the coefficient for SA (skin abrasion), we obtain $e^{(4.67941)}$ – STATA syntax: `disp exp(4.67941) = disp exp(4.67941) = 107.70651.`

STATA Syntax: logit DWI SA AGE SEX RBC CS, or

```
Logistic regression                               Number of obs   =         35
                                                  LR chi2(5)      =      21.66
                                                  Prob > chi2     =     0.0006
Log likelihood = -12.258271                       Pseudo R2       =     0.4691
```

DWI	Odds Ratio	Std. Err.	z	P>|z|	[95% Conf.	Interval]
SA	**107.7065**	216.934	2.32	**0.020**	**2.078823**	**5580.41**
AGE	.6467029	.1921335	-1.47	0.142	.3612562	1.157695
SEX	1.75591	1.986799	0.50	0.619	.1911497	16.12986
RBC	.9931053	.0032967	-2.08	**0.037**	**.9866649**	**.9995878**
CS	1.004606	.002525	1.83	0.067	.9996696	1.009568

The reduced model is run without the interaction term as indicated above. And after running this model, we used the STATA syntax, `lrtest, using (1)`. This syntax compares the full model with the interaction term SAA. The reduced model is termed the model without interaction.

```
. lrtest, using(1)
Likelihood-ratio test          LR chi2(1)  =   1.60
(Assumption: nested in LRTEST_1)   Prob > chi2 = 0.2055
```

The chi-square statistic with one degree of freedom is 1.60, which is statistically nonsignificant, $p = 0.20$. Therefore, we can present the result without interaction since there is no significant difference between the model with and that without interaction.

9.6.1 Types of logistic regression techniques

Logistic regression can also be used in addressing relationships involving matched pairs as seen in unconditional logistic regression (STATA syntax: `clogit`), ordinal logistic when the dependent variable is ordered (STATA syntax: `ologit`), and polytomous as well as multinomial when the dependent variable has many levels (STATA syntax: `mlogit`), correlated dichotomous data (STATA syntax: `xtgee`), and survey data (STATA syntax: `slogit`). The application of these specific logistic models is beyond the level of this book, which is intended to provide clinicians with a simplified guide on how to conduct and interpret results for valid statistical inference as well as clinical relevance to the evidence from the data. Further reading from these survey logistic or specialized logistic models could be assessed from intermediate and advanced biostatistics texts in this topic. Please note that unless otherwise specified or qualified, logistic regression refers to the unconditional logistic model. With sparse data, exact logistic is used to compensate for small sample size, and with repeated measure and binary outcome, repeated logistic regression model remains a suitable technique to assess such data.

9.7 Survival analysis: Time-to-event method

Survival analysis is used for time-to-an-event analysis, where the dependent, response, or outcome variable (time to an event or failure) is binary and one or more of the independent, predictor, or explanatory variables is measured on a discrete (binary or categorical) or continuous scale. This analysis uses the life table, Kaplan–Meier survival estimates, log-rank and similar tests for equality of survival, and the Cox proportional hazard model, also termed the Cox regression model.

This method, as mentioned earlier in Section 9.1, involves *censored observations* or data, where subjects have been observed unequal lengths of time and the outcome is not yet known for all subjects. Censoring could be (a) left and (b) right. Censoring is termed left-censored if the episodes started before the period of observation and right-censored if the episode ended after the period of observation.[14] Survival analysis assesses the effect of independent variables on the event (what terminates an episode, such as death in a clinical trial of drug or other therapeutics) in question. Simply, survival analysis examines the simultaneous effect of several variables (covariates) on length of survival.

9.7.1 What is a life table?

Consider a retrospective cohort study to determine the survival of older women diagnosed with cervical cancer and treated for the disease. If the investigators wanted to examine the survival by 5-year interval, a life table could be used to examine the survival experience of this cohort. The STATA statistical package is used to generate a life table with the following syntax: `ltable time vital, graph survival intervals(5)`. This syntax produces the interval, the number at risk as a beginning total, deaths, loss, and survival, as well as the standard error and the 95% CI. However, before commencing this analysis, the data must be first set on survival using the STATA syntax: `stset time, failure (vital)`, where `time` is the time variable and `vital` (dead or alive) is the failure variable.

STATA syntax: `ltable time vital, graph survival intervals(5)`

Interval		Beg. Total	**Deaths**	Lost	**Survival**	Std. Error	[95% Conf.	Int.]
0	**5**	**1426**	263	57	0.8118	0.0105	0.7903	0.8313
5	10	1106	129	0	0.7171	0.0121	0.6926	0.7401
10	15	977	109	0	0.6371	0.0130	0.6111	0.6619
15	20	868	72	0	0.5843	0.0133	0.5577	0.6098
20	25	796	49	0	0.5483	0.0134	0.5216	0.5742
25	30	747	44	0	0.5160	0.0135	0.4892	0.5421
30	35	703	32	0	0.4925	0.0135	0.4658	0.5187
35	40	671	33	0	0.4683	0.0135	0.4416	0.4945
40	45	638	24	0	0.4507	0.0134	0.4241	0.4768
45	50	614	21	23	0.4350	0.0134	0.4085	0.4611
50	55	570	16	43	0.4223	0.0134	0.3959	0.4484
55	60	511	19	22	0.4062	0.0134	0.3799	0.4323
60	65	470	11	31	0.3964	0.0134	0.3701	0.4225
65	70	428	9	28	0.3878	0.0134	0.3615	0.4140
70	75	391	17	21	0.3705	0.0134	0.3441	0.3968
75	80	353	8	31	0.3617	0.0135	0.3353	0.3881
80	85	314	10	34	0.3495	0.0136	0.3230	0.3761
85	90	270	3	23	0.3454	0.0136	0.3189	0.3721
90	95	244	9	29	0.3319	0.0138	0.3050	0.3590
95	100	206	8	17	0.3185	0.0140	0.2911	0.3461
100	105	181	3	23	0.3128	0.0142	0.2853	0.3407
105	110	155	10	30	0.2905	0.0148	0.2618	0.3197
110	115	115	4	16	0.2796	0.0152	0.2502	0.3097
115	120	95	4	17	0.2667	0.0158	0.2362	0.2981
120	125	74	2	25	0.2580	0.0165	0.2263	0.2907
125	130	47	2	13	0.2453	0.0179	0.2109	0.2811
130	135	32	2	16	0.2248	0.0215	0.1841	0.2681
135	140	14	0	11	0.2248	0.0215	0.1841	0.2681
140	145	3	0	3	0.2248	0.0215	0.1841	0.2681

Time-to-event analysis or duration modeling is (a) parametric, where the shape of the baseline hazard function is assumed (e.g., Weilbull model), or (b) semiparametric, where there is no assumption of the baseline hazard function shape but focus is on predicting the hazards ratio (e.g., Cox regression or proportional hazards model).[15] *Proportional hazard model (Cox regression)* refers to the baseline hazard ratio remaining constant over time, which does not mean the *same* over time as it is often misinterpreted.

Cox regression: hazard rate (not survival time) is the function of the independent covariates.

$$\boldsymbol{H(t) = H_0(\mathrm{t}) \times \exp(b_1X_1 + b_2X_2 + b_3X_3 + \ldots\ldots\ldots\ldots.. + b_mX_m)}$$

$X_1 \ldots X_m$ are predictor variables or covariates, and $H_0(t)$ is the baseline hazard at time t.

$$\text{Hazard ratio (HR)} = \ln[(H(t)/H_0(t)] = b_1X_1 + b_2X_2 + b_3X_3 + \ldots\ldots b_mX_m$$

$H(t)/H_0(t)$ = HR—Hazard is the probability of the end point, death. The following assumptions are required: (a) *proportionality*—given two observations with different values for the independent variables, the ratio of the hazard functions for these two observations does not depend on time, (b) *log-linearity*—there is a log-linear relationship between the independent variables and the underlying hazard function. This is Cox regression assumption: a violation may either overestimate or underestimate the point estimate (hazard ratio). The survival function $[S(t)]$ is the cumulative frequency of the proportion of the sample not experiencing the event by time t (alive or surviving observations). Mathematically, it appears as follows: $S(t) = 1 - F(t)$, which is the probability that the event will not occur until time t, which also implies the proportion of participants surviving beyond any given time t.[16]

9.7.2 Selected terms definition

The definition of terms used in the measure of effects in survival is essential in the understanding of the survival model and its interpretation.

- *Hazard* is the event of interest occurring (e.g., death or biochemical failure in a clinical trial of a therapeutic agent).
- *Hazard rate* at a given time is the probability of the event given that the dependent = 1, occurring in that time period, given survival through all prior time intervals.
- *Hazard ratio*, also termed hazard function, refers to the estimate of the ratio of the hazard rate in group A (treatment group) to the hazard rate in group B (placebo group).
- *Survival function plot* enables the comparison of the survival rates of two or more groups in a study.
- *Statistic* includes (1) the likelihood ratio test for the model (sometimes *score statistic* is used), (2) regression coefficients (β) for the statistical significance of individual independent variables or covariates in the model, and (3) log-rank test for the equality of survival function.

9.7.3 What is the Kaplan–Meier survival estimate?

Kaplan–Meier (KM) survival analysis, also termed *product-limit method*, refers to a nonparametric method of generating tables and plots or graphs of survival, failure, or hazards functions for time-to-event data.[17] The KM survival estimates involve the following: (a) the assumption of the method is that the event must be dependent on time, (b) the plotting of survival function on a linear scale, and (c) it is not designed to assess the effect or influence of covariates on the time-to-event status variable. The success or effectiveness of a treatment is measured in terms of the time that some desirable outcome is maintained. Such analysis (time-related patterns of survival) techniques originated from the life table procedures. Kaplan–Meier, also termed the product limit method, is more commonly used in biomedical and public health research compared to the actuarial method. Kaplan–Meier product limit and actuarial methods are commonly used to estimate the survival experience of samples. The methods are similar except that time since entry in the study is not divided into intervals for analysis in the Kaplan–Meier product limit method. Two or more life table curves could be tested to determine if they are significantly different. The *z* test for proportion is used for the actuarial curves while the log-rank test is used for Kaplan–Meier curves.

9.7.4 How are KM estimates derived or computed?

Consider a retrospective cohort study to examine the overall and cancer-specific survival of older women diagnosed with cervical cancer and for the disease, as well as the effect of treatment on survival. The Kaplan–Meier survival curve is feasible for addressing these overall and cause-specific survivals of the entire cohort and by the treatment received. Because the data have already been set to survival, the KM estimates could be obtained using appropriate STATA syntax. The following is the STATA command used to construct the KM survival estimate graph (Graph 9.4).

```
STATA syntax: sts graph, risktable risktable(, failevents
title(Numbers at risk and failure)) ytitle(Survival probability)
xtitle(Follow-up in months)
```

```
STATA syntax: sts graph, by(n_treat) (risktable risktable(,
failevents title(Numbers at risk and failure)) ytitle(Survival
probability) xtitle(Follow-up in months)
```

The Kaplan–Meier survival curve here is used to compare the survival of older women diagnosed with cervical cancer and treated for the disease (Graph 9.5). The KM shows the population at risk and the failure (dead from

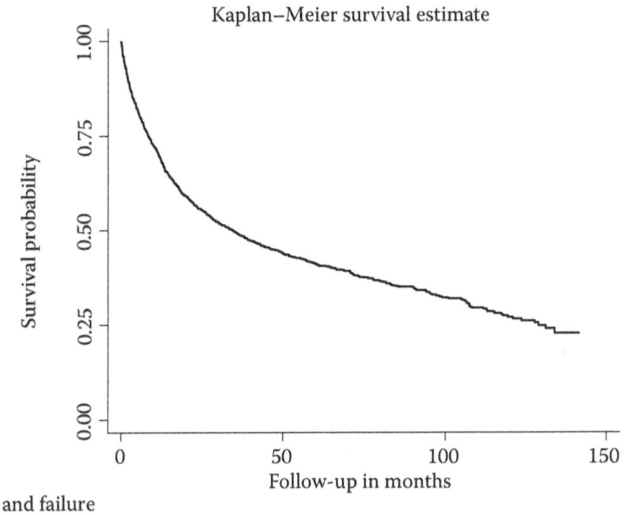

Numbers at risk and failure

1347	(754)	570	(110)	181	(27)	0

Graph 9.4 Kaplan–Meier survival estimate of survival probability.

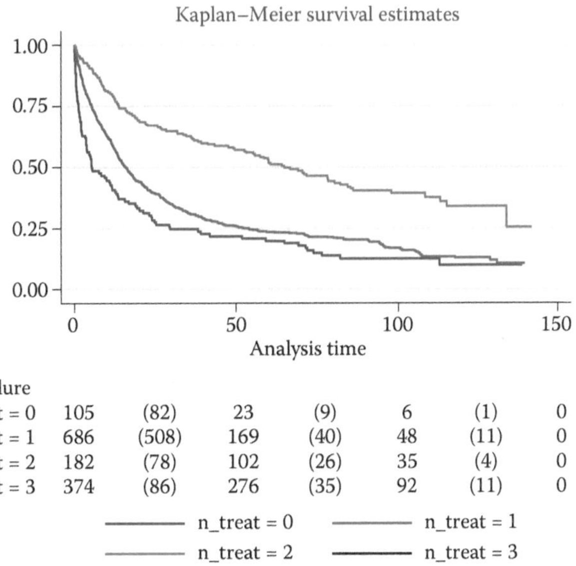

Numbers at risk and failure

n_treat = 0	105	(82)	23	(9)	6	(1)	0
n_treat = 1	686	(508)	169	(40)	48	(11)	0
n_treat = 2	182	(78)	102	(26)	35	(4)	0
n_treat = 3	374	(86)	276	(35)	92	(11)	0

Graph 9.5 Kaplan–Meier survival estimate by treatment type.

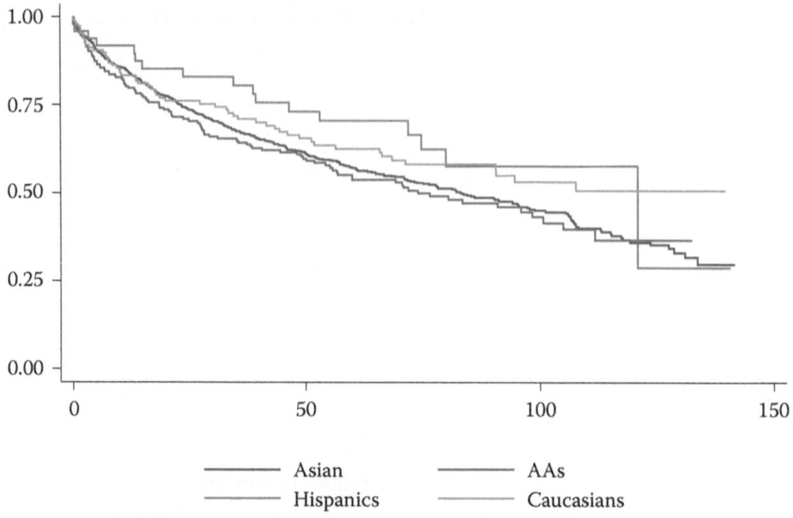

Graph 9.6 Kaplan–Meier survival estimate by race/ethnicity.

overall cause). The survival advantage is shown with treatment 3 (highest curve), while the lowest survival is shown by treatment 0 (lowest curve).

```
STATA syntax: st graph, by (race)
```

Graph 9.6 shows the Kaplan–Meier survival estimates by race/ethnicity. The curve indicates the crossing of hazards, indicating that the proportional hazard PH assumption is not met by race. This assumption states that the HR is constant over time, meaning that the hazard for one individual is proportional to the hazard for any other individual, where the proportionality constant is dependent on time. The Hispanics demonstrate the best survival in the unadjusted survival estimate, while blacks show the worst survival. Because the PH is not met, these curves must be interpreted with caution.

```
STATA syntax: sts graph, by(race) adjustfor tstage income comorbid
gscore surg XRT chemo ADT
```

The KM could be plotted for a covariate of interest, such as race, adjusting for other covariates (Graph 9.7). The STATA syntax including `adjustfor` allows this survivor function to be plotted.

9.7.5 What is the test for equality of survival?

The log-rank test is an approximate chi-square test and compares the number of observed deaths in each group with the number of deaths that would be expected from the number of deaths in the combined groups, implying that group

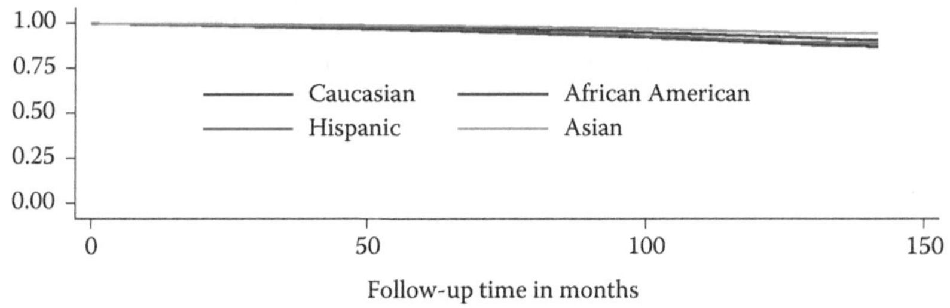

Graph 9.7 Kaplan–Meier survival estimate by race/ethnicity controlling for confounding.

membership or distinction did not matter. The null hypothesis is that there is no group difference in survival. The log-rank test is also referred to as the Cox–Mantel log-rank statistic or the Mantel log-rank statistic. The log-rank test, as may be incorrectly interpreted, does not involve ranking, nor does it employ logarithm in its computation of the survival differences of two or more groups.[18]

9.7.6 How is the log-rank test estimated?

The log-rank test, also termed the Cox–Mantel log-rank test, is used to determine the equality of survival (survival function test) between two or more groups.[19] The test is based on the alternative hypothesis that at least the survival of one of the groups is distinct. Consider a study to examine the survival of women diagnosed with cervical cancer and treated for the disease. If the investigators wanted to determine the survival experience of the cohort by the treatment received, the log-rank test is an appropriate test and is most commonly used in such situations. The following is the STATA output on the test of equality of survival. The output shows four treatment groups, with the intent to determine if the observed difference in the treatment groups shown by KM above is statistically significant.

```
STATA syntax: sts test n_treat
Log-rank test for equality of survivor functions
```

	Events	Events
n_treat	observed	expected
0	92	42.74
1	559	359.47
2	108	140.89
3	132	347.90
Total	891	891.00
	chi2(3) =	**319.02**
	Pr>chi2 =	**0.0000**

The *p* value above shows that at least one of the treatment groups is statistically significantly different. Other tests for the equality of survival function include (a) Wilcoxon—STATA syntax: *sts test n_treat, Wilcoxon*; (b) Tarone–Ware test—STATA syntax: *sts test n_treat, tware*; and (c) Peto–Peto–Prentice test—STATA syntax: *sts test n_treat, peto.*

9.7.7 *How is Cox regression computed?*

The Cox regression method is a distribution-free regression model but is classified as semiparametric, which allows for the assessment of the factors or covariates that affect survival. Consider the previous example on cervical cancer survival; race/ethnicity, treatment received, tumor stage, tumor histology, and age at diagnosis could be assessed individually (univariable Cox) or simultaneously (multivariable Cox) using this model.

In the above syntax, `xi` allows for the entry of the categorical variables into the model, with the lowest group used as the referent. The STATA output presents the hazard ratio, standard error, *z* statistic, and the *p* value as well as the 95% CI for the HR. The output shows the hazard ratio (HR), comparing the survival between treatment, tumor stage, and histology. Compared to treatment 0, patients with cervical cancer who received treatment 2 had a significant—49% (1.00 − 0.51)—decrease in the risk of dying, HR = 0.51, 95% CI = 0.38–0.68, $p < 0.001$. In contrast, compared with women who received treatment 0, those who received treatment 1 had an insignificant (12%) decrease in the risk of dying, HR = 0.88, 95% CI, 0.70–1.10. Please note the inclusion of 1.00 in the 95% confidence interval for the statistically nonsignificant result, where 1.00 means null or no association.

```
STATA Syntax: xi:stcox i.n_treat  i.n_stage i.n_cell
No. of subjects =            1347              Number of obs    =      1347
No. of failures =             891
Time at risk    =     61196.87354
                                               LR chi2(10)      =    620.42
Log likelihood  =      -5630.8466              Prob > chi2      =    0.0000
```

_t	Haz. Ratio	Std. Err.	z	P>|z|	[95% Conf.	Interval]
_In_treat_1	.8819597	.1015311	-1.09	0.275	.7038151	1.105195
_In_treat_2	**.513251**	.0752499	-4.55	0.000	**.3850628**	**.6841134**
_In_treat_3	.2700747	.0390126	-9.06	0.000	.2034824	.3584601
_In_treat_1	.1819678	.0209182	-14.82	0.000	.1452595	.2279528
_In_treat_2	.2406867	.0278555	-12.31	0.000	.1918402	.3019705
_In_treat_3	.3565025	.0398821	-9.22	0.000	.2863111	.4439018
_In_treat_4	.5083186	.0562702	-6.11	0.000	.409175	.6314847
_In_cell_1	1.134993	.1769257	0.81	0.417	.8361914	1.540568
_In_cell_2	.6853448	.0830986	-3.12	0.002	.5403813	.8691964
_In_cell_3	.8948169	.1245704	-0.80	0.425	.6811387	1.175527

9.7.8 How is Cox regression interpreted?

Hazard ratio (HR), sometimes termed the odds ratio, is given by the exponent (β); thus, HR = e^{β}. Using the prostate cancer study by Holmes et al.[20] on the effectiveness of ADT on survival, if HR = 1.0, this means that the covariate (e.g., androgen deprivation therapy, or ADT in the model) has no effect or impact on the time to event for the status or dependent variable (e.g., death from prostate cancer). If HR > 1.0, this indicates that ADT increases in the risk of dying given the use of ADT. Inversely, if HR < 1.0, this means that ADT diminishes or decreases the risk of dying on the subjects placed on ADT relative to those who are not.

Some researchers think that the end of statistical hypothesis testing is to establish a statistically significant difference. This is however an appropriate way of interpreting test results. Consider the effect of the treatment groups on cervical cancer survival of women diagnosed with all stages of cervical cancer and treated for the disease; the risk of dying associated with the types of treatment cannot be solely based on the treatment effects only without considering the bias and confounding, which statistical stability does not take into consideration. Therefore, a valid interpretation must consider the role played by bias, as well as possible explanation by confounding (tumor stage, age at diagnosis, comorbidities, tumor grade, extent of disease, and sex). These factors, which are prognostics, unless balanced between the treatment groups, may serve as confounders to the observed effect of treatment received and survival. Therefore, illustrating statistically significant difference alone does not constitute a valid scientific investigation of the role of the treatment received on cervical cancer survival, since without a sound design and bias minimization, treatment inference cannot be adequately drawn.

9.8 Poisson regression

What sorts of data are suitable for Poisson regression? Poisson regression is an example of a generalized linear model, such as logistic regression and Cox regression. Consider the distribution of the number of fractures attributed to osteoporosis over a long period of time, for example, 5 years. Assuming that the probability of a new fracture from osteoporosis in any one month is very small and that the number of cases reported in any two distinct periods of time are independent random variables, then the number of fractures over a 5-year period will follow a Poisson distribution. What is the distribution of the number of fractures due to osteoporosis from time 0 to time t, where t in this example is 5 years?

What assumptions should be made about the incidence of fractures attributed to osteoporosis? We must assume that (a) the probability of observing one fracture is directly proportional to the length of the time interval Δt and that Pr(1 fracture) = $\lambda \Delta t$ for some constant λ, (b) the probability of observing 0 fractures over Δt is approximately $1 - \lambda\Delta t$, and (c) the probability of observing more than one fracture over the time interval is 0. In addition, the following assumptions are necessary for Poisson probability distribution: (1) the number of fractures per unit time is the same throughout the time interval t, and (2) if a fracture occurs within one time subinterval, it has no bearing on the probability of a fracture in the next time subinterval. Also, it is essential to note that Poisson regression is not a good fit for the data if the mean and variance are different, indicative of overdispersion.

Poisson regression is appropriate if events occur independently with constant probability; then, counts over a given period of time follow a Poisson distribution. Let r_j represent the incidence rate. Mathematically, it appears as follows: r_j = count of events (numerator)/number of time event could have occurred (denominator). Since the denominator or exposure is often measured in person-time, such as person-years, r_j = counts of events/person-years observation multiplied by 1000. We can model the logarithm of the incidence rate as a linear function of one or more explanatory or independent variables: $\ln(r_j) = \beta_0 + \beta_1\chi_1 + \beta_2\chi_2 + \beta_3\chi_3 \ldots \ldots \ldots \beta_k\chi_k$.

What are the uses of Poisson regression? Consider an investigation to examine the presence of pediatric blunt trauma in Newcastle, Delaware; if 100 cases were observed over a period of 2 years where 50 cases would normally be expected, could Poisson regression be used for statistical inference? Poisson distribution can be used to calculate the probability of 100 or more cases, if Delaware's rates for pediatric blunt trauma were present in Newcastle. If the probability is smaller than the established significance level or type I error tolerance, then investigators will conclude that Newcastle has excessive number of fractures relative to the state of Delaware.

9.8.1 What is an example of Poisson regression?

Suppose a study was conducted to examine the increase in death rate associated with radiation level, and the following data were available (Table 9.1); is there a statistically significant effect? Using the data given here, let us examine the use of Poisson regression in statistical inference:

The following is the STATA output of the Poisson regression analysis. We tested the hypothesis on whether death rate increases with exposure to radiation in this cohort of patients with nonoperable meduloblastoma (fictitious study). The event count is mortality (deaths), which is the response or dependent variable, while radiation level is the predictor or independent variable. The Poisson "exposure" is the person-time in each radiation category or level. Using the STATA command below, we tested the hypothesis on whether or not radiation increases death rate in this cohort: `Poisson deaths rad, exposure(ptime) irr`.

Table 9.1 Hypothetical study of the effect of radiation level on mortality

Age group	*Radiation level*	*Deaths*	*Person-time*
<45	1	0	29,901
45–49	1	1	6521
50–54	2	4	5251
55–59	1	3	4126
60–64	4	3	2778
65–69	5	1	1607
70–74	3	2	3700
75–79	1	3	5520
80–84	1	2	29902
85–89	6	4	2330
90–94	1	1	1256

Note: The age groups (11) have more than one subject, not shown in the summary (hypothetical data for the illustration of Poisson distribution [11 categories for age and 6 categories for radiation]).

```
. poisson  Death Rlevel, exposure( P_Time) irr

Iteration 0:   log likelihood = -25.940721
Iteration 1:   log likelihood = -25.933184
Iteration 2:   log likelihood = -25.933182
Iteration 3:   log likelihood = -25.933182

Poisson regression                                Number of obs   =        11
                                                  LR chi2(1)      =     18.43
                                                  Prob > chi2     =    0.0000
Log likelihood = -25.933182                       Pseudo R2       =    0.2622

------------------------------------------------------------------------------
       Death |        IRR   Std. Err.      z    P>|z|     [99% Conf. Interval]
-------------+----------------------------------------------------------------
      Rlevel |    1.64447    .1644658    4.97   0.000      1.35175    2.00058
       _cons |   .0000986    .0000334  -27.20   0.000     .0000507   .0001917
  ln(P_time) |          1  (exposure)
------------------------------------------------------------------------------

. estat gof
         Deviance goodness-of-fit =  25.13191
         Prob > chi2(9)           =    0.0028

         Pearson goodness-of-fit  =  28.61376
         Prob > chi2(9)           =    0.0008
```

The STATA output indicates a 64% increase in the mortality rate with each increase in radiation level. The probability value shows a statistically significant rate ratio, $p < 0.0001$.The coefficient of determination is 26%, which is not very impressive, thus requiring a goodness-of-fit test. This test compares the Poisson model's predictions with the observed counts. The STATA command for this test is `poisgof (used after the regression computation)`. This test is a chi-square test with $n - 2$ degrees of freedom. The goodness-of-fit test, $\chi = 25.13$, df = 9, $p = 0.003$, implies that the Poisson model's predictions are significantly different from the actual count (model does not fit the data). To obtain a better model, we included age and found no change in the coefficient of determination or in the goodness of fit, $p = 0.002$ (rejection of the model). Finally, we checked the variance of the response variable, death from radiation for the proximity to the mean, and found that the variance (1.76), differed from the mean (2.18) but was not highly indicative of overdispersion. A large difference in variance relative to the means is suggestive of the use of negative binomial regression (more appropriate in cases of overdispersion), which could be easily performed using the STATA command: `bnreg death, rad`. This test uses the likelihood ratio test of the overdispersion parameter alpha. When the overdispersion parameter is zero, the negative binomial distribution is equivalent to a Poisson distribution. When alpha is significantly different from zero, this results in the rejection of the Poisson model for the data—appropriate application of Poisson distribution. The likelihood ratio test obtained in this case showed a probability value >0.05, implying that Poisson model is appropriate (alpha parameter is not significantly different from zero) for the data on the effect of radiation level and mortality.

```
. poisson  Death Rlevel numn_agegrp, exposure( P_Time) irr

Iteration 0:   log likelihood = -25.768359
Iteration 1:   log likelihood = -25.751968
Iteration 2:   log likelihood =  -25.75196
Iteration 3:   log likelihood =  -25.75196

Poisson regression                          Number of obs   =        11
                                            LR chi2(2)      =     18.80
                                            Prob > chi2     =    0.0001
Log likelihood = -25.75196                  Pseudo R2       =    0.2674
```

Death	IRR	Std. Err.	z	P>|z|	[99% Conf.	Interval]
Rlevel	1.593905	.1755274	4.23	0.000	1.284472	1.977881
numn_agegrp	1.041627	.0704774	0.60	0.547	.9122611	1.189338
_cons	.0000832	.0000378	-20.71	0.000	.0000342	.0002025
ln(P_Time)	1	(exposure)				

```
. estat gof

         Deviance goodness-of-fit =  24.76947
         Prob > chi2(8)           =    0.0017

         Pearson goodness-of-fit  =  28.42559
         Prob > chi2(8)           =    0.0004
.
```

9.9 Summary

This chapter discussed several statistical techniques in providing scientific evidence from the data, thus explaining how statistical methods are used to test scientific hypotheses involving relationships or associations. We stated the assumptions required for the selection of a specific test or statistical method. Essentially, these studies considered the analytic situations involving making predictions about the response variable, given the predictor or explanatory variable/s. Like with other methods discussed earlier, we stressed the use of samples to estimate the population in establishing a statistical inference (drawing conclusions about populations based on data from limited samples). We must assume that our sample is representative of the entire population (unbiased sample) in order for the conclusions drawn from our sample to be generalized to the targeted population or larger group. To achieve this objective, a random sample is required, implying that every subject in the population has an *equal and independent chance* of being selected for the sample. Equal chance implies that all subjects are listed in the sampling frame, while independent chance means that the probability of selecting a subject is not affected by the subject selected before that subject.

Hypothesis testing involving associations commonly use the following statistical methods: (a) correlation coefficient, (b) simple and multiple linear regression, (c) logistic and binomial regression (termed *generalized linear models* [GLM]), (d) Cox regression for time-to-event data, and (e) Poisson regression, also a GLM. The correlation coefficient is used to test the hypothesis of relationship where there is no specified independent and dependent variable. Both parametric and nonparametric tests are used, depending on whether or not there is shape assumption (Pearson correlation coefficient) (Figure 9.6). When data are ordered or nonnormal, the Spearman rank correlation coefficient is appropriate. A linear relation, simple or multiple, is appropriate if there is a straight line relationship in the intent of the statistical inference and independent and response variables are prespecified. The logistic and binomial regressions are used when predicting the outcome or response variable by the independent variable/s and the response or outcome variable is measured on a binary scale. The Poisson regression is appropriate in determining the incidence rate of interest when groups are compared and involves count data. When time-to-event data are involved and the outcome variable is measured on a binary scale, while the independent variables/s are measured on a mixed scale (binary, discrete, continuous), the Cox regression (also termed the *proportional hazard method*) is used to examine the effects of the covariates on survival. Also, Kaplan–Meier's (KM) survival estimates are useful in examining the survival curve, while the log-rank test is adequate in testing the equality of survival.

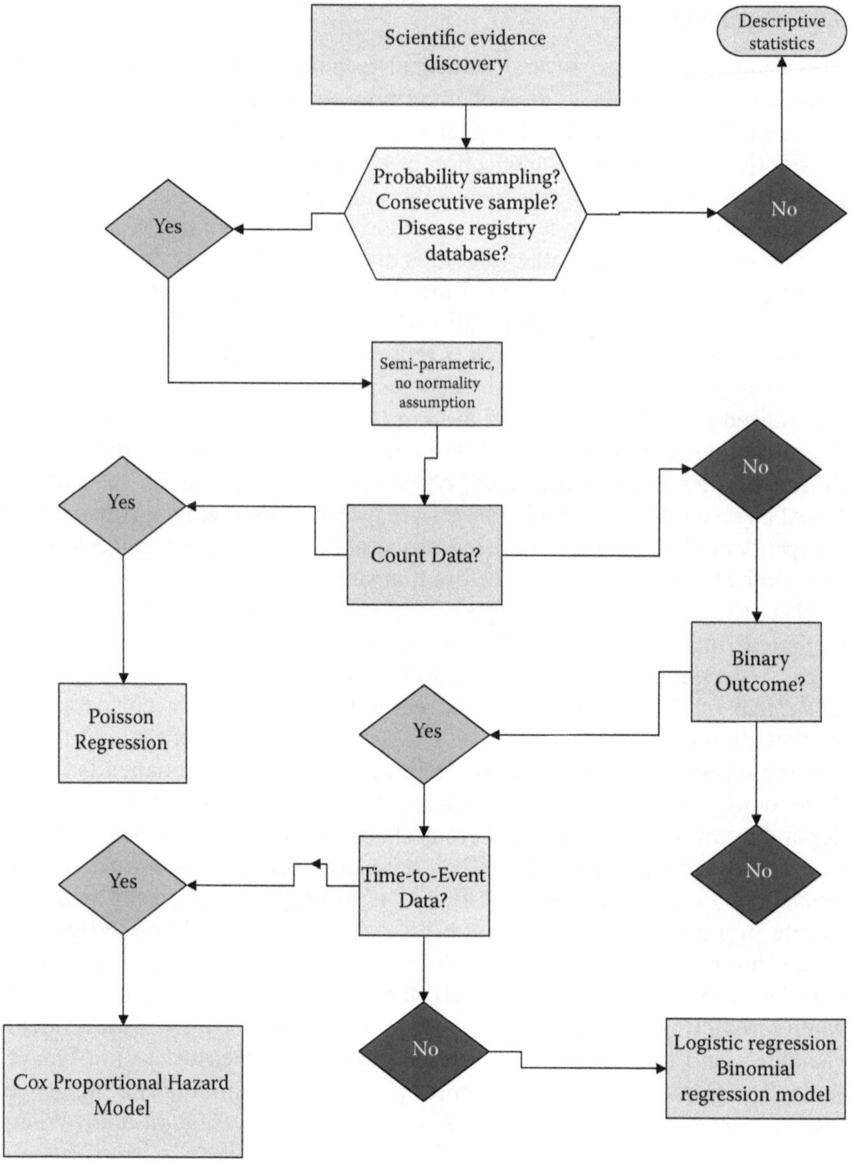

Figure 9.6 Hypothesis testing involving relationships—nonparametric and semiparametric models.

Questions for discussion

1 Read the study by L. Holmes et al., The impact of androgen deprivation therapy (ADT) on ethnic/racial variance in the survival of older men treated for locoregional prostate cancer, *Cancer Control* 16 (2009):176–185. (a) Comment on the design used in this study. (b) Do you agree with the statistical inference used in this study? (c) The study size is considered relatively large. Comment on the use of 5% as the significance level. (d) Do you think that the conclusion drawn supports the data used in this study?

2 Suppose you are conducting a double-blinded randomized clinical trial to examine the efficacy of lidocaine combined with triamcinolone, and Botox, with the third arm receiving placebo in reducing sciatica among women, aged 45 to 75 years. (a) Discuss the randomization process. (b) What will the measure of effect be? (c) What sort of analysis will be appropriate assuming that the follow-up period is 24 months and there is nondifferential loss to follow-up of 15%?

3 Consider this to be hypothetical data on the relationship between colorectal cancer incidence and consumption of vegetables and fruits among men, 40 to 50 years old. Among current consumers, there were 13 cases and 4761 number of person-years, past consumers had 164 cases and 121,091 number of person-years, while never consumers had 113 cases and 98,091 number of person-years. (a) Compare the incidence density of colorectal cancer in current consumers versus never consumers. What can you conclude from these data? (b) Compare the incidence density of colorectal cancer in the past versus never consumers of vegetables and fruits. What can you conclude from these data? (c) Estimate the rate ratios in (a) and (b), and comment the 95% confidence interval for these estimates.

4 Poisson regression is used in counting data. Comment on the use of this GLM in statistical inference. (a) What are the assumptions for the use of Poisson regression? (b) When is negative binomial regression an appropriate alternative to Poisson regression? (c) What is the interpretation of the goodness-of-fit test for Poisson regression and the likelihood ratio test for the negative binomial regression?

References

1. B. Dawson-Saunders and R. G. Trap, *Basic and Clinical Biostatistics*, 2nd ed. (Norwalk, CT: Appleton & Lange, 1994); W. D. Dupont, Statistical Modeling for Biomedical Researchers (Cambridge, UK: Cambridge University Press, 2003); B. C. Cronk, *How to Use SPSS. A Step-by-Step Guide to Analysis and Interpretation*, 3rd ed. (Glendale, CA: Pyrczak Publishing, 2004); T. D. V. Swinscow and M. J. Campbell, *Statistics at Square One*, 10th ed. (Spain: BMJ Books, 2002).
2. D. A. Freedman et al., *Statistics*, 4th ed. (New York: Norton, 2007).

3. B. Dawson-Saunders and R. G. Trap, *Basic and Clinical Biostatistics*, 2nd ed. (Norwalk, CT: Appleton & Lange, 1994); T. D. V. Swinscow and M. J. Campbell, *Statistics at Square One*, 10th ed. (Spain: BMJ Books, 2002).
4. B. Dawson-Saunders and R. G. Trap, *Basic and Clinical Biostatistics*, 2nd ed. (Norwalk, CT: Appleton & Lange, 1994); P. Armitage and G. Berry, *Statistical Methods in Medical Research*, 3rd ed. (Oxford, UK: Blackwell Scientific Publishing, 1994).
5. B. Dawson-Saunders and R. G. Trap, *Basic and Clinical Biostatistics*, 2nd ed. (Norwalk, CT: Appleton & Lange, 1994).
6. P. Armitage and G. Berry, *Statistical Methods in Medical Research*, 3rd ed. (Oxford, UK: Blackwell Scientific Publishing, 1994); D. W. Hosmer and S. Lemeshow, *Applied Logistic Regression Analysis*, 2nd ed. (New York: Wiley, 1989); D. G. Kleinbaum and M. Klein, *Logistic Regression*, 2nd ed. (New York: Springer, 2002); J. F. Jekel, L. Katz, and J. G. Elmore, *Epidemiology, Biostatistics, and Preventive Medicine* (Philadelphia: Saunders, 2001); H. A. Khan and C. T. Sempos, *Statistical Methods in Epidemiology* (New York: Oxford University Press, 1989); D. G. Kleinbaum and M. Klein, *Survival Analysis*, 2nd ed. (New York: Springer, 2005); M. A. Cleves, W. W. Gould, and R. G. Gutierrez, *An Introduction to Survival Analysis Using STATA* (College Station, Texas: STATA Press, 2004).
7. H. A. Khan and C. T. Sempos, *Statistical Methods in Epidemiology* (New York: Oxford University Press, 1989); D. G. Kleinbaum and M. Klein, *Survival Analysis*, 2nd ed. (New York: Springer, 2005); M. A. Cleves, W. W. Gould, and R. G. Gutierrez, *An Introduction to Survival Analysis Using STATA* (College Station, Texas: STATA Press, 2004); J. H. Abrahamson, *Making Sense of Data*, 2nd ed. (New York: Oxford University Press, 1994).
8. D. G. Kleinbaum and M. Klein, *Survival Analysis*, 2nd ed. (New York: Springer, 2005); M. A. Cleves, W. W. Gould, and R. G. Gutierrez, *An Introduction to Survival Analysis Using STATA* (College Station, Texas: STATA Press, 2004).
9. D. G. Kleinbaum and M. Klein, *Survival Analysis*, 2nd ed. (New York: Springer, 2005); M. A. Cleves, W. W. Gould, and R. G. Gutierrez, *An Introduction to Survival Analysis Using STATA* (College Station, Texas: STATA Press, 2004).
10. B. Dawson-Saunders and R. G. Trap, *Basic and Clinical Biostatistics*, 2nd ed. (Norwalk, CT: Appleton & Lange, 1994); B. C. Cronk, *How to Use SPSS. A Step-by-Step Guide to Analysis and Interpretation*, 3rd ed. (Glendale, CA: Pyrczak Publishing, 2004); T. D. V. Swinscow and M. J. Campbell, *Statistics at Square One*, 10th ed. (Spain: BMJ Books, 2002).
11. J. H. Abrahamson, *Making Sense of Data*, 2nd ed. (New York: Oxford University Press, 1994).
12. B. Dawson-Saunders and R. G. Trap, *Basic and Clinical Biostatistics*, 2nd ed. (Norwalk, CT: Appleton & Lange, 1994); W. D. Dupont, Statistical Modeling for Biomedical Researchers (Cambridge, UK: Cambridge University Press, 2003); B. C. Cronk, *How to Use SPSS. A Step-by-Step Guide to Analysis and Interpretation*, 3rd ed. (Glendale, CA: Pyrczak Publishing, 2004).
13. B. Dawson-Saunders and R. G. Trap, *Basic and Clinical Biostatistics*, 2nd ed. (Norwalk, CT: Appleton & Lange, 1994); D. A. Freedman et al., *Statistics*, 4th ed. (New York: Norton, 2007).
14. 30,31
15. 31,32
16. 30,32
17. D. G. Kleinbaum and M. Klein, *Survival Analysis*, 2nd ed. (New York: Springer, 2005); M. A. Cleves, W. W. Gould, and R. G. Gutierrez, *An Introduction to Survival Analysis Using STATA* (College Station, Texas: STATA Press, 2004).

18. L. Holmes, *Basics of Public Health Core Competencies* (Sudbury, MA: Jones and Bartlett Publishers, 2009); J. P. Klein and M. L. Moeschberger, *Survival Analysis—Techniques for Censored and Truncated Data*, 2nd ed. (New York: Springer, 2003); L. Holmes, W. Chan, Z. Jiang, and X. L. Du. Effectiveness of androgen deprivation therapy in prolonging survival of older men treated for locoregional prostate cancer, *Prostate Cancer and Prostatic Diseases* 10 (2007):388–395.
19. D. G. Kleinbaum and M. Klein, *Survival Analysis*, 2nd ed. (New York: Springer, 2005); M. A. Cleves, W. W. Gould, and R. G. Gutierrez, *An Introduction to Survival Analysis Using STATA* (College Station, Texas: STATA Press, 2004).
20. L. Holmes, W. Chan, Z. Jiang, and X. L. Du. Effectiveness of androgen deprivation therapy in prolonging survival of older men treated for locoregional prostate cancer, *Prostate Cancer and Prostatic Diseases* 10 (2007):388–395.

10 Special topics in evidence discovery

10.1 Introduction

The emergence of "big data," complexities in disease etiology and therapeutics, and the reliability and validity issues in evidence discovery signals some departure from traditional foundation of statistics as a tool in data collection, processing, analysis, and interpretation. With these challenges, biostatistics needs to critically examine the following: (i) *Big data and its implication in clinical decision-making in improving care and safety*, (ii) *reality is statistical modeling of clinical and translational research data,* and (iii) *tabulation/stratification versus regression model.*

"Big data," as the name implies, reflects the accumulation of large information nationally and globally via online and recently social media with the intent to influence decision-making in retail, education, manufacturing, government and banking, and so on. With this technology and management of this large stream of information, a real-time analysis is feasible, and with its proper analytics, decision is supported in improving services and products. The availability of "big data" reflecting large data size but not sample size raises the question on how large is large enough as well as the traditional foundation of statistic, implying sampling. With big data, the era of sampling is over, and hence the notion of statistics drifting from sampling to "population." This departure raises another question on population estimate from a "representative sample."

With large or legacy data that have resulted in the "big data" approach to evidence discovery, we need to revisit the notion of hypothesis testing and the level of type I error tolerance, clinical and biologic relevance of our data, effect size (δ), and, more importantly, findings generalization for clinical decision-making and other decisions such as policies around healthcare and population health.

Without doubt, the big data concept and application portray benefits to evidence discovery if properly utilized. For example, consider a study conducted to examine the cost-effectiveness of hip replacement in older patients treated for locoregional prostatic adenocarcinoma, the assessment of a national registry on hip replacement with respect to cost and health outcomes is more likely to result in a useful inference in terms of clinical guidelines and recommendations relative to a few center studies. The down side on the other hand involves inaccurate interpretation of findings from legacy or big data that ignores clinical or biological relevance of the study. To illustrate this, assume a prospective cohort study ($n = 95{,}656$) with a 5-year survival advantage of 0.5% in a new antihypertensive agent compared to a standard of care, HR, 1.05, 95% CI, 1.03–1.08, $p < 0.0001$. Does this imply a change in clinical guidelines for HTN treatment based on the new data?

The larger the sample studied, the more likely it is that very small effect difference or size and clinically irrelevant findings become statistically significant, which raises the question: How large is large enough?

Public health, epidemiology, translational and clinical research, as well as biomedical sciences have a unique issue in evidence discovery, mainly sampling insufficiencies since most data in these fields are not probability samples. The problem in using these data without random variable reflects the inherent problem with inference. Therefore, by emphasizing reality in the statistical modeling of clinical and translational science data, researchers must consider elements of sampling and its relevance in evidence discovery. Further, the perpetual failure of researchers to process data, visualize, and apply tabulation/stratification analysis before regression requires a revisitation of such vital statistical concept and application in evidence discovery.

This chapter reflects on the "big data" concept and application in clinical medicine and public health, hypothesis testing and statistical significance, and biological relevance as effect size, namely, absolute and relative measures of evidence. Additionally, the ongoing research myths and realities of p value as a measure of evidence in the pseudo-notion of statistically significant is described. Also covered in this chapter is the reality in the statistical modeling of translational and clinical research data. Attempts are made in this special topic section to introduce models and model specification and describe the elements of model building in hypothesis testing as well as appropriate selection of a model that fit the data. This section also delves into assumptions and the rationale behind models and their conformation to biologic and social realities in evidence discovery. Further, the last section explains in detail the differences in the application of tabulation, stratification, and regression model. Very importantly, the section describes and provides guidelines on when and when not to use regression model and provides example with a large-size data set.

10.2 Big data and implication in evidence discovery

10.2.1 Big data: Concept and application

While there are several notions of the big data concept that tends to vary from industry to industry, and business to business, this notion basically reflects the acquisition, storage, and analysis of large and complex data. This process of accumulating and storing large volume of information for subsequent analysis is not as new as currently perceived. However, the technologies and management of such data remain novel and hence the "big data" notion as used today. With current technological advances, volume, velocity, variety, variability, and complexities had been used to characterize big data.[1,2] Since data continue to accumulate every second, and hence big data, the importance of the concept shifts to application, implying the importance.[3] Therefore, the appropriate application of analytic tool to make sense of discovery from such data in supporting decision-making remains an important consideration in applied statistics.

What are the main sources of big data? Big data emerge from data streaming, social media, and publicly available or public access data. Within clinical medicine and public health, US government data as illustrated with the National Cancer Institute (NCI), Surveillance Epidemiology and End Result (SEER) cancer patients data represent such public access data. Like disease registry, research scientists should consider this sample (data) to be representative of the population of children with cancer in the United States. With this consideration, evidence discovery requires the treatment of such samples as probability sample, hence the justification for the quantification of random error in hypothesis testing situation. Another example of big data is the use of the genome-wide data set for the assessment of genomic instability and the related issues in genetic aberration and variance. Specific analysis in this example include (1) the detection of differentially expressed genes, which is a common goal in DNA microarray experiments, implying genes detection with differential expression across two or more biological conditions,[4] and (2) the identification of exonic splicing enhancers, short oligonucleotide sequences that enhance pre-mRNA splicing when present in exons.[5]

Social media data such as mHealth are gaining place in health research especially in surveys and disease prevalence assessment. These data are massive and voluminous, and could provide reliable inference on issues pertaining to those who participate in social media. However, researchers must be very cautious in drawing inferences from such data. For example, using social media such as Facebook to determine the prevalence of flu and symptoms severity by person, place, and time is unrepresentative of the populations at most risk, namely, elderly (declined/compromised immune responsiveness) and children (immature immune response).

Despite the inference limitation of some "big data," if properly managed, these data are reliable and valid in assessing health situations: (a) less expensive as preexisting data compared to data collection by researchers, (b) storage capacity availability, and (c) faster processing capability. With needed resources to operate on big data, the analysis and dissemination provided additional advantage relative to "non-preexisting data." These advantages include, though not limited to, parallel processing, clustering, cloud computing, high connectivity, and high throughputs.

10.2.2 Statistical analysis consideration

The value of big data in medical, biomedical, and public health discoveries requires a careful understanding of model specification, analysis, and interpretation: (1) the types of scales used in the measurement of the several variables in the data set, which is very important in determining the statistic with respect to hypothesis testing; (2) appropriate estimator of effect or a predictive model, implying averaging many predictive models together using such approaches as a bootstrapping sample (test utilized in sampling with replacement as well as when a parametric test is inappropriate and standard error is difficult to estimate), bagging involving bootstrap aggregation (*procedure involving the generation of multiple versions of a predictor, and averaging these predictor versions to obtain an aggregate predictor*), and random forests; (3) multiple comparison or testing when assessing multiple hypothesis as observed in genome-wide analysis—departure from traditional or classical hypothesis testing with 5% type I error tolerance to *false discovery rate (FDR)*—concept applied to type I error rate, while testing multiple hypothesis as observed in multivariable model that utilize multiple comparison, and FDR controlling tends to minimize such FDR; (4) data smoothing, a form of regression using smoothing splines, hidden Markov models, moving or rolling averages especially when such data are measured over space, distance, or time; (5) data plotting before model fitting, which allows for the visualization of big data with MA plot (derivation of Bland–Altman plot—difference plot) used in genomics; the plot transforms data onto M (log ratio) and A (mean average) scales and then plots these values as seen in DNA microarray gene expression and high-throughput sequencing data; (6) interactive process implying the use of random sample by rendering big data, small and increasing the efficiency, speed, and accuracy in handling such data volume-enhanced inherent veracity; (7) determining the real sample size, since data size differs from sample size; for example, in genome-wide data, the data size reflects the number of reads measured and not the sample size, which reflects the number of individuals that contribute to the reads; (8) assessing the data for potential confounders even if randomization process was utilized at the design phase, and if feasible, effect measure modifier; (9) determination of the statistical tool/method through rationale and assumption behind the data and the hypothesis to be tested such as parametric, nonparametric, or semi-parametric; this approach based in part on decision theory limits data exploration or fishing, which has an adverse effect on inference; (10) providing access to the syntax and code utilized for the analysis as well as data availability to colleagues; (11) considering tabulation analysis before predictive model, probit, logit, and so on; and (12) avoiding regression model as a universal approach and only using this model when appropriate (assumptions and rationale) and reliable as a predictive model, and in confounding adjustment.

10.3 Reality in statistical modeling of translational and clinical science data

During the past six decades, researchers in public health and medicine have applied inference, meaning the quantification of random error in a nonprobability sample. However, such practices are justified if consecutive samples and the entire disease registry are utilized in evidence discovery. The reality in statistical modeling requires specification and model selection. These requirements are dependent on several aspects of discovery, namely: (a) research question that specifies primary and secondary outcome variables if any; (b) hypothesis or multiple hypotheses; (c) sound biologic or social understanding of the research phenomenon of interest; (d) appropriate sample size to ensure the statistical power of the study, implying the ability to correctly reject the null hypothesis if indeed the null is true; (e) assessment and controlling for confounding; (f) assessing for effect measure modifier and result presentation at the level of the stratum; (g) utilization of the effect size as the measure of evidence in the data; and (h) precise quantification of random error and not as a cutoff ($p > 0.05$ or $p < 0.05$), as well as the use of confidence interval as the measure of precision in the data.

The statistical reasoning surrounding the measure of outcomes as primary or secondary evolves around the scales of measurement of the variable, measurement error, sample size, and the adequacy of such measure as primary or secondary outcome. For example, if a study is conducted to assess a new anti-neoplastic agent in prolonging survival of men with prostate cancer, the primary end point could be death from all causes, while the secondary end point or outcome could be PSA level. A good research question for the primary outcome could be: Does chemotherapy X reduce mortality in men with stage 3 prostate cancer compared to the standard of care and observational management (watchful waiting)? With respect to the second outcome or end point, researchers could ask: Does chemotherapy X lower PSA level of men with stage 3 prostate cancer relative to the standard of care and watchful waiting? These measures differ based on the end points specified. While the primary end point is measured by a binary scale, which will require a logistic or binomial regression model, the secondary end point involved an interval or ratio scale as a cardinal scale measure, requiring a different predictive model, specifically the analysis of variance, ANOVA, and, if applicable, given the presence of a covariate, ANCOVA.

10.3.1 Statistical modeling: Basic notion

What model is acceptable for the discovery of truth or evidence from clinical and translational research data? Conventional model of data analysis or inference is based on randomization and random error assumptions. Simple tabulation and graphic methods are sufficient and adequate if only few variables for example age, sex, treatment are assessed. Such analysis include the Pearson chi-square and Mantel–Haenszel odds ratio using the 2 × 2 table. However, given the complexities of disease etiologies and genetic heterogeneity of human animals that tend to influence the validity and reliability of studies, statistical modeling that aligns data to these realities is necessary in evidence discovery involving care, therapeutics, diagnostics, morbidity, and mortality.

10.3.2 Why model?

Models remain an explicit construct (with or without theoretical basis but background and significance of health issues and problems) that aligns health data to clinical and social realities, but with the disadvantage that model specification and interpretation may not be understood by investigators as well as the audience (researchers and readers). Because of the expected explicitness of a model, accurate evidence discovery that aims at care and safety improvement in health and healthcare requires an applied and replicable model.

10.3.3 What is a model in clinical and translational research?

A model is a simplified, concise, or structural representation of system or phenomenon. Simply, a model could be described as a pattern of something to be made or something such as a construct used to visualize or explore something else including, though not limited to, data, treatment, or therapeutic and diagnostic framework.

A statistical model thus represents a parameterized set of probability distribution, and all such models make assumptions about the data. Examples include Cox proportional hazard (with hazard ratio [HR] estimate) − Cox, 1972, logistic (odds ratio [OR] estimate), binomial (risk ratio [RR] estimate), and Poisson regressions (incident rate ratio [IRR] estimate). Extremely helpful devices for making estimates of treatment effects, testing hypothesis about those effects, and studying the simultaneous influence of covariates and confounding on outcome (multivariate—more than one response variable and multiple independent variables; multivariable—one response variable and multiple independent variable models). Since the basic tabular methods are limited in the number of variables that can be examined simultaneously, the reality of clinical, translational, and population-based data analysis requires that reliable evidence be obtained through accurate application of predictive or regression models.

10.3.4 Minimal model

A model that is compatible with available information and does not conflict with background information remains a desired model in accurate evidence discovery. However, in structural equation modeling, there is a requirement of a theory-based model in a multivariate analysis setting.

10.3.5 What sort of background information?

To be credible, a selected model to examine our data must flow from the background information or solid scientific literature of the study/research questions. A scientific knowledge of the topic guides the scales of measurements of the variables, which is suggestive of the credible and reasonable model.

10.3.6 Why reality in statistical modeling?

Data present with language, and we must explore this language before model specification: (a) shape of the distribution of data: normal or distribution-free assumption; (b) scale of measurement of the variables: discrete or continuous; (c) probability sampling and random variable assumption must be assessed. Power and sample size estimations are necessary since absence of evidence does not imply evidence of absence. The statistical power of a study can be increased not only by increasing the sample size but also by reducing the measurement error (SD). Small-size studies are likely to yield negative results, and such results should not be reported with statistical significance without the power estimation.

Descriptive statistics should be applied when data violate sampling assumption. One should simply describe the data without random error quantification (*p* value) and/or precision (CI).

Researchers should use a nonparametric test when data are distribution-free and when study size is small even with ratio or interval scale data (cardinal or continuous variables). It is meaningless to apply a *p* value to studies that did not apply probability sampling in the selection of study participants and hence did not assess random variables, except when disease registry or consecutive patients were used as the sample, implying a representative sample of the target population. Other exceptions are large sample claims/administrative data and research registries, since these data are assumed to be representative of the population of interest.

The probability value (*p*) should not be overemphasized in the presentation of clinical and translational study findings. The *p* value, no matter how small, does not rule out alternative explanation to the obtained results—bias and confounding. Additionally, *p* values do not measure evidence but partially reflect the size of the study.

The interpretation of biologic and clinical relevance of the findings precedes statistical inference or stability. Researchers and clinicians working in research settings should examine the magnitude of effect or point estimate and provide a clinical/public health interpretation before random error quantification. Clinical and translational research results should be presented with the point estimate such as hazard ratio (HR), risk or rate ratio (RR), odds ratio (OR) or relative odds (RO), and confidence interval (CI)—lower and upper 95% or 99%. Why the preference for CI to *p* value in reporting precision or random variability?

10.4 Tabulation versus regression analysis: When and when not to use regression

The ongoing conflicting results in basic sciences, clinical medicine, and population-based studies are indicative in part of sampling bias and inadequate statistical technique as well as inappropriate confounding adjustment used in evidence discovery. For translational, clinical, and epidemiologic research to be accountable, we must clearly understand the distribution of our response (outcomes—cure, control, survival) and main independent variables (exposure—treatment, medication, surgery, follow-up) as well as the patterns in the data, since regression models per se are less effective in providing these details. Tabulation (contingency)/stratification analysis provide an excellent opportunity to uncover these details, rendering these methods equally effective in modeling provided the assumptions are maintained! Since nothing explains everything in research implying the role of confounding, which model do we use to address the complexities in disease etiology and therapeutics in order to improve the care of our individual patients as well as the health of the population that we serve?

Hypothesis testing with a given test statistic requires the computation of probability distribution of the statistic over repetition of the study when the test hypothesis is true. The validity assumptions include the following: (a) only chance produces differences between repetitions, and (b) absence of bias or no biases are operating (selection, information, Berksonian, etc.) and that the statistical method used to derive the distribution is accurate. Within this context of p-value interpretation, a high p value implies that the observations are far from what will be expected under the test hypothesis, while a low p value reflects the closeness or proximity of the observations to this expectation.

10.4.1 Selection of test statistic

How should one select a statistic Y as the basis for testing and estimation? If we examined outcome of Ebola viral infection on patients treated with plasma transfusion from Ebola-free patients as absence of viral load, implying favorable outcome denoted by A, as test statistic Y, then $Y = A$. Also, we could select: $Y = \ln(A)$ or $Y = \text{logit}(A/N) = \ln[A/(N - A)]$ as test statistic for normal approximation. Why choose Y to be the viral load?

Precision—for reasonable-sized samples and reasonable parameter values, a valid and precise interval has an average width over the repetitions that is no greater than other valid intervals. The validity and precision reflect accuracy criteria. The availability of computational formulas for its mean and variance: In $Y = \text{logit}(A/N)$ above, approximate means and variance apply. We can select Y = viral load as a compromise between accuracy and simplicity.

10.4.2 Essential stages in scientific evidence discovery

Once data had been gathered from clinical and translational research, such data require the following:

1. Data editing/cleaning—review of collected data for accuracy, consistency, and completeness
2. Data summary/data reduction—descriptive analysis
   a. Graphic exploration of distributions—scatterplots, box plots, histogram
3. Estimation—data modeling involving statistical hypothesis testing
   a. Estimation stage involves the consideration of unmeasured factors that might have influenced subject selection, measurement/observation bias, confounding, as well as statistical inference issues
4. Results interpretation—descriptive and inferential

10.4.3 Tabulation analysis: Basic concept and application

Tabulation analysis is performed by contingency tables that demonstrate the frequency of subjects or units of observation with specific combination of variable values with the key variable of interest. For example, the description of study characteristics investigating the prevalence of colon cancer screening by race is indicative of the application of this process in evidence discovery. In this case, tabulation analysis involves the frequency or summary of the categorical/discrete variables by race.

10.4.4 Rationale and assumption

Tabulation analysis allows one to appraise all the data because it contains all the relevant information in the data. It reflects the contingency table (2×2) and allows for estimation, and displays relations among the main study variables. For variables such as systolic blood pressure (SBP), erythrocyte sedimentation rate (ESR), estimated blood loss (EBL), and age measured on continuous scales, besides summary statistics utilizing the mean, SD/SEM or median, and IQR, scatterplots, box plots, and histograms provide further insights to evidence discovery. The contingency tables and visual displays of the data serve as a check for validity of regression models.

The application of tabulation or stratification analysis as it is sometimes interchangeably used assumes marginal confounders and effect measure modifiers. The model so to state is inappropriate as a sole model when assessing relationship involving many confounders, where regression model is an appropriate choice. In such situation, the regression model remains a justifiable and efficient approach to evidence discovery.

Consider a study conducted using National Children Health Survey (2012) data on the relationship between autism and race/ethnicity (Table 10.1). The frequency is used to illustrate the distribution of autistic spectrum disorder

Table 10.1 Tabulation analysis illustrating the association between race/ethnicity and autistic disorder prevalence, NSCH, 2012

Autistic disorder	Race/Ethnicity Categories					
,	Hispanic	White, No	Black, No	Multi-rac	DK/REF/SY	Total
YES	10,939	53,788	7852	8942	1994	83,515
	11,069.9	53,578.5	7746.9	9118.2	2001.5	83,515.0
	1.5	0.8	1.4	3.4	0.0	7.2
	13.10	64.41	9.40	10.71	2.39	100.00
	86.26	87.63	88.47	85.60	86.96	87.29
Ever told, BDNH	39	214	38	44	8	343
	45.5	220.0	31.8	37.4	8.2	343.0
	0.9	0.2	1.2	1.1	0.0	3.4
	11.37	62.39	11.08	12.83	2.33	100.00
	0.31	0.35	0.43	0.42	0.35	0.36
NO	147	1139	123	186	29	1624
	215.3	1041.9	150.6	177.3	38.9	1624.0
	21.6	9.1	5.1	0.4	2.5	38.7
	9.05	70.14	7.57	11.45	1.79	100.00
	1.16	1.86	1.39	1.78	1.26	1.70

Pearson chi2(20) = 157.5930 Pr = 0.000

Notes and abbreviations: Race/ethnicity is classified as Hispanic (column 2); White, non-Hispanic (column 3); Black, non-Hispanic (column 4); and multiracial (column 5), while Don't know (DK), Refuse to answer (REF), and System missing (SY) are in column 6. Chi2 is the chi-square with 20 as the degree of freedom, while pr is the p value, <0.0001.

by race/ethnicity. Do we observe any pattern from these data? What further evidence do we wish to present?

10.4.5 Confounding and covariates: What is a confounding variable?

One of the issues in validating a translational and clinical research is to assess whether associations between exposure and disease derived from the observed data are of a factual nature or not (due to systematic error, random error, or confounding). A covariate differs from a confounding variable though interchangeably used in the statistics community. This concept is described in an ANOVA model in epidemiology text (Holmes). Confounding refers to the influence or effect of an extraneous factor(s) on the relationship or associations between the exposure and the outcome of interest (Figure 10.1). Nonexperimental studies are potentially subject to the effect of extraneous factors, which may distort the findings of these studies.

The assessment of confounding is discussed in detail in epidemiologic text (Holmes, Rothman, and Greenland). To be a confounding, the extraneous variable must be (1) a risk factor for the disease being studied and (2) associated with the exposure being studied but is not a consequence of exposure. Consequently, confounding occurs (a) when the effects of the exposure are mixed together with the effect of another variable, leading to a bias or biased estimate, and (b) if exposure X causes disease Y, Z is a confounder if Z is a

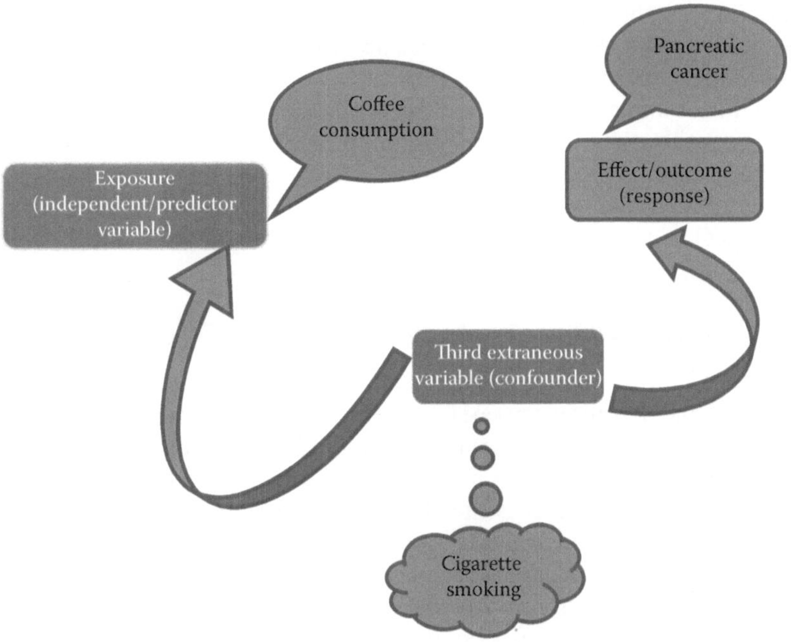

Figure 10.1 Confounding by cigarette smoking in the relationship between coffee consumption and pancreatic neoplasm. A greater percentage of those who drink coffee also smoke, implying the observed relationship to be confounded by smoking, a known carcinogen. In effect, unless coffee or exposure is stratified by smoking and nonsmoking, the relationship between coffee and pancreatic neoplasm will remain nonfactual, implying the need for stratification analysis to control for confounding.

known risk factor for disease Y, and Z is associated with X, but Z is not a result of exposure X.

10.4.6 Stratification analysis

This is an extension of tabulation or cross-tabulation analysis, implying the cross-tabulation of data on exposure (ionizing radiation via CT) or treatment (medication—chemotherapy/surgery/behavioral therapy/physiotherapy) and disease (childhood leukemia) or outcome (tumor remission or mortality) by categories or strata of one or more variables assessed to be potential confounders. It is an efficient and simple means of controlling for confounding such as smoking in the association between coffee consumption and pancreatic neoplasm.

10.4.7 Rationale and assumption

Stratification into categories allows for the assessment of confounding and effect measure modifier also termed interaction/product term in statistical arena. This method allows for the generation of subgroups to assess the differences in confounding factor, if any, and *t* permits the refinement of point estimate from the crude estimate. If variables are random as anticipated from probability samples, it allows for the application of inference and random error quantification. However, only one potential confounding variable is required in the method for practical purpose of revealing several interesting aspects of the data. Consequently, stratification analysis is ineffective and impractical in controlling for more than one confounding variable.

10.4.8 Addressing for confounding: How?

In assessing for confounding, researchers should note that if within the categories of the stratification variable there is no meaningful variability, then the variable is a potential confounder. In addition, the effect being estimated is constant across strata, with each stratum providing a separate point estimate—stratum-specific estimate. Is the effect measure modifier implicated if the stratum-specific estimate differs substantially between strata but there is not much variability with the crude or unadjusted point estimate? With continuous variable, such transformation into several categories may result in less variability of the continuous confounding variable such as age. Assessing for the magnitude or degree of confounding is relevant to stratified analysis. There are practical issues when it comes to confounding, namely: (1) What should we do if the potential confounding variable presents with very little or marginalized effect on the association? (2) How do we evaluate or assess for potential confounders? (3) What do we do if a variable is both a confounder and an effect measure modifier? (4) Should we use a significance test to determine whether the unconfounded point estimate differs from the crude point estimate with some difference in magnitude? These issues are addressed in detail in major textbooks of epidemiology (Rothman and Greenland).

Consider an example of a study conducted to examine the relationship between race/ethnicity and developmental disorders (DD), with sex and age as potential confounding variables (Table 10.2). How are these two potential confounders assessed before stratification? Can stratified analysis provide us with meaningful and reliable information with simultaneous stratification by these two variables (2 [sex] × 4 [race] = 8 categories)?

In this sample (NSCH, 2012), the stratified analysis by sex varied from the crude estimate, and with a difference in magnitude of at least 10%, confounding is expected by sex, given also no substantial difference in DD by sex-specific stratum. However, while stratified by age (age categories: 2–5 years = 1, 6–10 years = 2, 11–14 years = 3, and 15–17 years = 4), the stratified point estimate for DD differed substantially from the crude estimate, and there is a sizable difference between age-specific stratum for DD. This observation is indicative of age as an effect measure modifier as well and a confounder in the association between race and developmental disorder in children. Therefore,

Table 10.2 Crude analysis of the association between race and developmental disorder, NSCH, 2012

race	cases	controls	odds	[95% Conf.	Interval]
1	338	10,584	0.03193	0.02866	0.03559
2	2002	51,631	0.03878	0.03708	0.04055
3	336	7517	0.04470	0.04007	0.04986
4	364	8545	0.04260	0.03836	0.04731

```
Test of homogeneity (equal odds): chi2 (3) = 21.94
                    Pr (chi2) =  0.0001
Score test for trend of odds:    chi2(1) =   16.38
                    Pr (chi2) =  0.0001
```

Notes: Race/ethnicity was defined by Hispanic, 1; non-Hispanic white, 2; non-Hispanic black, 3; and multiracial, 4.

given this heterogeneity by age, the data on race and DD association should be presented by age group, thus minimizing errors on global/crude association between race and DD.

10.4.9 Regression as a predictive model

Since tabular and stratification methods are limited owing to the number of variables that could be controlled simultaneously, the regression method presents an efficient alternative. Even with the sparse-strata method of Mantel–Haenszel, there remains a methodological flaw as more variables and categories are applied in stratification, resulting in empty strata with zeros (0) and ones (1). The regression method has an advantage over tabular and stratification methods; although the regression method has explicit advantages, it may be difficult to be understood by the scientific audience and sometimes by investigators who depend on this method for their results or evidence, implying the ability to interpret the results as well as to understand the scientific context of the model.

The regression equation is presented as

$$Y = \alpha + \beta_1 X_1 + \ldots\ldots \beta_k X_k + \varepsilon$$

This equation fits into binary, multiple or multivariable linear, exponential risk models; logistic models—logit transformation, logistic model extension: polytomous, ordinal, multinomial; as well as rate models, namely, (a) incidence–time and hazard model, and (b) generalized linear model—Poisson.

Statistical tests are based on assumptions regarding the variables used in the analysis, with the violation of such assumptions resulting in biased estimates. But few researchers ever test the assumptions that their test is based on, implying potentials for biased conclusion and inference from the data! Translational and clinical research must be more consequential by testing assumptions and examining the rationale behind the data.

Regression Method Assumption

$$Y = \alpha + \beta_1 X_1 + \ldots\ldots \beta_k X_k + \varepsilon$$

The validity of regression model depends on the following: (a) Normality—variables are normally distributed. Regression assumes that variables have normal distributions. Nonnormally distributed variables (highly skewed or kurtotic variables, or variables with substantial outliers) can distort relationships and significance tests. Exceptions are other generalized linear models that are semi-parametric and hence distribution-free (e.g., logistic regression, Cox proportional hazard model). (b) Linear relationship or approximately linear, implying that the independent and dependent variable must be linearly related. Single and multiple linear regression can only accurately estimate the relationship between dependent and independent variables if the relationships are linear in nature. (c) None or marginalized measurement errors—variables are measured without errors. In simple correlation and regression,

Table 10.3 Regression model of the association between race/ethnicity controlling for sex and age

```
xi:logistic DD sex i.race i.n_age
i.race            _Irace_1-4           (naturally coded; _Irace_1 omitted)
i.n_age           _In_age_1-40         (naturally coded; _In_age_1 omitted)
Logistic regression                              Number of obs  =     81,317
                                                 LR chi2(7)     =     377.93
                                                 Prob > chi2    =     0.0000
Log likelihood = -12,784.442                     Pseudo R2      =     0.0146
```

DD	Odds Ratio	Std. Err.	z	P>|z|	[99% Conf.	Interval]
sex	.5091094	.0199495	-17.23	0.000	.4714729	.5497503
_Irace_2	1.244359	.0746333	3.65	0.000	1.106351	1.399582
_Irace_3	1.428749	.1124493	4.53	0.000	1.22451	1.667054
_Irace_4	1.361277	.1049411	4.00	0.000	1.170381	1.583309
_In_age_20	1.112351	.0583836	2.03	0.042	1.00361	1.232873
_In_age_30	1.023837	.051301	0.47	0.638	.928068	1.129488
_In_age_40	.7730633	.0453263	-4.39	0.000	.6891399	.867207
_cons	.0823965	.0067816	-30.33	0.000	.0701215	.0968203

Notes: The STATA syntax is used in the analysis of the data with the regression model. As indicated earlier, this model restricts details on the sample compared to tabular or stratification models. The reference groups are allocated OR = 1.00 in the model (male = 1 and female = 2 for sex, with male being referent), and type I error tolerance is set at 1% (0.01) due to multiple comparison and false discovery rate (FDR) for more accuracy or precision.

unreliable measurement causes relationships to be underestimated, increasing the risk of type II errors. In the case of multiple regression or partial correlation, effect sizes of other variables can be overestimated if the covariate is not measured accurately. (d) Homoscadasticity—the variance of errors (ε) is the same across all levels of the independent variable. Therefore, meeting these assumptions results in increased accuracy of the estimates.

Consider the regression model of the association between race/ethnicity and DD controlling for age and sex (Table 10.3). The model assumptions are as follows: (a) Random variable implying probability sampling or consecutive sample—Health/Disease Registry or national survey (b) more than one confounding variable (age and race) to control for—simultaneous adjustment for multiple confounding. The point estimates (OR) and precision (99% CI) are comparable in either stratified or regression models.

10.4.10 Tabular and stratification models: Benefits and limitations

The benefits of tabulation and stratification models include (a) visualization of exposure (risk, treatment), disease (outcome, response), and confounding variables that are usually obscured in multivariable regression; and (b) fewer assumptions needed, minimizing the potentials for obtaining a biased results. The difficulties to provide accurate, mutually unconfounded coefficient estimates (β_1, β_2, β_3) of two or more predictive/confounding factors such as smoking and family history in the association between coffee drinking and pancreatic malignancy, renders stratification analysis in preference of regression model: $Y = \beta_0 + \beta_1 X_1 + \beta_2 X_2 + \beta_3 X_3$ (logit transformation of general linear model allows for the fitting of logistic regression line).

10.4.11 Regression model: Benefits and limitations

Regression as a predictive model is based on information from risk predictors and remains efficient if properly utilized in evidence discovery. For example, values of predictor variables such as fever, history of travel from infected region, contact with symptomatic Ebola, and direct contact with patient saliva could be inserted into logit (logistic transformation) to predict the risk of Ebola virus. Controlling for multiple confounding variables for individual estimate of risk and for causal inference requires a regression model. This model provides an accurate, mutually unconfounded coefficient estimates (β_1, β_2, β_3) of two or more predictive/confounding factors such as smoking and family history in the association between coffee drinking and pancreatic neoplasm: $Y = \beta_0 + \beta_1 X_1 + \beta_2 X_2 + \beta_3 X_3$ (logit transformation of general linear model allows for the fitting of logistic regression line). Many assumptions are needed, increasing the potentials for obtaining a biased result with unexamined assumptions and rationales. In addition, regression obscures the visualization of exposure, outcome, and confounding variables, which is extremely necessary in observing data patterns. In effect, the regression model should never be utilized unless data are visualized and tabulated for detail assessment before model specification and building as a predictive model.

10.5 Summary

The emergence of "big data" signaled a threat to the very foundation of statistics, sampling, implying a representative sample that mirrors the population characteristics or attributes. Since statistics rarely studies the population but draws sample judged to be representative from the population, the sample parameter such as the mean remains an approximation of the population mean, hence the notion of estimate or estimation. The use of big data reflects volume, variability, veracity, and velocity. In general, streaming, social media, and public access data remain the source of big data. With big data, approach to evidence discovery varies from the traditional method utilized in making sense of data. Researchers handling big data should attempt at the combination of novel with traditional approaches. These guidelines to processing and analysis of big data include (a) generation of multiple versions of predictor and averaging these predictor versions to obtain an aggregate predictor, (b) smoothing, (c) adjustment for multiple comparison by assessing false discovery rate (FDR), (d) MA plot utilization for data visualization, (e) application of tabulation before regression model fitting, (f) avoidance of regression as a universal model, (g) addressing and controlling for confounding, (h) determining real sample size from data size, and (i) application of data reduction by obtaining random sample from big data.

Reality in statistical modeling of clinical and translational research data reflects the ability to provide sound background knowledge of the research entity of interest, appropriate sampling, internal and external validity of the study, effect size, application for measure of association or effect, and the application of confidence interval to determine data precision.

The utilization of the regression model should be handled with caution. As a predictive model, regression provides explicit measure of effect and prediction when assumptions are met. However, the violation of these assumptions renders this model inadequate to fit the data. As a rule, researchers should avoid the regression model unless the tabulation model and data visualization are performed before selecting regression. In controlling for confounding when more than one confounding is assessed, regression remains an efficient model.

Questions for discussion

1 (a) Discuss the advantage and disadvantage of using "big data" in assessing the outcome of hip replacement surgery associated with private insurance. (b) Using big data, discuss the relevance of type I error tolerance in this context. (c) What is bagging? Explain the importance of applying this tool in big data scenario.

2 Supposing you are conducting a study on the effect of chemotherapy X on acute lymphocytic leukemia using SEER data, discuss how you will discover evidence on the benefit of this drug (n = 72,000). What will be type I error tolerance? If multiple comparison is involved, how will you determine false discovery rate?

3 Visit https://wwwn.cdc.gov/Nchs/Nhanes/2011-2012/DR1IFF_G.htm and obtain the codebook and the data to describe the demographics of the participants and correlate between micronutrients and poverty level. Using effect size, determine whether it is feasible from the data policy formulation to address racial/ethnic variability in micronutrients in this sample.

4 Wald tests and confidence interval are based on Wald's (1934) comment on the use of Wald statistics in regression models. The association between cancer and alcohol is often confounded by age and smoking. Comment on overestimation or underestimation of the joint effect of these two risk factors and discuss the relevance of utilizing an interaction term in such a model.

5 While using simple linear regression, we model the value of a response variable as a linear function of a single independent variable or explanatory variable. Suppose we have observations on n patients, construct a multiple linear regression model. Comment on the importance of the multiple regression model in an attempt to improve the ability to predict a response variable with several explanatory variables. Comment on the accuracy of multiple regression parameter estimates.

6 The null hypothesis allows us to completely specify the distribution of a relevant test statistic, while the alternate hypothesis includes all possible distributions except the null. The probability value (p) as indicated in the text is the probability of obtaining a sample mean that is at least as unlikely under the null hypothesis as the observed value of x (hypothetical). Discuss the importance of p value as the measure of evidence (true mean, point estimate) in clinical, translational, and population-based studies.

References

1. Big data definition. Available at https://www.technologyreview.com/s/519851/the-big-data-conundrum-how-to-define-it/ (accessed March 29, 2017).
2. Big data description. Available at https://www.sas.com/en_us/insights/big-data/what-is-big-data.html (accessed March 21, 2017).
3. Big data pioneer and concept. Available at: http://controltrends.org/building-automation-and-integration/05/john-wilder-tukey-the-pioneer-of-big-data-and-visualization/ (accessed March 23, 2017).
4. D. K. Slonim, From patterns to pathways: Gene expression data analysis comes of age. *Nat Genet* 32 (2002):502–508.
5. W. G. Fairbrother, R. Yeh, P. A. Sharp, and C. B. Burge, Predictive identification of exonic splicing enhancers in human genes. *Science* 297 (2002):1007–1013.

Appendix

Making sense of evidence discovery—hypothesis testing, scale of measurement, sample, and statistical technique

Hypothesis	*Design*	*Scale of measurement*	*Statistical technique*
Single sample (noncorrelated)—Examines mean/median/proportion difference between sample and known population mean	Cross-sectional (snapshot data)	Cardinal, interval, ratio (continuous); normality test required	Single sample t test (t value, mean difference, SEM, SD, p, CI)
		Ordinal, continuous but normality assumption violated, small sample size	Sign ranked test (median, z value, p)
Single sample (correlated)—Examines mean/median/proportion difference between baseline/pre-intervention mean and post-intervention means (before and after, correlated, repeated measures)	Longitudinal (repeated measure, test and retest, pre- and post-test, correlated sample, dependent sample)	Cardinal, interval, ratio (continuous); normality test required as well as equality of variance assumption	Paired t test, repeated-measure analysis of variance (RANOVA) (F, df, p)
		Ordinal, Likert scale, continuous but normality assumption violated, small sample size	McNemar's test, Wilcoxon sign-rank test, Friedman's statistic (multiple repeated measures)
Two independent sample (noncorrelated)—Examines the mean/median/proportion/difference between two samples that are independent and not correlated	Cross-sectional, retrospective, prospective, case–control, etc.	Cardinal, interval, ratio (continuous); normality test required as well as equality of variance assumption	Independent sample t test (with and without equal variance assumption), ANOVA (F, df, p)
		Ordinal, Likert scale, continuous but normality assumption violated, small sample size	Mann–Whitney, Kruskal–Wallis
		Nominal, categorical, discrete	Chi-square statistic; Fisher's exact test, Yates correction

(*Continued*)

Making sense of evidence discovery—hypothesis testing, scale of measurement, sample, and statistical technique

Hypothesis	*Design*	*Scale of measurement*	*Statistical technique*
Mixed effect (random/fixed) applicable also to >2 samples	Random effect variable	Cardinal (continuous)	Mixed-model ANOVA
> Two independent samples (noncorrelated)—Examines the mean/median/proportion difference between two samples that are independent and not correlated	Cross-sectional, retrospective, prospective, case–control, etc.	Cardinal, interval, ratio (continuous); normality test required as well as equality of variance assumption	ANOVA, ANCOVA, (*F* value, df, wmean, SEM, SD, *p*, CI)
		Ordinal, continuous but normality assumption violated, small sample size	Kruskal–Wallis (median, *z* value, *p*)
Relationship (linear assumption)—Examines the linear association between one independent and one dependent variable	Longitudinal (prospective/concurrent cohort), retrospective, ecologic, etc.	Cardinal, interval, ratio (continuous); normality test required but robust analysis is appropriate upon violation	Simple linear regression model (β coefficient, constant, p, R^2)
Examines the linear association between one dependent and > one independent variable			Multiple linear regression (β coefficient, constant, p, R^2)
Examines the linear association between > one dependent and > one independent variable		.	Multivariate linear regression analysis (β coefficient, constant, p, R^2)
Relationship (linear assumption)—Assesses the linear association between two variables	Correlation design (no predetermined independent or dependent variable)	Cardinal, interval, ratio (continuous); normality test	Pearson correlation coefficient (r), p

(*Continued*)

Making sense of evidence discovery—hypothesis testing, scale of measurement, sample, and statistical technique

Hypothesis	*Design*	*Scale of measurement*	*Statistical technique*
Assesses the linear association between two variables		Cardinal, ordinal (normality not assumed)	Spearman rank correlation (rho), *p*
Relationship (nonlinear)—Binary outcomes	Longitudinal (prospective/ concurrent cohort), retrospective, ecologic, etc.	Mixed scale (binary outcome and mixed independent variables)	Logistic/binomial regression model (crude effect size)
One dependent and > one predictor variable			Multivariable model (adjusted effect size)
Relationship involving count data		Count data (area incidence)	Poisson regression
Survival (time to event) analysis		Binary outcome and mixed independent	KM, Cox proportional hazard, life table
Repeated measures		Binary outcome	Repeated logistic regression model

Notes: (1) These techniques apply to random sample, implying that all subjects or participants in the study have an equal probability of being selected (random sample), the exception being the use of registries and consecutive patients as representative sample. (2) Type I error is committed if we reject a true null hypothesis. (3) Type II error is committed if we accept a false null hypothesis, and the alternate hypothesis is true.

Index

A

Absolute risk (AR), 21–22
Accuracy, diagnostic/screening tests, 15–17
Acute lymphocytic leukemia (ALL), 67, 70
Acute myeloid leukemia (AML), 70–71
Adenocarcinoma, metastatic prostatic, 110
Adolescent idiopathic scoliosis (AIS), 6
ADT (androgen-deprivation therapy), xxvii, 237
African-American women (AAW), 134
Age-adjusted rate, 36
Alcohol consumption, 39, 40
Allergies, 72
Analysis
  bivariable, 93, 191
  correlation
    defined, 93–94
    result of, 94–95
  discriminant, 96
  linear regression, 95
  log-linear, 96
  MANCOVA, 173
  multivariable/multivariate, 93, 191
  preanalysis screening, 77
  regression, *see* Regression analysis, tabulation *vs.*
  research questions, 93–94, 96
  statistical, consideration, big data, 250
  stratification, 257
  survival, *see* Survival analysis
  techniques, in clinical research data, 93–94
  time series, xxviii
  univariable, 93, 191
Analysis of covariance (ANCOVA), 93, 183
Analysis of variance (ANOVA), 173–188
  assumptions, 174
  computation, 174–177
  feasibility, 173
  hypothesis and possible computation, 173
  Kruskal–Wallis
    statistic, 172
    test, computation, 188
  MANCOVA, 173
  normality test, xxvi
  null hypothesis in, 173, 174, 175
  one-sample, 142–145
  one-way, nonparametric alternative to, 187–188
  other hypothesis tests, 182–188
  overview, 172, 173
  post hoc/posteriori comparison, 177–182
  RANOVA, xxvi
  repeated-measure, 126, 142–143
    appropriate, 143
    defined, 142
    one-way, nonparametric equivalent of, 144–145
    results, interpretation, 143–144
    used as test statistic, 143
  test, 92–93
  two-way, 182–185
  variability, measurement, 172
ANCOVA (analysis of covariance), 93, 183
Androgen deprivation therapy (ADT), xxvii, 237
ANOVA, *see* Analysis of variance (ANOVA)
Antagonism, 38
Antibiotics, erythromycin, 69
Apoptosis, in transgenic mice, 6

Applications
big data, 248–249
CI in assessing evidence, xxxi–xxxiv
inferential statistics, 125
probability model, 77
significance level, 125
stratification analysis, 255
tabulation analysis, 255
Applied biostatistics
binary outcome, xxvi–xxvii
CI, *see* Confidence intervals (CIs)
confounding, *see* Confounding
data, *see* Data
design process, *see* Design(s)
errors, types, *see* Errors
hypothesis testing, *see* Hypothesis testing
inference, *see* Inferences
null hypothesis, *see* Null hypothesis
poolability, fixed and random effect, xxviii
p value, *see* Probability (*p*) value
sampling, *see* Sample and sampling
statistical power, *see* Statistical power
statistical significance, *see* Statistical significance
survival analysis (time-to-event data), *see* Survival analysis
time series analysis, xxviii
ARD (absolute risk difference), 21
ARR (absolute risk reduction), 21–22
Asbestos, 40
Associations, statistical inference involving, 191–240
correlation and correlation coefficients, 202–209
appropriate, 203
computation, 204–208
defined, 202
interpretation, 208–209
overview, 202–203
STATA syntax, 202–203
logistic regression technique, 219–222
computation, 220, 222
defined, 219–220
feasibility, 220
unconditional, 220, 226, 229
model building and interpretation, 222–229
backward technique, 223, 225–228
logistic regression, types, 229
overview, 222–225
multivariable/multivariate linear regression, 197, 217–219
computation, 217–219
defined, 217
feasibility, 217
overview, 191–202
Poisson regression, 237–240
example, 238–240
overview, 237–238
uses, 238
simple linear regression, 209–217
computation, 211–216
defined, 209
feasibility, 209
interpretation, 216–217
survival analysis, time-to-event method, 229–237
Cox regression, computation, 236
Cox regression, interpretation, 237
definition of terms, 231
equality of survival, test for, 234–235
KM estimates, derivation/ computation, 232–234
KM survival estimates, 232
life table, 229–231
log-rank test, estimation, 235–236
overview, 229
Association study, 113
Asthma, 47, 49
Autistic spectrum disorder, 255–256
Autoimmune disorders, race/ethnicity and, 165, 166

B

Back pain, 33
Backward stepwise elimination, 98
Backward technique, model building using, 223, 225–228
Baclofen, 28
Balancing, benefits and harmful effects in medicine, 21–22
Baseline hazard, 201
Bayesian theorem, 12, 20
Bayes's theorem, PPV, 12
Bell-shaped curve, defined, 132
Benefits
balancing benefits, in medicine, 21–22
diagnostic tests, 14–15, 18
regression model, 261–262
screening tests, 14–15, 18–19
tabulation and stratification models, 261

Bernoulli trial, 80
Beta error rate, defined, 10
Biases
in disease screening and detection, 19
handling, 36–37
lead-time, 19
length, 19
research design, 36–39
Big data, 248–250
concept and application, 248–249
sources of, 249
statistical analysis consideration, 250
Binary/dichotomous variable, 83
Binary outcome, xxvi–xxvii
Binomial distribution model, 72, 83
Binomial regression, 80–82
defined, 80
use, 80–82
Biomedical and clinical research, 3–22
balancing benefits and harmful effects in medicine, 21–22
conducting, 5–6
diagnostic (confirmation) tests, 8–21; *see also* Diagnostic tests
generalization, 7–8
overview, 3–4
sample size and power estimations, 8
sampling, 7
screening (detection) tests, 8–21; *see also* Screening tests
standardized distribution, *z* score statistics, 68
study subjects, 6
subject selection, 6–7
Biostatistical inference, 45
Biostatistical modeling
evidence discovery, *see* Evidence discovery
overview, 75
statistical considerations, in clinical research, *see* Statistical considerations
statistical inference, *see* Statistical inference
statistical power estimations, *see* Statistical power
Biostatistical reasoning
defined, 45
involvement, 45–46
overview, xxxi–xxxii, 45–46
purpose, 48–49
statistical *vs.*, 49
Biostatistics, populations, 45–47
Bivariable analysis, 93, 191
Bivariate association, defined, xxii
Bland–Altman plot, 250
Blood pressure (BP), dopamine in, 139, 140, 141
Body mass index (BMI)
descriptive/summary statistics, 52
normality test for distribution, 51
Bonferroni correction, 203
Bonferroni procedure, 177, 180
Bootstrapping, sample, 250
Botulinum toxin, 28
Box plot
central tendency and dispersion, measures of, 60–65
of median SBP, 180
Breast cancer, diagnosis, 153–154

C

Calcium supplement, 152
Cancers
breast, diagnosis, 153–154
cervical, *see* Cervical cancer
colorectal, 191
endometrial, 198
hepatocellular carcinoma, 195
locoregional prostatic adenocarcinoma, 247
lung, 40
oral, 39, 40
prostate, *see* Prostate cancer
Cardinal variable, 136–137
Cardiomyopathies, 91
Case–control studies
nonexperimental design, type of, 31
sample size estimation for, 121–122
sampling, 35
Censored data, 199–200, 229
Central location, measurement, 50
Central tendency, measurement, 49–68
choice of, 51
defined, 50
descriptive/summary statistics, BMI, 52
median, 53–55
mode, 55–56
normality tests
for distribution of BMI, 51
SK and SBP, 53
skewness/kurtosis test, 57
SK of 31 subjects with SBP, 54
overview, 49–53

quartiles and interquartile range and box plot, 60–65
range, 56–60
SBP and, 54, 55
variance, standard deviation, and SEM, 66–68
Cerebral palsy
curve deformities in, 45
deep wound infection, 77, 163
equinus foot deformity, 166, 171, 200
follow-up, 144
population, sample and, 84–85
postoperative infection in, 22
recurrent surgery and, 166, 168
spine fusion in, 77, 163, 171
types, 136, 166, 168
Cervical arthrodesis, 78–79, 80, 119
Cervical cancer
diagnosis, 82, 232–234
survival, 237
treatment, 237
Cervical spine instability, 126
Cervical stability, on SKD pediatric patients, 80
Characteristics
confounding, 39–40
ROC curve, 17–18
Characterization, sample size, 110
Chemoprophylaxis, for urticaria, 141–142
Chemotherapy, leukemia, 161, 162
Chi-square statistics, 79–80
assumptions, 91
defined, 79
use, 79–80
Chi-square test
disadvantage of, 152
of independence, xxv
proportions in two groups, 164–168
assumptions, 166
compare proportions, 166
computation, 166–168
defined, 164–165
hypothesis testing, 165
overview, 164
types, 164–165
Chronologic age, 40
Clinical phase, early disease detection, 18
Clinical reasoning, 20–21
Clinical research
data
analysis techniques in, 93–94
statistical modeling of, xxxi
statistical considerations in, *see* Statistical considerations
Clinical science data, statistical modeling of, 251–253
Clinical trials
conducting, 33
cost, 32–33
defined, 27
minimum detectable difference in, 107
parallel design in, 112
phases, 34
prospective cohort/two-group comparison in, 120–121
randomized crossover, 33
randomized placebo-controlled, 33–34
RCT, 33–34
sample size in, 110
Clubfoot, surgically treated, 191–192
Cobb angle, 77, 220
Cohort studies, 31, 35
Colorectal cancer, 191
Computation
paired *t* tests, 139–141
sample size, 110, 112–114
Conditional probability, 70–71
Conducting
biomedical and clinical research
diagnostic test, 9
reasons, 5–6
clinical trials, 33
Confidence intervals (CIs)
application, in assessing evidence, xxxi–xxxiv
biostatistical reasoning and, 49
influence on, 86
overview, xxiii–xxiv
precision and, xxx–xxxi
Confirmation tests, 8–21; *see also* Diagnostic tests
Confounding
addressing for, 258–259
assessment, 257–258
defined, xxix, 39, 256
elements and characteristics, 39–40
overview, xxviii–xxix
p value and measure of evidence, xxix
research design, 39–41
role of random error, xxix–xxx
in translational and clinical research, 256–257
variables, 256–257

Continuous variables, 83
Convenience sampling, 48
Correlation analysis
  defined, 93–94
  result of, 94–95
Correlation and correlation coefficients, 202–209
  appropriate, 203
  computation, 204–208
  defined, 202
  interpretation, 208–209
  null hypothesis for, 204, 205
  overview, 202–203
  Pearson, xxvi, 191, 192, 202, 203, 204
  Spearman, 191, 194, 202, 203, 205
  Spearman rank (rho), xxvi
  STATA syntax, 202–203
Corticosteroids, in racial/ethnic disparities, 49
Costs
  clinical trials, 32–33
  hip replacement, 247–248
Covariates
  research design, 39–41
  in translational and clinical research, 256–257
Cox–Mantel log-rank tests, 235
Cox proportional hazard model, xxvii–xxviii, 199, 201
Cox regression
  computation, 236
  in failure-time model, 199
  interpretation, 237
  proportional hazard model, 199, 200, 201, 202, 229, 231
Critical point, defined, 18
Crossover study, 112–113
Cross-sectional studies, 35
Cystitis, 69

D

Data
  censored, 199–200, 229
  clinical research, analysis techniques in, 93–94
  one-sample, statistical test for, 146
  for Poisson regression, 237
  social media, 249
  statistical modeling of biomedical and clinical research, xxxi
  time-to-event, xxvii–xxviii
  translational and clinical science, statistical modeling, 251–253
  visualization, xxiii
Deep-vein thrombosis (DVT), 13
Deep wound infection
  development, 198, 199, 220, 222
  model building, 222–223
  predictors, 222
Dental disorders, pediatric, 118, 119
Dependent *t* test, 89
Dependent variables
  coding, 226
  defined, 220
  levels, 229
  logit of, 96–97
  scale of measurement, 78–79, 220
Descriptive statistics
  BMI, 52
  in clinical research, 125
Design(s)
  epidemiologic
    defined, 27
    study, 28–29
  experimental
    nonexperimental *vs.*, 34–35
    overview, 32–34
  nonexperimental
    experimental *vs.*, 34–35
    overview, 30–32
  one-sample group, 130
  parallel, 112
  process
    biomedical and clinical research, *see* Biomedical and clinical research
    research design, *see* Research design
  randomized block, 183
  repeated measures, 187
  study, *see* Study designs
Detectable preclinical phase, early disease detection, 18
Detection tests, 8–21; *see also* Screening tests
Developmental disorders (DD), 258–259
Diabetes
  diagnosis, 9
  diagnosis of, 71
  implication, 118, 119
  prevalence, educational status and, 47
  renal insufficiency and, 22
  underestimation/overestimation, 47
Diabetic keto-acidosis (DKA), 162–163

Diagnosis
  bacterial cystitis, 9
  breast cancer, 153–154
  cervical cancer, 82, 232–234
  diabetes, 71
Diagnostic tests, 8–21
  accuracy/validity, 15–17
  advantages and disadvantages, 18
  biases, 19
  clinical reasoning, 20–21
  conducting, 9
  disease prevalence, 11, 12, 18
  issues in early disease detection, 18–19
  likelihood ratio (LR), 12–14
  measures of, 10–11
  multiple/sequential testing, 14
  overview, 8–9
  possible results, 9–10
  predictive values in, 11–12, 18
  principles, advantages, and limitations, 14–15
  ROC curve, 17–18
Dichotomous variables, 83
Dimensional variables, 83
Discrete variables, 83
Discriminant analysis, 96
Disease association/effect, measures of, 36–37
Disease detection, issues in, 18–19
Disease prevalence, relationship
  predictive values, 11, 12, 18
  sensitivity, 11, 12
  specificity, 11, 12
Dispersion, measurement, 49–68
  median, 53–55
  mode, 55–56
  overview, 49–53, 56
  quartiles and interquartile range and box plot, 60–65
  range, 56–60
  variance, standard deviation, and SEM, 66–68
Distribution(s)
  free tests, 141
  normal distribution of BMI, 51
  probability, *see* Probability distributions
  probability, random variables and, 82
  standardized, 68
Dopamine, 139, 140
Doppler ultrasound study, 13
Dot plot, SBP, 180, 181
Dunnett's procedure, 178
Dunn's multiple-comparison procedure, 177

E

Ebola virus, 254, 261
Effect measure modifier, research design, 40–41
Effect size, defined, 108
Elbow ligament thickness, 67
Elements, confounding, 39–40
Endometrial carcinoma/cancer, 198
Epidemiologic designs
  defined, 27
  study, 28–29
Epidemiology, defined, 28
Equality of survival, test for, 234–235
Equal variances, test for, 157, 159
Equinus foot deformity, 200
Equipoise, 31
Error bars, 153–154
Error rate, false-negative/false-positive, 10, 11, 17
Errors
  random, *see* Random errors
  type I and II, hypothesis testing and, 86, 87
  types of, xxx–xxxiv, 38
Erythromycin, 69
Escherichia coli, 9
Ethnicity
  autistic spectrum disorder and, 255–256
  autoimmune disorders and, 165, 166
  developmental disorders (DD) and, 258–259
  disparities, 49
  KM survival estimates by, 234–235
Event rate in control (ERC), 21
Event rate in treatment (ERT), 21
Events, independent, 84
Evidence discovery, 247–262
  big data, 248–250
    concept and application, 248–249
    sources of, 249
    statistical analysis consideration, 250
  making sense of, 266–268
  overview, 247–248
  statistical modeling, 251–253
    background information, 253
    basic notion, 251–252
    in clinical and translational research, 252

minimal model, 252
overview, 251
reality in, 253
tabulation *vs.* regression analysis, 254–262
basic concept and application, 255
benefits and limitations, 261–262
confounding and covariates, 256–257, 258–259
overview, 254
rationale and assumption, 255–256, 257–258
regression as predictive model, 259–261
scientific, essential stages, 255
stratification analysis, 257
test statistics, selection of, 254
Experimental designs
nonexperimental *vs.*, 34–35
overview, 32–34
Explanatory variables, 220, 229, 238
External-beam radiation (EBT), 110
External validity, 37

F

Facebook, 249
False discovery rate (FDR), 250
Fasting serum cholesterol level (FSCL), 134
Feasibility
ANOVA, 173
logistic regression technique, 220
multivariable/multivariate linear regression, 217
simple linear regression, 209
Fisher's exact test, 91, 152, 166, 168
Fixed effect, xxviii
Forward technique, model building, 223
Fraction, sampling, 85
Fractures, 237–238
Frame, sampling, 85
Francia and Shapiro's method, 53, 54
F ratio, 175
Friedman test, 92, 144
F tests, 92, 174, 175
F value, 143–144

G

Gastroesophageal reflux disease (GERD), 182
Gaussian distribution, defined, 132
Generalization, biomedical and clinical research, 7–8
Generalized linear model (GLM), 97, 98–99
Gleason score, 82
Glycosylated hemoglobin, 139
Gold standard, defined, 33

H

Harmful effects in medicine, balancing, 21–22
Hazard, defined, 231
Hazard function, defined, 232
Hazard rate, defined, 231
Hazard ratio (HR), 49, 230, 231, 236, 237
Heel impulse, 191–192
Hepatocellular carcinoma, 195
High-density lipoprotein (HDL), 183–185, 186, 187
Hip fracture, probability of, 20
Hip replacement, in older patients, 247–248
Homogeneous variance, defined, 154
Homoscadasticity, 261
Honestly significant difference (HSD), Tukey's, 178
Hypothesis
ANOVA, 173
defined, 91
statement, 130
Hypothesis testing, 87–99
analysis techniques in clinical research data, 93–94
appropriate test, 88–89
chi-square statistics, 165
in clinical research, 79
correlated/paired sample, xxv
defined, 87–88
evidence discovery, 266–268
independent sample, xxv
involving binary outcomes, 221
involving linear relationship, 210
involving relationships, 242
linear relationship, xxvi
more-than-two-samples, xxv
nonparametric tests in, 136–137
one-sample, 147, 151
one-sample *t* test, 130
in one-way between-subject ANOVA, 92
other, ANOVA, 182–188

overview, 87–88
paired *t* tests in, 139
random error and, 108
single-/one-sample proportion, 114–115
single-sample *t* test, 126
steps in, 127–128
technique, xxiii
two-sample, xxv
data, 168
examples of, 152
type I and II errors, 87, 113, 114
types, 38–39
z distribution and, 90
Hypothetico-deductive reasoning, 20

I

Incidences
fractures, 237
prostate cancer, 152
Independence
concept, 47
probability, 71
in sampling, 47
Independent events, 84
Independent samples, 151–169
chi-square test of proportions in two groups, 164–168
assumptions, 166
compare proportions, 166
computation, 166–168
defined, 164–165
hypothesis testing, 165
overview, 164
types, 164–165
defined, 151, 153
overview, 151–152
terms explanation, 153–154
two-sample (*t* test), 89, 152–162
appropriate, 154
assumptions, 154–155
computation, 155–157
defined, 154
equal variances, test for, 157, 159–161
nonparametric alternative, 161–162
overview, 152–153
two-sample hypothesis tests, examples of, 152
z test, two independent proportions, 162–164
computation, 163–164
defined, 163
formula for, 163
use, 163
Independent variables
categorical, 174
chi-square statistic, 79, 80
continuous and/or binary/categorical, 97
different values for, 231
effect of, 229
measurement, 82, 219–220, 229
radiation level, 238
random variables, 237
Inferences
biostatistical, 45
from nonnormal population, one-sample *t*-test, 136–138
nonparametric alternative, 136–137
sign test, 137–138
overview, xxi–xxiii
statistical, *see* Statistical inference
Inferential statistics, application, 125
Information
for sample size, 108–109, 112, 117
statistical power, estimations, 108–109
Insulin, 22
Interaction
RAD and GERD, 182
research design, 39–41
Interaction/product term, 257–258
Intermediate variate, defined, 40
Internal validity, 37, 38
Interpretation
logistic regression result, 98
repeated-measure ANOVA, results, 143–144
simple linear regression, 216–217
Wald test in logistic regression, 98
Interquartile range, 60–65
Issues, in early disease detection, 18–19

K

Kaplan–Meier (KM) survival estimates
derivation/computation, 232–234
function, 199–200
survival analysis, 229
Knee flexion, peak, 206, 207, 211–217
Kruskal–Wallis statistics, 172
Kruskal–Wallis test, xxvi, 92, 188
Kurtosis
defined, 51
normality test, 57, 217

L

Lead time
  bias, 19
  early disease detection, 18
Least squares regression, 95
Length bias, 19
Leukemia, 161, 162
Leukodystrophy, types, 166
Levene test, for equal variances, 159
Life table, 229–231
Likelihood ratio (LR)
  overview, 12–13
  positive and negative tests, 13, 17
    measure of separation, 13–14
  test, 98, 226
Likert scale, 136
Limitations
  regression model, 261–262
  screening and diagnostic test, 14–15
  tabulation and stratification models, 261
Linear regression(s)
  analysis, 95
  model
    multiple, xxvi
    simple, xxvi
  multiple/multivariable, 95, 96
  multivariable/multivariate, 197, 217–219
    computation, 217–219
    defined, 217
    feasibility, 217
  results, 95–96
  simple, *see* Simple linear regression
Locoregional prostatic adenocarcinoma, 247
Logistic regression (LR)
  overview, 96–99
  techniques, 219–222
    computation, 220, 222
    defined, 219–220
    feasibility, 220
    types, 229
    unconditional, 220, 226, 229
Logit transformation, 96, 97
Log-linear analysis, 96
Log-rank test
  defined, 235
  estimation, 235–236
  Mantel, 235
Low density lipoprotein (LDL), 186–187
Lung cancer, 40

M

MANCOVA (multiple analysis of variance), 173
Mann–Whitney test, xxv, 90, 152–162
Mantel log-rank test, 235
Mean
  population, 88
  population parameter, 46, 47
  sample, 67
Mean life expectancy, for independent samples, 157, 158
Measurements
  dependent/response variable, 78–79
  diagnostic/screening tests, 10–11
  disease association/effect, 36–37
  of evidence, *p* value and, xxix
  separation between LR positive and negative tests, 13–14
  variables, scales in, 83
Measurements, central tendency and dispersion, 49–68
  choice of, 51
  defined, 50
  descriptive/summary statistics, BMI, 52
  median, 53–55
  mode, 55–56
  normality tests
    distribution of BMI, 51
    SK and SBP, 53
    skewness/kurtosis test, 57
    SK of 31 subjects with SBP, 54
    utilizing Francia and Shapiro's method, 53, 54
  overview, 49–53
  quartiles and interquartile range and box plot, 60–65
  range, 56–60
  SBP and, 54, 55
  variance, standard deviation, and SEM, 66–68
Median, 53–55
Median survival time, 200
Metastatic prostatic adenocarcinoma, 110
mHealth, 249
Migration index (MI), 49
Minimum detectable difference, 107
Mixed scale, defined, 199
Mode, 55–56
Model building and interpretation, 222–229
  backward technique, 223, 225–228

logistic regression, types, 229
overview, 222–225
Models/modeling
binomial distribution model, 72
biostatistical, *see* Biostatistical modeling
Cox proportional hazard, xxvii–xxviii, 199, 201
cross-sectional time-series data analysis/modeling, xxviii
data analysis/modeling, panel/ longitudinal/cross-sectional, xxviii
GLM, 97, 98–99
longitudinal time-series data analysis/ modeling, xxviii
mouse models, 6
multiple linear regression model, xxvi
multivariable Cox regression proportional hazard model, xxvii–xxviii
null model, 98
panel time-series data analysis/ modeling, xxviii
proportional hazard model, 199, 201, 231
robust simple linear regression model, xxvi
simple linear regression model, xxvi
statistical, *see* Statistical modeling
testing, 98
univariable Cox proportional hazard, xxvii–xxviii
ZIP regression model, 99
Mortality
chemotherapy, 251
prostate cancer, 5
radiation level on, 239–240
Mouse models
apoptosis, 6
n34 mice, 6
Multiple analysis of variance (MANCOVA), 173
Multiple/multivariable linear regression, 95, 96
Multiple testing, 14
Multiplication rule, 84
Multivariable analysis, 93, 191
Multivariable/multivariate linear regression, 197, 217–219
computation, 217–219
defined, 217
feasibility, 217
Mutually exclusive events, 84
Myocardial infarction, 40, 72

N

National Cancer Institute (NCI), 154, 249
National Children Health Survey, 255–256
National Study of Nutrition (NSN), 88, 130, 131
Negative binomial regression, 99
Negative predictive value (NPV), 12
Nested designs, 187
Neuromuscular scoliosis
Cobb angle in, 220
curve deformities, correcting, 197–198
deep wound infection, 154, 199
posterior spine fusion, 114, 154, 197–198, 199, 222
prevention of infection in, 114
n34 mice, 6
Nominal variables, 83, 136
Nonexperimental designs
experimental *vs.,* 34–35
overview, 30–32
Nonnormal population, inference from, 136–138
nonparametric alternative, 136–137
sign test, 137–138
Nonnormal statistical inference tests, 141
Nonparametric alternatives
computation, STATA statistical software, 142
defined, 92
Kruskal–Wallis test, 92
Mann–Whitney *u* test, 152–162
one-sample *t* test, 136–137
one-way ANOVA, 187–188
paired *t* tests, 141
Pearson correlation, 94
to Pearson correlation coefficient, 191, 202
two-sample *t* test, 161–162
Nonparametric equivalent, of one-way repeated-measure ANOVA, 144–145
Nonparametric procedures, 90, 92, 94
Nonparametric tests, 113, 136–137, 141
Nonprobability sampling, 47–48
Norm, defined, 88
Normal curve, defined, 127
Normal distribution, 83, 132

Normality tests
  ANOVA assumptions, 174, 175, 176
  data for, 204
  distribution of BMI, 51
  peak knee flexion, 207
  for SK and SBP, 53, 54
  skewness/kurtosis test, 57
  on two variables of interest, 192
  utilizing Francia and Shapiro's method, 53, 54
Null hypothesis
  in ANOVA, 173, 174, 175
  application of CI in assessing evidence, xxxi–xxxiv
  CI and precision, xxx–xxxi
  for correlation coefficient, 204, 205
  evidence against, 125
  overview, xxx
  rejection, 128–129, 134, 140, 164, 165, 192–193, 205, 217
  significance level, xxx, 140
  types of errors and, 38
Null model, 98
Number needed to harm (NNH), 21–22
Number needed to treat (NNT), 21–22

O

Obesity, 40
Observations, censored, 229
Odds ratio (OR)
  approximation of, 13
  case–control study, 121
  disease frequency, measures of, 36
  interpretation of logistic regression result, 98
  Mantel–Haenszel, 252
  measure of effect, 49
  in STATA output, 223, 226–227, 228
Older patients, hip replacement in, 247–248
One-sample analysis of variance, 142–145
  data, statistical test for, 146
  hypothesis testing, 147
  repeated-measure, 142–145
    appropriate, 143
    defined, 142
    one-way, nonparametric equivalent of, 144–145
    results, interpretation, 143–144
    used as test statistic, 143
One-sample estimation, of sample size
  with outcome mean, 116–117
  proportion hypothesis testing, 114–115
One-sample group design, 130
One-sample tests, illustrations, 127
One-sample *t*-test, 130–131
  appropriate test statistic, 130–131
  formula for, 131
  inference from nonnormal
    population, 136–138
    nonparametric alternative, 136–137
    sign test, 137–138
  power of, 135
  purpose, 131
  result, interpretation, 133
  statistical power, estimation, 133–134
  type of test, 89
One-way ANOVA
  between-subject ANOVA, 92–93
  nonparametric alternative to, 187–188
  repeated-measure ANOVA, 144–145
Oral cancer, 39, 40
Oral contraceptives, 40
Ordinal variables, 83, 136, 137
Organophosphates, 97
Osteoporosis, 20, 237–238

P

Paired *t* tests, 138–139
  assumptions, 139
  computation, 139–141
  defined, 127, 138–139
  formula for, 139
  in hypothesis testing, 139
  nonparametric alternative, 141
  in pre- and post-test measurements, 126
  samples, 89
Pancreatitis, postoperative, 182
Parallel design, 112
Parallel testing, 14
Parametric tests, 113
Peak knee flexion, 206, 207, 211–217
Pearson correlation, 94, 191, 192, 202, 203, 204
Pearson product moment, defined, 203
Pediatric dental disorders, 118, 119
Pedobarographic measure, 191–192, 193
Pedographic measure, 192
Pelvic osteotomy, 49
Point estimates
  precision, 49
  quantification, 49

Poisson distribution, 83
Poisson regression, 237–240
  example, 238–240
  overview, 237–238
  statistical method, 99
  uses, 238
Polycystic ovarian syndrome (POS), diagnosis, 198
Polynomial regression, 96
Poolability, xxviii
Population mean, defined, 88
Populations, 45–47
  biostatistical notion, 46–47
  overview, 45–46
  parameters, 45
  sample and, 84–85
  standard deviation, 153
Positive predictive value (PPV), 12
Post hoc/posteriori comparison, ANOVA, 177–182
Power, statistical, *see* Statistical power
Power estimations, sample size and, 8
Preanalysis screening, defined, 77
Precision, 36–39
  confidence interval and, xxx–xxxi
  defined, 37, 38
  enhancing, 38
  estimation, 36–37
  influence by, 37
  of point estimate, 49
Preclinical phase, early disease detection, 18
Predictive model, regression as, 259–261
Predictive values, 11–12
  defined, 11
  disease prevalence, relationship between, 11, 12, 18
  sensitivity, relationship between, 11, 12
  specificity, relationship between, 11, 12
  types of, 12
Predictor variables, 220, 222, 229, 231, 238
Prevalence, of disease, *see* Disease prevalence, relationship predictive values
Principles, screening and diagnostic test, 14–15
Probability
  conditional, 70–71
  independence, 71
  model, application of, 77
  notion, basic, 69
  rules, types, 84
  simple and unconditional probability, 69–70
  uses of, 84
Probability distributions, 83–84
  defined, 83, 111
  overview, 72
  random variables and, 82
  types, 83–84
Probability sampling
  requirement for, 7
  type of sampling, 47
  types of, 85
Probability (*p*) value
  clinical and translational study findings, 253
  interpretation, 175–176
  likelihood ratio test, 226
  measure of evidence and, xxix
  overview, xxi–xxviii
  significance level, 111
  two-sample *t* test, 192, 194
  for Wald test, 226
Product-limit estimator, 201
Product-limit method, defined, 232
Prognostic marker
  in hepatocellular carcinoma, 195
  STATA output, 195
Proliferative marker
  in hepatocellular carcinoma, 195
  STATA output, 195
Proportional hazard model
  Cox, 199, 201
  defined, 231
Prospective cohort, clinical trials, 120–121
Prostate cancer
  ADT, effectiveness of, 237
  anti-neoplastic agent, 251
  calcium supplement, 152
  cause-specific mortality, 5
  population of US males, 46
  probability of developing, 96–97
  prognosis, reliable marker of, 9
  radical prostatectomy for, 82
  screening/diagnostic tests, 8–9
  screening program, 19
  Swedish prospective cohort study, 5
Prostate-specific antigen (PSA), 8–9, 152
Prostatic adenocarcinoma, metastatic, 110
Proton-beam therapy (PBT), 110
Pseudoarthrosis, 9

Purposes
one-sample *t* test, 131
sample size, 110

Q

Quality of life (QOL), 161–162
Quartiles range, 60–65
Quota sampling, 48

R

Race
autistic spectrum disorder and, 255–256
autoimmune disorders and, 165, 166
developmental disorders (DD) and, 258–259
disparities, 49
KM survival estimates by, 234–235
Radical prostatectomy, for prostate cancer, 82
Radiographic measure, 192
Random errors, 36–39
CI by, xxx–xxxi
defined, 37
handling, 36–37
hypothesis testing and, 108
minimizing, 38
rates, sample size equation formula and, 116
role, 38
role of, xxix–xxx
Randomized block designs, 183
Randomized controlled clinical trial (RCT), 33, 109, 110
Randomized crossover clinical trial, 33
Randomized factorial design, 183
Random samples/sampling
defined, 47
error, minimizing, xxix–xxx
overview, xxiii, xxx
population of patients, xxxiii
simple, 48, 77
systematic, 48
of systolic blood pressure, 133
Random variables, 125–126
defined, 47, 82
probability distributions, 82
Range
measure of dispersion, 56–60
as quantity and interval, 57
quartiles and interquartile, box plot and, 60–65
RANOVA, *see* Repeated-measure ANOVA (RANOVA)
Reactive airway disease (RAD), 182
Receiver operating characteristic (ROC) curve, 17–18
Rectus femoris transfer surgery, 144
Referral bias, defined, 19
Regression analysis, tabulation *vs.*, 254–262
basic concept and application, 255
benefits and limitations, 261–262
confounding and covariates, 256–257, 258–259
overview, 254
as predictive model, 259–261
rationale and assumption, 255–256, 257–258
scientific evidence discovery, essential stages, 255
stratification analysis, 257
test statistics, selection of, 254
Regressions
analyzing time-to-event data, 199
Cox, *see* Cox regression
function, defined, 198
least squares, 95
linear, 95, 96, 97–98
multivariable/multivariate, *see* Multivariable/multivariate linear regression
simple, *see* Simple linear regression
linear regression analysis, 95
logistic regression (LR), 96–99
logistic regression technique, 219–222
computation, 220, 222
defined, 219–220
feasibility, 220
unconditional, 220, 226, 229
multiple/multivariable linear regression, 95, 96
Poisson, *see* Poisson regression
robust, STATA output, 195, 197, 198, 213
types, 96
Relationships, statistical inference involving, 191–240
correlation and correlation coefficients, 202–209
appropriate, 203
computation, 204–208
defined, 202
interpretation, 208–209

overview, 202–203
STATA syntax, 202–203
logistic regression technique, 219–222
computation, 220, 222
defined, 219–220
feasibility, 220
unconditional, 220, 226, 229
model building and interpretation, 222–229
backward technique, 223, 225–228
logistic regression, types, 229
overview, 222–225
multivariable/multivariate linear regression, 197, 217–219
computation, 217–219
defined, 217
feasibility, 217
overview, 191–202
Poisson regression, 237–240
example, 238–240
overview, 237–238
uses, 238
simple linear regression, 211–217
computation, 211–216
defined, 209
feasibility, 209
interpretation, 216–217
survival analysis, time-to-event method, 229–237
Cox regression, computation, 236
Cox regression, interpretation, 237
definition of terms, 231
equality of survival, test for, 234–235
KM estimates, derivation/computation, 232–234
KM survival estimates, 232
life table, 229–231
log-rank test, estimation, 235–236
overview, 229
Relative risk (RR), 21–22, 36
Renal failure, 163
Renal insufficiency, 22
Repeated-measure ANOVA (RANOVA)
appropriate, 143
defined, 142
one-way, nonparametric equivalent of, 144–145
overview, xxvi, 126
results, interpretation, 143–144
used as test statistic, 143
Repeated measures design, 187
Representative sample, defined, xxi
Requirements
paired *t* test, in hypothesis testing, 139
sample size estimation, 108–109, 112, 117
Research
biomedical and clinical, *see* Biomedical and clinical research
design, *see* Research design
Research design, 27–41
biases, 36–39
clinical trials, 32–34
confounding, covariates, effect measure modifier, interaction, 39–41
disease association/effect, measures of, 36–37
epidemiologic study designs, 28–29
experimental designs
nonexperimental *vs.*, 34–35
overview, 32–34
nonexperimental designs
experimental *vs.*, 34–35
overview, 30–32
overview, 27–28
precision, 36–39
random error, 36–39
validity, estimation, 36–37
Research questions
analysis of, 93–94, 96
defined, 87, 130
examples of, 90–91, 165
hypothesis testing, *z* distribution and, 90
overview, 87
Response variables, 78–79, 219, 220, 222, 229, 238, 240
Results
interpretation, statistical inference and, xxxii
linear regressions, 95–96
logistic regression, 98
one-sample *t*-test, interpretation, 133
possible, screening tests, 9–10
repeated-measure ANOVA, interpretation, 143–144
sign test, interpretation, 138
Risk difference, defined, 21
Robust regression, 213
R-Plus, statistical software, 174

S

Sample and sampling
biomedical and clinical research, 7

characterization, xxiii
convenience, 48
correlated/paired sample, xxv
design, 45
evidence discovery, 266–268
fraction, frame, and scheme, 85
independent, *see* Independent samples
mean, SEM, SE, and sample size, 67
more-than-two-samples hypothesis testing, xxvi
nonprobability, 47–48
overview, xxiii–xxiv, 45–46
population and, 84–85
probability, *see* Probability sampling
quota, 48
random, *see* Random samples/sampling
sample/study size, estimation, 86
selection, 47
simple random, 48, 77
single, *see* Single sample statistical inference
size, effect size, and variability, xxiv
size and power, 8, 84–87
statistics, 45
strategies, 47–48
stratified, 48
systematic random, 48
technique, 85
three/more samples, statistical inference, *see* Statistical inference
unit/element, 85
Sample size
effect size and, xxiv
elements influencing size and, 135
estimation, 86
increasing, SEM reduction with, 67, 68
power estimations and, 8
power of test by, 135–136
Sample size, estimation, 107–123
case–control studies, 121–122
characterization, 110
in clinical trials, 110
computation, 110, 112–114
determining, 109
equation formula and random error rates, 116
factors affecting, 114, 115
factors associated, 107
information required for, 108–109, 112, 117
one-sample
with outcome mean, 116–117
proportion hypothesis testing, 114–115
overview, 107–109
prospective cohort/two-group comparison in clinical trials, 120–121
purpose, 110
requirements, 108–109, 112, 117
for single-sample proportion hypothesis testing, 114–115
two independent group, defined, 119–120
two independent samples
computation, 117–119
proportions, 117–119
requirements, 117
Sampling fraction, defined, 48
SAS, statistical software, 174
Satterthwaite's test, 157
SBP, *see* Systolic blood pressure (SBP)
Scale of measurement, evidence discovery, 266–268
Scales, in measuring variables, 83
Scheffe's procedure, 177, 178, 179
Scheme, sampling, 85
Scientific evidence discovery, essential stages, 255
Scoliosis
cerebral palsy with, 22
neuromuscular, *see* Neuromuscular scoliosis
types, 173
Scores, standardizing, 68
Score statistics, 231
Screening preanalysis, defined, 77
Screening tests, 8–21
accuracy/validity, 15–17
advantages and disadvantages, 18
benefits, 18–19
biases, 19
clinical reasoning, 20–21
defined, 9
disease prevalence, 11, 12, 18
issues in early disease detection, 18–19
likelihood ratio (LR), 12–14
measures of, 10–11
multiple/sequential testing, 14
possible results, 9–10
predictive values in, 11–12, 18
principles, advantages, and limitations, 14–15

PSA, 8–9
ROC curve, 17–18
Sensitivity
defined, 10, 15–16
predictive values, disease prevalence, and specificity, 11
Sequential testing, 14
Serial testing, 14
Sex-adjusted rate, 36
Significance level
application, 125
for null hypothesis, 140
p value, 111
test statistics, 38–39
Sign test, 137–138
applying, 137
appropriate, 137
computation, 137–138
defined, 127, 136
feasibility, 137
result, interpretation, 138
Simple linear regression, 95, 211–217
computation, 211–216
defined, 209
feasibility, 209
interpretation, 216–217
Simple probability, 69–70
Simple random sampling (SRS), 48, 77
Single sample proportion hypothesis testing, 114–115
Single sample statistical inference, 125–145
drawing and stating conclusion, 128–129
hypothesis statement, 130
one-sample
group design, 130
tests, illustrations, 127
one-sample *t*-test, inference from
nonnormal population, 136–138
nonparametric alternative, 136–137
sign test, 137–138
overview, 125–126
steps in hypothesis testing, 127–128
test statistics, 130–136
defined, 130
one-sample *t* test, 130–131
one-sample *t*-test result, interpretation, 133
power of test, sample size and, 135–136
statistical significance, 131–136
test assumption, 132
test techniques, 126–127
t test
computation of, 128
one-sample analysis of variance, 142–145
paired *t* test, 138–139
types, 138–145
Wilcoxon signed-rank test, 141–142
Single-sample *t* test, 126, 127
Skeletal dysplasia (SKD), 78–79, 119
Skewness
defined, 51
tests, for normality, 57
Smoking, 39, 40
Social media, 249
Sources of variation (variability), variables and, 82–84
Sparse-strata method, 259
Spastic cerebral palsy, 28
Spearman correlation coefficient, 191, 194, 202, 203, 205
Spearman rank correlation coefficients, 94
Spearman Rho, 191
Specificity
defined, 11, 16
predictive values, disease prevalence, and sensitivity, 11
Sphericity
test of, 187
S-Plus, statistical software, 174
SPSS, statistical software, 174
Standard deviations (SD)
estimation, 66
population, 153
population parameter, 46, 47
sample, 67
two independent group, 119
unequal, 157
vitamin C intake, 88
Standard error (SE), 131
Standard error of estimate, 95
Standard error of mean (SEM), 66–68
Standardized distribution, *z* score statistics, 68
Standardized rate, defined, 36
Standard normal (*z*) distribution, 84
STATA statistical software
ANOVA, computation, 174, 175, 176, 179
Bonferroni correction, 203
central tendency and dispersion, measures of, 52, 53, 56, 58–59
equality of survival, test of, 234, 235

error line/bars of SBP, 180, 181
hazard ratio, 236
independent *t* test using, 155
KM estimates, 232–234
life table, generating, 230
likelihood ratio test, 227–228
logistic regression, 220, 223, 224, 226
mortality rate, 239–240
multiple linear regression, 218
nonparametric alternative, computation, 142
normality, test of, 204
paired *t* test using, 140
for Pearson correlation coefficient, 202, 204
Poisson regression analysis, 238–240
power of study, 135–136
proliferative and prognostic markers, 195
robust regression, 197, 213
sample, estimation, 118, 120
sample number, 116
sample size, computation, 112
SBP, normality test for, 53, 59
Scheffe's multiple comparisons, 179, 180
sign test, computation of, 137–138
single sample, 126, 128
two-sample/independent-sample *t* test, 192–193
two-way ANOVA, 182–183

Statistical analysis, consideration, big data, 250

Statistical considerations, in clinical research, 77–101
application of probability model, 77
binomial regression, 80–82
Chi-square statistic, 79–80
hypothesis testing, *see* Hypothesis testing
notion of statistics, 78
overview, 77–82
research questions, *see* Research questions
sampling, sample size and power, 84–87
fraction, frame, and scheme, 85
population, 84–85
power, 86–87
probability, 84
probability sampling, types of, 85
sample/study size, estimation, 86
technique, 85
statistical inference, 87–99
variables
in clinical research, 83
dependent/response/independent, 78–79, 80, 82, 97
measuring, scales in, 83
probability distribution, 83–84
random, probability distributions, 82
sources of variation (variability) and, 82–84
types, 82, 83

Statistical inference
ANOVA, *see* Analysis of variance (ANOVA)
appropriate, 111
in clinical research, 87–99
independent samples, *see* Independent samples
involving relationships/associations, 191–240
correlation and correlation coefficients, 202–209
logistic regression technique, 219–222
model building and interpretation, 222–229
multivariable/multivariate linear regression, 197, 217–219
overview, 191–202
Poisson regression, 237–240
simple linear regression, 211–217
survival analysis, time-to-event method, 229–237
overview, 171–172
results interpretation and, xxxii
single samples, *see* Single sample statistical inference
test selection for three/more samples, 189
in three/more samples, 171–189

Statistical modeling, 251–253
background information, 253
basic notion, 251–252
biomedical and clinical research data, xxxi
in clinical and translational research, 252
minimal model, 252
overview, 251
reality in, 253

Statistical power
defined, 86

estimations, 107–123
elements influencing power, 134
graphical illustration, 119
information required for, 108–109
in one-sample *t* test, 133–134
overview, 107–109
for prospective/clinical trials, 120
sample size and, 135–136; *see also* Sample size
significance and, 122
factors influencing, xxiv
Statistical reasoning, biostatistical *vs.*, 49
Statistical significance, 131–136
defined, 111, 125
overview, xxi–xxiii
statistical power and, 122
Statistical technique, evidence discovery, 266–268
Statistics
Chi-square, 79–80
notion of, 78
score, 231
test, for ANOVA, 92–93
Stiff knee, 144
Strategies, sample and sampling, 47–48
Stratification analysis, 257
Stratified sampling, 48, 85
Student's *t* test, *see* *t*-tests
Study designs
epidemiologic, 28–29
experimental (clinical trials), 32–34
nonexperimental, 30–32
Study subjects, 6
Subject(s)
selection, 6–7
study, 6
Summary statistics
BMI, 52
defined, 50
Surrogate confounders, defined, 40
Surveillance Epidemiology and End Results (SEER), 153, 249
Survival analysis, 229–237
Cox regression
computation, 236
interpretation, 237
definition of terms, 231
equality of survival, test for, 234–235
KM survival estimates, 232
derivation/computation, 232–234
life table, 229–231
log-rank test, estimation, 235–236
overview, xxvii–xxviii, 229
Survival function plot, defined, 231
Synergism, 37–38
Systematic error, handling, 36–37
Systematic random sampling, 48
Systematic sampling, 85
Systolic blood pressure (SBP)
age on, 52
box plots, 60–65, 180
central tendency of 31 subjects with, 54
confounding effect of HDL on, 183
distribution of, 175
dopamine in, 139, 140
dot plot, 180, 181
linear relationship between, 192
lowering, treatment in, 142
mean values with error line/bars, 180, 181
minimum difference in, 135
mode, 55–56
normality tests, 53
Francia and Shapiro's method, 53, 54
SK of 31 subjects with, 54
post hoc comparison, 180, 181
quartiles, 65
random sample, 133
spread of, central tendency, 54
variance of, 66

T

Tabulation, regression analysis *vs.*, 254–262
basic concept and application, 255
benefits and limitations, 261–262
confounding and covariates, 256–257, 258–259
overview, 254
rationale and assumption, 255–256, 257–258
regression as predictive model, 259–261
scientific evidence discovery, essential stages, 255
stratification analysis, 257
test statistics, selection of, 254
Talo-calcaneal angle, 191–192
t distribution, 88, 89–90
Test assumption, 132
Testing
chi-square test, *see* Chi-square test
Cox–Mantel log-rank tests, 235

diagnostic/confirmation tests, *see* Diagnostic tests
equality of survival, 234–235
equal variances, 157, 159
Fisher's exact test, 91, 152, 166, 168
Friedman, 92, 144
F tests, 92, 174, 175
hypothesis, *see* Hypothesis testing
Kruskal–Wallis test, xxvi, 92, 188
Levene test, for equal variances, 159
log-rank test, 235–236
Mann–Whitney test, xxv, 90, 152–162
multiple, 14
nonnormal statistical inference, 141
nonparametric, 113, 136–137, 141
normality, *see* Normality tests
one-sample tests, illustrations, 127
parallel, 14
parametric tests, 113
Satterthwaite's test, 157
screening/detection tests, *see* Screening tests
sequential, 14
serial, 14
sign test, *see* Sign test
skewness tests, for normality, 57
sphericity, 187
t-tests, *see* *t*-tests
Wald, 98, 226
Wilcoxon rank-sum test, xxv, 141, 152, 162, 169
Wilcoxon signed-rank test, 90, 92, 127, 141–142, 152
z test, *see* *z* test
Test statistics, 130–136
ANCOVA, 93
ANOVA test, 92–93
correlation analysis, result of, 94–95
defined, 130
GLMs, types of, 98, 99
linear regression analysis, 95
logistic regression, 96–99
model testing, 98
multiple/multivariable linear regression, 95, 96
nonparametric procedures, 90, 92, 94
one-sample *t* test, *see* One-sample *t*-test
other, 90
power of test, sample size and, 135–136
regressions, types of, 96
repeated-measure ANOVA used as, 143
results of linear regressions, 95–96
selection of, 101, 254
statistical significance, 131–136
test assumption, 132
t test, 88, 89–90; *see also* *t*-tests
Wald statistic tests, 98
z test, 90
Test techniques, single-sample, 126–127
Thoraco-lumbar kyphosis progression, 113
Time-to-event method, 229–237
Cox regression
computation, 236
interpretation, 237
data, xxvii–xxviii
definition of terms, 231
equality of survival, test for, 234–235
KM survival estimates, 232
derivation/computation, 232–234
life table, 229–231
log-rank test, estimation, 235–236
overview, 229
Translational data, statistical modeling of, 251–253
t-tests, 88, 89–90
formula, 131
for independent groups, 152–162
appropriate, 154
assumptions, 154–155
computation, 155–157
defined, 154
equal variances, test for, 157, 159–161
nonparametric alternative, 161–162
overview, 152–153
one-sample, *see* One-sample *t*-test
one-sample analysis of variance, 142–145
repeated-measure, 142–145
paired, *see* Paired *t* tests
single-sample, 126, 127
computation, 128
types, 138–145
Wilcoxon signed-rank test, 141–142
Tukey's HSD, 178
Tumor prognostic marker, 197
Tumor proliferative marker, 197
Two-group comparison, in clinical trials, 120–121
Two independent group, defined, 119–120

Two independent samples
  computation, 117–119
  proportions, 117–119
  requirements, 117
Two-sample hypothesis testing
  examples, 152
  overview, xxv
Two-sample *t* test, 152–162
  appropriate, 154
  assumptions, 154–155
  computation, 155–157
  defined, 154
  equal variances, test for, 157, 159–161
  nonparametric alternative, 161–162
  overview, 152–153
Two-way ANOVA, 172–185
Two-way scatterplot, defined, 211

U

Uncertainty, defined, 111
Unconditional logistic regression, 220, 226, 229
Unconditional probability, 69–70
Unequal standard deviations, 157
Unicameral bone cyst, 5, 17
Univariable analysis, 93, 191
Univariate distribution pattern, defined, xxii
Unordered variables, 83
Urticaria, chemoprophylaxis for, 141–142
US National Health Interview Survey, 31
U test, Mann–Whitney, 152–162

V

Validity
  components, 37
  defined, 37
  diagnostic/screening tests, 15–17
  estimation, 36–37
  external, 37
  internal, 37, 38
Variability, 82–84
Variables
  binary/dichotomous, 83
  cardinal, 136
  in clinical research, 83
  confounding, 256–257
  continuous, 83
  defined, 82
  dependent, *see* Dependent variables
  dichotomous, 83
  dimensional, 83
  discrete, 83
  explanatory, 220, 229, 238
  independent, *see* Independent variables
  measuring, scales in, 83
  nominal, 83, 136
  ordinal, 136
  predictor, 220, 222, 229, 231, 238
  probability distribution, 83–84
  random, 125–126
    defined, 82
    probability distributions, 82
  response, 78–79, 219, 220, 222, 229, 238, 240
  sources of variation (variability) and, 82–84
  types, 82, 83
  unordered, 83
Variance, SBP, 66
Variation, sources of, 82–84
Violation, of normality assumption, xxv
Vitamin C, 88, 131

W

Wald tests, 98, 226
Wilcoxon rank-sum test, xxv, 141, 152, 162, 169
Wilcoxon signed-rank test, 90, 92, 127, 141–142, 152

X

X-ray imaging
  pedobarograph and, correlation, 195
  SKD patients, 78–79
  solid fusion based on, 80
xtbreg, xxviii
xtpois, xxviii

Z

z distribution, 153
Z distribution, hypothesis testing and, 90
Zero-inflated Poisson (ZIP) regression model, 99
z score, 68, 89
z test, for two independent proportions, 162–164
  computation, 163–164
  defined, 163
  formula for, 163
  use, 163